REVIEW OF **Dental assisting**

February 13th - pictures - 9:00
bring cups & wear uniforms

Call Kuhn
about next extern sight

REVIEW OF
Dental assisting

EDITED BY

BETTY A. LADLEY, C.D.A., R.D.A., B.S., M.S.

Instructional Coordinator, Dental Assisting Program,
Washtenaw Community College, Ann Arbor, Michigan

SHIRLEY A. WILSON, C.D.A., R.D.A.

Assistant Professor; formerly Director,
Dental Assisting Program, University of Detroit
School of Dentistry, Detroit, Michigan

with 222 illustrations

The C. V. Mosby Company

ST. LOUIS • TORONTO • LONDON   1980

The C. V. Mosby Company
11830 Westline Industrial Drive, St. Louis, Missouri 63141

Library of Congress Cataloging in Publication Data

Main entry under title:

Review of dental assisting.

  Bibliography: p.
   1. Dental assistants—Examinations, questions, etc.
2. Dentistry—Examinations, questions, etc. I. Ladley,
Betty A., date.   II. Wilson, Shirley A.
RK60.5.R48   617.6'0076   79-18921
ISBN 0-8016-2806-7

GW/M/M 9 8 7 6 5   03/C/367

Contributors

Marian R. Algarda, C.D.A., R.D.H., B.S., M.S.Ed.

Associate Professor, Department of Dental Assisting, St. Louis Community College at Meramec, St. Louis, Missouri

Elizabeth Gorman Allen, C.D.A, A.A.S., B.S.

Director, Dental Assisting Program, Trenholm State Technical College, Montgomery, Alabama

Daniel R. Balbach, D.D.S., M.S.

Orthodontist, Ann Arbor, Michigan; Visiting Lecturer, Faculty of Dentistry, University of Western Ontario, London, Ontario, Canada

Richard W. Brand, B.S., D.D.S., F.A.C.D.

Associate Professor of Anatomy, Washington University School of Dental Medicine; Instructor in Dental Science, St. Louis Community College at Meramec, St. Louis, Missouri

Carol M. Brobst, C.D.A., B.A.

Coordinator, Dental Assisting Program, Department of Health Sciences, Hawkeye Institute of Technology, Waterloo, Iowa

Roslyn M. Cidado, C.D.A., B.S., M.Ed.

Formerly Assistant Professor, Dental Assistant Program, Boston University School of Graduate Dentistry, Boston, Massachusetts

Robert G. Craig, Ph.D.

Professor and Chairman, Department of Dental Materials, The University of Michigan School of Dentistry, Ann Arbor, Michigan

Ann Ehrlich, C.D.A., M.A.

Director of Dental Services for Practice Productivity, Incorporated, Atlanta, Georgia

John P. Gobetti, D.D.S., M.S.

Professor, Department of Oral Diagnosis and Radiology, The University of Michigan School of Dentistry, Ann Arbor, Michigan

Felice Levine Hirsch, C.D.A., A.S., B.S., M.Ed.

Assistant Professor, Department of Dental Assisting, Medical University of South Carolina, College of Allied Health Sciences, Charleston, South Carolina

Evelyn R. King, C.D.A., R.D.A., B.A., M.A.

Coordinator, Dental Assisting Program, C. S. Mott Community College, Flint, Michigan

Betty A. Ladley, C.D.A., R.D.A., B.S., M.S.

Instructional Coordinator, Dental Assisting Program, Washtenaw Community College, Ann Arbor, Michigan

Judith A. McKay, A.A., C.D.A., B.S., M.A.

Health Occupation's Instructor, Phymouth Canton Community School District, Plymouth, Michigan

Marsha N. Meyer, A.A., C.D.A.

Supervisor, Health Service Dental Clinic, The University of Michigan School of Dentistry, Ann Arbor, Michigan

John A. Molinari, Ph.D.

Associate Professor and Chairman, Department of Microbiology and Biochemistry, University of Detroit School of Dentistry, Detroit, Michigan

Elizabeth Ochoa, C.D.A., M.A.T.

Associate Professor and Program Director, Dental Assisting Program, Medical University of South Carolina College of Allied Health Sciences, Charleston, South Carolina

Jerry Crowe Patt, B.S.

Instructor, Secretarial/Office Department, Washtenaw Community College, Ann Arbor, Michigan

Pamela M. Peters, C.D.A., B.S., M.Ed.

Instructor, Department of Dental Ecology, The University of North Carolina at Chapel Hill School of Dentistry, Chapel Hill, North Carolina

Michael J. Phillip, M.Sc., Ph.D.

Professor, Department of Microbiology and Biochemistry, University of Detroit School of Dentistry, Detroit, Michigan

Nancy A. Polcyn, A.A., C.D.A., R.D.A.

Instructor, University of Detroit School of Dentistry, Detroit, Michigan

Janice A. Schweitzer, C.D.A.

Office Manager in private practice, West Allis, Wisconsin

Joni A. Self, R.D.H., B.S., M.S.

Assistant Professor, Department of Dental Hygiene, Loma Linda University School of Dentistry, Loma Linda, California

Jack Ellis Showley, D.D.S.

Assistant Professor; Expanded Functions for Dental Auxiliary Education Project Director, Indiana University School of Dentistry, Indianapolis, Indiana

Susan Harper Van Steenhouse, C.D.A., R.D.A., R.D.H., M.A.

Assistant Professor, Delta College, University Center, Michigan

Marilyn A. Westerhoff, C.D.A., B.S.

Coordinator, Dental Assisting Department, Elgin Community College, Elgin, Illinois

Shirley A. Wilson, C.D.A., R.D.A.

Assistant Professor; formerly Director, Dental Assisting Program, University of Detroit School of Dentistry, Detroit, Michigan

Frank B. Womer, B.A., B.Ed., M.A., Ph.D.

Professor of Education; Director, Michigan School Testing Service, Bureau of School Services, The University of Michigan, Ann Arbor, Michigan

Betty H. Zendner, C.D.A., R.D.A., R.D.H., B.S., M.A.

Associate Professor, Department of Dental Assisting, Loma Linda University School of Dentistry, Loma Linda, California

To

all dental assistants

who desire to prove competency
through a credentialing examination

Preface

Recently, the profession of dental assisting has changed and gained recognition as an integral part of the dental care delivery system. Consequently, the need to maintain high standards has resulted in the credentialing of dental assistants on both a state and a national level.

As editors we have recognized the need for a comprehensive review so that individuals preparing for a credentialing examination will have an overview of the basic sciences and the practice of dentistry. This information has been identified by a group of contributors who represent a broad professional and geographic spectrum within the dental profession.

We have selected a format that should facilitate preparation for a credentialing examination. The text begins with an introduction on how to prepare for an examination and progresses through a review of major topics common to credentialing examinations. We believe that the expertise of the contributing authors overshadows the necessity for consistent flow from chapter to chapter. Furthermore, we believe that Chapter 15 on expanded functions will give the reader insight into a rapidly changing segment of the profession. This chapter is unique in that the author has provided an introductory review of the evolution of expanded functions.

The chapters are organized around two types of questions, one that provides information in short narrative answer form and another that provides an opportunity for the student to demonstrate understanding in multiple-choice form. Since this is a review text, the reader will note that not all multiple-choice questions are covered by the narrative. In addition, the illustrations provide visual support to the narrative.

The combined efforts of many friends have made this project a reality. We wish to give special recognition to all the contributors for preparing their respective portions of the manuscript and for meeting the many deadlines. Special thanks are extended to our colleagues who made it possible for us to complete the manuscript and continue our teaching responsibilities. We wish to thank Jan Newman, Nancy Polcyn, and Dean James Smudski of the University of Detroit and Claudia Allard, LaRuth Edwards Martin, Dr. William Nevers, Donna Swatz, and Associate Dean Roger Bertoia of Washtenaw Community College.

We are grateful to Dr. George Goodis and Dr. Ralph Nothhelfer for reviewing and critiquing portions of the manuscript and to Loretta Santana and Suzanne Spencer for typing the manuscript. To Charles Finkbeiner, Jim and Jerry Patt, Margaret and Norman Rieger, Toni and Woody Wilson, Nel Workman, Mildred Hayden, and the West family we give our warmest appreciation for their patience and encouragement.

Betty A. Ladley
Shirley A. Wilson

Contents

REVIEW OF **Dental assisting**

CHAPTER 1

Preparing for an examination— guidelines for the student

FRANK B. WOMER

■ **What is the most important thing a student should do to prepare for an examination?**

a. Get a good night's sleep before the examination and eat only a light breakfast.

b. Take two aspirin before entering the examination room to ward off the distraction of a possible headache.

c. Develop an attitude of cautious optimism, that is, "I believe I will pass this examination."

d. Develop a thorough understanding of the body of knowledge and concepts to be covered by the examination.

If you chose the fourth alternative, "D," you are off to a good start in getting yourself ready for any examination, particularly ones like the "Certification Examination for Dental Assistants" or a registry examination. There is only one way to "beat" a well-developed examination—to know the answers to most of the questions. The "trick" to getting good test scores is primarily to retain and apply the knowledge and skills learned in formal course work and in clinical applications. Various ways of helping you develop this "trick" will be discussed.

If you chose "C" in answer to the question, you chose an important response but not the "best" one. It *is* important to go into any examination with a positive attitude and with minimal anxiety, but such an attitude is realistic only if you do have a good command of the subject.

If you chose "A," then perhaps you interpreted the words "prepare for an examination" to mean only those things that should be done on the day before and the day of an examination. But preparation for any examination begins on the day you learn the first vocabulary word or the first concept associated with any area of learning. Examinations are just one phase in the total ongoing learning process.

Alternative "B" in the opening example should have been a "throwaway" response for everyone unless you are one of those unusual individuals who does suffer physically while taking an exam. Even then, it should be obvious that neither aspirin nor any other drug can compensate for knowledge.

■ **If you were asked to develop a certification or registry examination for dental assistants, what would it be like? What topics would be covered? What type of item(s) would be used? How would it be like a classroom test and how would it be different?**

Credentialing examinations for dental assisting are developed by persons who know about how different types of tests are developed for different purposes; but most of all they are developed by persons knowledgeable about dentistry. So, one should think first about potential topics that may be covered in a certification examination.

When you sign up to take a credentialing examination, you will receive an outline of the material to be covered in the examination. Pay close attention to the content outline *and* to the number of questions to be asked on each topic. That information should serve as a guide for your examination preparation. If 50 questions are going to be asked on one topic, that topic deserves more of your study time than a topic to be covered by 5 questions.

Following is the descriptive outline of one state-wide licensing examination. Some outlines will be even more detailed than this one.

FORMAT OF EXAMINATION

The examination consists of two sections, a written section and a clinical section.

I. Written section
   The written examination consists of 150 multiple-choice questions covering the following areas:
   A. General section—100 questions
      1. Oral anatomy
      2. Instrumentation and use of dental materials
   B. Five specific categories—10 questions per section
      1. Mouth mirror inspection
      2. Rubber dam application
      3. Application of topical fluorides
      4. Sizing and removal of temporary crowns and bands
      5. Radiography
II. Clinical section
   The clinical examination will test the candidate's ability to perform the following tasks:
   A. Chart conditions of the oral cavity
   B. Apply topical fluoride
   C. Place and remove an intracoronal temporary filling and an aluminum shell crown
   D. Mount a full-mouth set of radiographs
   E. Identify anatomic landmarks and radiologic processing errors
   F. Apply and remove rubber dam

In addition to knowing the content to be covered, it is important to know that written certification examinations are usually multiple-choice examinations. All questions are apt to be in that format with *one* best answer for each question. Many multiple-choice questions are written with distractors (responses that are *not* the answers) that are partially correct or that are correct but are not the *best* answer.

Some critics of multiple-choice tests claim that one can score well on such a test by memorizing facts and by learning some tricks to answering such questions. That may be true when taking a multiple-choice test that is developed by a classroom teacher who is unskilled in writing such tests and who inadvertently lets "cues" to the answers creep into the test. However, such criticism is *not* true for any well-

developed national or state certification or registry examination. The examination you take will have been prepared by test specialists as well as by content specialists. Each test question will have been tried out in regular testing situations with students in classes for dental assistants. The poor questions will have been eliminated. You will be taking a great risk if you assume that skillful "guessing" will produce a passing score on such an examination.

No written examination can test one's ability to *apply* the knowledge or the understanding that one must possess to function as a dental assistant. Credentialing examinations also are apt to include a practical or clinical test, a test in which you will be asked to "demonstrate" what you have learned by doing such things as selecting the instruments necessary for a given task or taking an x-ray film or processing it. Any of the chairside or other office tasks that you have learned to do may serve as a "situational" test in which your actual performance is observed and graded.

The purpose of any credentialing examination is to determine as well as possible the extent to which each candidate has mastered the knowledge, concepts, and skills necessary to perform satisfactorily as a dental assistant. No examination, either written or practical, can be long enough to actually cover every concept or every skill. Therefore, test developers must develop questions and practical situations that are typical of the total body of knowledge and skills in dental assisting. As a candidate, you will not know what specific concepts and skills will be tested the year that you take the examination. The only solution is to be well prepared in all aspects of dental assisting.

■ **Think about some recent classroom examination that you have taken in which the instructor used multiple-choice questions. What are some good ways to study for an examination like that? Is it sufficient to memorize selected information for such an examination? Think about some recent practical classroom examination in which you were asked to demonstrate setting up equipment. What are some good ways to study for such an examination? Is it neces-**

sary to memorize which instruments to use for every possible situation?

For written examinations the multiple-choice test question is considered the most versatile. It is a good method of measuring vocabulary-type information, that is, knowledge of the technical vocabulary and specific information that dental assistants must have. It is also an effective method of measuring understanding of relationships and interrelationships (which things go together and which do not). It may be used for measuring students' application of knowledge to situations that are different from ones the students have experienced before.

About the only type of cognitive skill that is not measured well by the multiple-choice question or by any type of choice question is creativity. But credentialing examinations are designed to find out whether applicants have mastered the basic fundamental skills of a subject area; they are not designed to discover potential talent for creative innovations.

The practical part of such an examination is a direct method of measuring important dental assisting skills. It provides final evidence of whether or not a candidate can "put it all together" and function satisfactorily in a setting that simulates real life in a dental office.

On a certification or registry examination you will be examined on how well you have acquired and internalized the basic language, concepts, and skills of dental assisting — those things that must become second nature to you as a practicing dental assistant.

GETTING READY

Before beginning to study for any type of examination, there are at least two things to do: (1) secure a set of behavioral objectives for the area or areas that the examination is designed to cover, and (2) secure a set of sample questions that are similar to the ones to be used on the examination for which you will be studying. Whether these two things will be readily available will vary with the examination. Typically, the information printed in an explanatory bulletin for a credentialing examination will contain some sample multiple-choice questions but will not contain a detailed set of behavioral objectives. If the explanatory material contains a content outline for the examination, that outline will be helpful, if not ideal. Knowing what a test is designed to measure and having sample items are the best possible ways to become familiar with the areas to which study should be directed.

If behavioral objectives and/or sample items are not available to you, the next best things to do are (1) to examine this text and others that cover the field of dental assisting, and (2) to ask your instructors for their judgment of what most important facts and skills probably will be covered in a credentialing examination.

The general purpose of any of these approaches is to make sure that you "zero in" on the key concepts and skills of dental assisting and that you spend major portions both of study time and of review time on these key concepts and skills.

STUDYING

The best preparation for a credentialing examination is good preparation for every class that you take which is aimed at preparing you in dental assisting. The required textbooks for courses in dental assisting should be studied carefully with an eye not only to immediate acquisition of knowledge, but particularly to internalization and *retention* of that knowledge. Many students find it helpful to underline key passages in a text or to go over them with a felt tipped marker that enables one to go back and skim those key passages easily. Sometimes the author(s) of a text will emphasize important points for you by paragraph headings or by italicized sentences. Acquisition *and retention* of important concepts require repetition for most people. Therefore taking the time during an initial reading to make review work easy is time well spent.

Taking good class notes is a very important study skill. Many instructors spend "some" time making key points and "quite a bit" of time illustrating these points. Most students are well-advised to concentrate on writing down the key points without trying to take notes verbatim. It may be helpful to write down some of your instructor's examples but only if these examples seem necessary to remember the discussion.

Some students face the problem of not understanding their own notes. This can be a real problem if a student waits to review class notes until a number of days after the class. Anyone's memory of a lecture or discussion is best immediately after that lecture or discussion. Thus the sooner a student can review class notes, the better. Some students find it useful to recopy notes, abstracting and highlighting the major points. Others can do this well in the original notes. Your decision may depend on how organized you are at notetaking and/or how organized your instructor is in presenting material. A key element here is timing—be sure that your original notes, edited notes, or rewritten notes include the important concepts. If any doubts remain or if you have unanswered questions, as soon as possible be sure to ask your instructor those questions. Although instructors are often busy, most of them do want their students to succeed and are willing and anxious to clear up ambiguities or misunderstandings.

In addition to identifying key concepts from textual materials, lectures, and notes, it is important to develop a thorough understanding of the vocabulary of dentistry. Every profession has its own vocabulary—not only the technical words that identify important materials, concepts, rules, and ideas, but also the words commonly used to communicate in that profession. Technical vocabulary will be tested, one can be sure, in any written or practical examination. But in addition to that, the questions that you will be asked on any credentialing examination will be worded in the day-to-day language of the dental classroom and the dental office. It is essential that you understand quickly and completely each question that you are asked on an examination. If you do not understand a question, it will be difficult to answer it correctly.

In addition to the general suggestions for learning and studying throughout your period of training, there are some things that may be helpful as you review material in preparation for a credentialing examination and/or any end-of-term examination. One of the most effective things to do is to develop cooperative study sessions with one or two friends. Such sessions are best conducted as much like a classroom situation as possible, that is, each person should have developed *prior* to the joint study session a series of questions to ask the other(s) along with the materials necessary to answer the questions. If your colleagues miss any of your questions, you should be prepared to explain the answers to them and vice versa. Teaching a concept or skill to someone else is one of the best learning techniques that we know of to acquire that concept or skill yourself. Therefore the best area for you to teach to others is your weakest area. Naturally, study sessions such as suggested here will not be directly comparable to a formal class, but they should be conducted in a businesslike fashion. If these study sessions become just socialization among friends, you may enjoy these sessions more, but they will not contribute much to your preparation for an examination.

An additional bonus that many students receive from joint study sessions is enhanced confidence in one's ability to do well in an examination. There is nothing that builds confidence as much as feeling that you have mastered some area of knowledge or skill so well that you can help others understand it.

FRAME OF MIND

Some people will caution you to prepare for an examination by being physically alert and healthy, that is, get 8 hours sleep, avoid coffee, avoid pep pills, etc. Certainly it is wise and prudent to be physically healthy, but keep in mind that any examination you take in dental assisting is going to measure your *mental* ability rather than your physical prowess. This does not mean that studying all night before an examination is recommended behavior—it is not. Physical fatigue can depress test taking efficiency. The best physical preparation for an examination is simply to avoid any major variation from your normal routine.

Of much greater concern is your "mental health." In the context of test taking, good mental health can be defined as a feeling of confidence that you have prepared yourself to take the examination and that you expect to do well. You may approach an examination with some degree of anxiety, like an athlete who enters a game desiring to play as well as possible. This is not necessarily bad. Research indicates that some test anxiety, as long as it is not severe, may help to produce a positive result. One can be fired up mentally to take an examination, just as one can be fired up to play basketball, tennis, or any other sport.

There is a myth abroad that large numbers of students "clutch" when taking examinations, particularly written examinations. No doubt there are some individuals who have developed psychologic blocks to taking tests, but it is my experience that many (probably most) of the students who claim that a low test score was caused by an inability to perform well on tests have not developed the requisite knowledge and skills to answer the questions.

If you are one of those few individuals who can demonstrate definitive knowledge of the material, perhaps by repeated personal testing by one of your instructors, but who panics in a formal written testing situation, you have a very serious problem that may or may not be solvable. You could ask the licensure board in your state to provide personal testing by some neutral party (probably at your own expense). Or you could seek professional help to overcome your test panic. Sometimes repeated practice on similar written examinations will be helpful; sometimes a skilled counselor can help. There is no easy solution to this problem. Perhaps the next section will be helpful if you are one of the individuals who have difficulty taking a test.

■ **Many persons believe that some students are better "test takers" than other students. What are some things that a "good" test taker will do during an examination to increase the chances of doing well?**

It cannot be stated too often that test-taking skills are no substitute for knowledge and skill in any learning area. However, it is possible to fail to maximize the opportunity to demonstrate what you really do know by "inefficiency" in test taking. "Good" test takers are those who have mastered the process of test taking so well that they are able to concentrate on the knowledge and skill called for by the test question.

When you enter the testing room, you may be assigned a seat or location or you may be able to choose your own seat. If you can choose, pick a spot that will be comfortable *for you*. Some people like to be in the front; others do not. There is no "best" location, but there may be poor locations, such as near a noisy fan or air duct.

Of much greater importance is initial concentration on developing a thorough understanding of the procedures and regulations for *that* testing session. *Read* carefully the printed directions given to you. *Listen* carefully to the verbal directions. Do not assume that just because you have previously taken many examinations that the directions for this one will be the same—they may be; they may not be. If the printed and/or verbal directions are not perfectly clear *to you,* ask the examiner in charge of your session to explain exactly what is required. Your first task is to understand thoroughly the mechanics that you are expected to follow during the examination.

In a practical examination, you may be expected to select instruments, arrange instruments, and/or perform some other task. The physical arrangements may or may not be identical to those used by your instructors. If they are not and yet it is clear how you are to proceed, there is no problem. If they are not the same or similar and the required procedures are not clear to you, be sure to ask for clarification. You do not want to begin a practical examination by making an error based on a misunderstanding of *how* you are to proceed.

In a written examination you probably will be given multiple-choice questions in a test booklet with a separate answer sheet for recording your choice of a, b, c, or d or whatever letters or numbers are used as an alternative response. The mechanics of recording your choice of the answer are simple; they just require *accurate* execution. Do not make responses hurriedly or carelessly. A test scoring machine reads responses exactly where you put them. If you put them on the wrong line or in the wrong column, there is no way that a machine can give you credit for a correct response.

When responding to multiple-choice questions it is important to keep in mind that you can arrive at the answer in two different ways, that is, by "knowing" the answer and finding it among the alternatives offered, or by eliminating incorrect responses by either knowing they are wrong or being able to figure it out. Both methods are perfectly legitimate. Both methods are based on knowing what is correct and/or what is incorrect. You must arrive at the one correct or one "best" answer by whatever method you use, or you must choose the one answer that seems *best to you*. Be sure to mark an answer for each question. Do not omit any. If you must, "guess" between two alternatives after eliminating two or three because you *know* they are wrong. Very few widely used tests apply a correction-for-guessing formula these days. And even if they do, the correction is only for completely random guessing across all alternatives offered. If you can eliminate any responses as incorrect based on your knowledge, you will *not* be guessing randomly but will be exercising "informed guessing."

It is wise to budget your time on any examination. Make a quick overview of the number of tasks required in a practical examination or the number of questions to be answered in a written examination and then think of the pace you will need to follow to allow appropriate amounts of time for each section. If part one has 10 questions and part two has 30 questions, in all probability you will need to spend more time on part two.

Even though you do think about budgeting your time, some tasks or some questions may require more of your time than other tasks or questions because they are more difficult. Therefore most test takers find it wise to work all the way through a written examination at a fairly rapid pace by answering first all the questions that they "know" or to which they can work out the answer fairly quickly. This method suggests skipping the tough questions the first time through and coming back to them.

There are several good reasons for doing this. You will build on your own success. This success can help lessen any fears or concerns that you may have about the testing situation. This method also leaves time available for the tougher questions for which you need more time. Sometimes the mere "reading of questions" in the middle or toward the end of an

examination may trigger your mind to respond with the answer or may provide an important cue for an earlier question. Mental "germination" is a process that seems to work for some people. They "know" the answer but cannot latch onto it immediately.

If you use the approach of moving through the test fairly rapidly and skipping some questions, you must be particularly cautious in locating accurately the answer space for each question on your answer sheet. Inaccuracies in spacing on your answer sheet could create a problem that you might not locate until later, and having to make spacing corrections is a time-wasting activity.

For some candidates, it is helpful to take a break every now and then. You will not be allowed to leave an examination for a leisurely cup of coffee, but there is no reason why you cannot put your pencil down, close your eyes, and relax for a few minutes. Your own personal style of working efficiently will dictate whether or not this technique is appropriate for you.

Some people say that it is best when answering a multiple-choice question to mark your first "hunch" and then stick with it. Others suggest that examinees should review questions carefully after finishing marking the answers to all questions. The rather limited research available suggests that "abler" students tend to increase their test scores "a bit" by carefully reviewing items, whereas lower scoring students do not. In my opinion, the appropriate procedure is to (1) mark responses to all questions that you "know" and (2) eliminate all wrong responses that you can for other questions and make your best estimate among the remaining choices. Go back over questions primarily to check that you have not made some obvious error in such things as reading or marking. Agonizing over choices does not seem to be a particularly profitable approach.

Occasionally a student will try to second-guess the authors of a test by looking for response patterns such as a "run" of answers in a particular response position (alternative c). Although it may be true that amateur test writers sometimes give students such cues inadvertently, professional authors of credentialing examinations will not fall in that trap. A credentialing examination is not a game of wits between you and the author; it *is* an attempt to allow you to demonstrate the knowledge and skill you have attained.

When taking a practical examination, many of the same principles apply. It is wise to proceed slowly and deliberately, making sure that you understand the task being presented and thinking about how to proceed before beginning. A review of your own efforts before indicating completion of your task is also appropriate. The task or tasks that you will be asked to perform will be designed to test your ability to perform successfully as a dental assistant. If you have learned those skills in your training, you should be able to demonstrate them in a formal testing setting.

■ **What major point has the author of this chapter tried to make to help examinees prepare to take a credentialing examination? Do you agree or disagree with that point?**

Any well-developed examination is an instrument designed to *allow* examinees to demonstrate knowledge and skills deemed essential for some important task. Any dental assisting examination is to help examinees who *are* ready to begin work in this profession show their pro-

ficiency. The examination is designed to bring into the profession those who are prepared to work. Therefore the examination will, of course, focus on a variety of skills that specialists already in the profession know to be important if one is to succeed. Think of the credentialing examination in dental assisting as an opportunity for demonstrating professional competency in your chosen field. Preparation for such an examination is preparation for your chosen profession.

SUGGESTED READINGS

Ebel, R. L.: Essentials of educational measurement, Englewood Cliffs, N.J., 1972, Prentice-Hall, Inc., Chapter 9.

Heston, J. C.: How to take a test, Chicago, 1953, Science Research Associates, Inc.

Manuel, H.: Taking a test, New York, 1956, Harcourt Brace Jovanovich, Inc.

Millman, J., and Paulk, W.: How to take tests, New York, 1969, McGraw-Hill Book Co.

Millman, J., Bishop, C. H., and Ebel, R.: An analysis of testiveness, Educational and psychological measurement **25**:707, 1965.

Rudman, J., et al.: How to pass dental aptitude tests; questions and answers, New York, 1964, College Publishing Corp.

Slakter, M. J.: The penalty for not guessing, Journal of Educational Measurement **5**:217, 1968.

Taking the SAT, Princeton, N.J., 1978, College Entrance Examination Board.

CHAPTER 2

The profession—history, organization, ethics, and jurisprudence

EVELYN R. KING

■ **Who is regarded as the "father of dentistry" and why?**

Pierre Fauchard (1678-1761) is recognized as the father of dentistry because of his research and work during the early eighteenth century. Far ahead of his time in thought and vision, he is credited with establishing the science of dentistry. In 1728 he published *Le Chirurgien Dentiste on Traite' des Dents*. This was the first complete treatise ever written on odontology and remains as an outstanding piece of dental literature today. Perhaps his greatest contribution was the sharing of his scientific knowledge and experience for the benefit of mankind and the encouragement he gave to others to share also. Thus was born the "profession."

■ **When and where was the first dental school established?**

The first dental school in the world was founded in November, 1840 in Baltimore, Maryland. At that time it was called the Baltimore College of Dental Surgery and had a class enrollment of five. The school is now a part of the University of Maryland.

■ **Who was G. V. Black, and why is he remembered?**

This "Grand Old Man of Dentistry" (1836-1915) was self-educated and renown as chemist, anatomist, histologist, and bacteriologist as well as pathologist, dentist, teacher, and lecturer. His books dealing with the structural anatomy of the teeth, operative dentistry, and oral pathology are classics in dental literature. His system of cavity classification and preparation are standard procedures that are still taught in dental schools. His influence on the standardization of manufacturing dental amalgam, of dental nomenclature, and of dental instruments has been, and continues to be, significant.

■ **When were x-ray films first used in dentistry?**

The first x-ray films of teeth were taken in 1896 by Dr. W. Koenig of Frankfort, Germany. In that same year the x-ray technique was demonstrated in New York by Dr. W. J. Morton at a meeting of the Odontological Society.

It is Dr. C. Edmund Kells of New Orleans, however, who is given credit for the first use of the x-ray machine in the United States. The dangers of x radiation were unknown at that time, and it was the use and development of this technique that finally cost Dr. Kells his life.

■ **When was the first national dental organization formed, and what was its purpose?**

The American Society of Dental Surgeons was founded in 1840 in New York. At this time the United States was recovering from a depression, and unemployment was high. Dentistry was open to anyone who chose to enter the field. In the 2 years following the depression, the number of dentists nearly doubled. There was much concern about the increasing number of incompetent persons who simply wanted to make as much money as possible without regard for professional standards or education.

The new professional organization set these goals: education of members of the profession, free exchange of scientific information and knowledge, and improvement in the respect and confidence of the public in the profession. The organization served well until it became embroiled in the "Amalgam War" and took an official position against the use of amalgam as a restorative material.

■ **How did the American Dental Association come into being?**

With the growth of the dental profession in the 1840s, many states began to form their own individual societies. In 1859 representatives from eight states met in Niagara Falls, New York, and the American Dental Association was organized. It was hoped that other states would join to form one association, but the Civil War intervened, and it was some time before the plan was realized.

In 1869 the Southern Dental Association was established, organized by the former confederate states. Although the advantages of joining together the American and the Southern Dental Associations were obvious, it was not until a new generation of leadership evolved that unity could occur.

Finally in 1892 the two organizations became one, and this new organization was named the National Dental Association. The organization was beset with problems, but in 1912 a plan was adopted that allowed the members to make a single payment of dues for membership in both the state and national associations. This strengthened the organization, and as it became more representative of the entire profession, more states joined.

In 1922 the name was changed back to the American Dental Association, and its official publication was named the Journal of the American Dental Association.

■ **When and by whom was the first dental assistant employed?**

Reportedly, the first dental assistant or "lady in attendance" began her career in the office of Dr. C. Edmund Kells of New Orleans in 1885. Quick to see the obvious benefits, this progressive dentist added two more assistants to his staff in a short while. At that time the employment of women as dental assistants was a highly controversial topic among dentists.

■ **When and by whom was the first organization for dental assistants formed?**

The first organization of assistants was formed in New York City in 1921 by Juliette Southard. It was called the Education and Efficiency Society, and its primary purpose was education. Several other dental assistant organizations were formed soon afterward, and Miss Southard envisioned a national organization that would unite the various groups for the common purpose of advancing dental assisting. To this end she and 14 others held the first meeting of the American Dental Assistants Association in Dallas, Texas in 1924.

■ **How did certification for dental assistants come into being and gain recognition?**

In 1930, under the leadership of Juliette Southard as president of the American Dental Assistants Association (ADAA), a curriculum committee was established to set guidelines for an educational program for dental assistants. The course of study that was established proved valuable, and plans were made to credential the "qualified" dental assistants.

In 1948 the Certifying Board of the ADAA was established and incorporated in La Porte, Indiana for the purpose of testing and credentialing those dental assistants who had completed the extension course of study. The educational system continually improved, and the demand for this program grew.

In 1960 The American Dental Association (ADA) accepted the requirements recommended by the Certifying Board, and the "certified dental assistant" became officially recognized by the dental profession. At that time dental assistants had to complete a 104 hour course of study and a specified amount of work experience to satisfy the requirements of certification. Since 1969 the requirement for certification has been graduation from a 1- or 2-year college program accredited by the Commission of Accreditation of the ADA.

In January 1979, a 3-year study was begun to assess the feasibility of permitting any dental assistant to sit for the certification examination. This study was undertaken to gather statistics on the work force of uncredentialed dental assistants who had acquired skills without benefit of formal education. The study is to identify and provide the means for credentialing those persons who have competencies that have been determined to be basic to dental assisting. A complete report of the commission's findings is to be made at the close of the study.

■ **What is the difference between a "certified" dental assistant and a "currently certified" dental assistant?**

A *certified* dental assistant is a dental assistant who has met the requirements for and successfully passed the certification examination. A *currently certified* dental assistant has accomplished the same goals but has, in addition, maintained this status with a current certificate each year by completing continuing education requirements and paying an annual renewal fee.

■ **What is a registered dental assistant?**

At this time, many states have changed or are in the process of changing their dental practice acts to allow dental auxiliaries, particularly dental assistants, to perform expanded intraoral functions. In three states—California, Minnesota, and Michigan—qualified dental assistants may sit for a state board examination on the expanded functions permitted in that state. On passing the examination, the dental assistant is licensed *in that state* as a *registered* dental assistant to perform the expanded intraoral functions outlined in that dental practice act.

■ **How are policies and goals established by the ADAA?**

Traditionally, policies and goals have been established by the membership-at-large who send representatives from each state to an annual meeting. These delegates elect officers and a board of trustees to carry out policies and goals until the next annual session. Because of the growth of the organization, a central office staff is now housed in Chicago, Illinois. The staff is responsible to the officers and board for day-to-day functioning of the organization. It is through this network that communication and representation have been established and are maintained at the national, state, and local

levels in professional matters of dental assisting.

■ **What are ethics, and how are they applied to a profession?**

Ethics is that part of philosophy that deals with conduct and moral judgments regarding right and wrong. All people have their own set of ethics or conscience by which they act and make decisions. Each profession has a "code of ethics" that is the common standard of moral judgment and conduct to which each member of the profession is expected to subscribe and observe.

■ **Is there a "code of ethics" for dental assistants?**

Absolutely! Although the code of ethics is too lengthy to print here, a copy may be obtained free by writing the American Dental Assistants Association, 666 North Lakeshore Drive, Suite 1130, Chicago, Illinois 60611. The code is also printed in various current dental assisting textbooks.

■ **What is jurisprudence?**

Jurisprudence is the law or system of laws by which we are governed. When law is applied to dentistry, it is called "dental jurisprudence."

■ **Can a situation arise in which the actions of a professional may be legal but unethical?**

Yes, laws are rules of society enforced by government, whereas ethics are voluntary standards of conduct. Oftentimes the code of ethics will require a higher level of conduct than the law requires. One example of this dichotomy might be a practitioner who places several gold restorations for a patient whose periodontal condition is questionable prior to doing thorough prophylaxis and securing x ray films of that patient.

■ **From where does our system of laws originate?**

In the United States laws originate from four basic sources; (1) the United States Constitution and federal laws enacted by the Congress,

(2) state constitutions and state laws established by the state legislatures, (3) judicial decisions that become part of the law as binding precedents, and (4) "common law," the body of statutory and case law in effect in Great Britain when the United States was established which became, and is still a part of our legal system.

■ Which laws primarily affect the practice of dentistry?

The practice of dentistry is primarily affected by laws of the state in which the practice occurs. Basically, state laws affecting the dental profession include the dental practice act that regulates the profession and the civil law that applies when one person sues another.

Civil law includes contract law and tort law. Contract law involves disputes between persons who have entered into an agreement together, and that agreement, whether implied or expressed has been violated. Tort law deals with the private enforcement of rights and duties of people toward each other and violations of those rights and duties. Claims involving civil law may be resolved by legal action brought to court.

■ What is a dental practice act, and how does it work?

Each state government has the power to regulate and control the practice of dentistry within its own jurisdiction. The dental practice act is a state law that specifies the requirements for and restrictions placed on the practice of dentistry within that state. It protects the public against incompetent or unscrupulous practitioners by providing for enforcement of these regulations.

■ Who is responsible for the administration and enforcement of the dental practice act?

Each state has created a board of examiners or board of dentistry to supervise the practice of dentistry and the enforcement of that state's dental practice act. Their responsibilities include establishing standards of education for dentists and auxiliaries, establishing examinations for eligible candidates, adopting new rules of practice to keep the act current with changing needs and envoking disciplinary action for violations.

■ Who is eligible to be a member of a board of examiners?

In general only dentists have been eligible to be members of a dental board. Many states have begun to appoint representatives of the public and of the dental assisting and dental hygiene professions. This depends, however, on the practice act of each state.

■ How are dental assistants affected by a dental practice act?

A practice act affects every dental assistant because it determines what constitutes the practice of dentistry. The act identifies what functions may or may not be delegated to and performed by dental auxiliaries and recognizes, or omits the recognition of, dental assistants. Practicing dental assistants should become familiar with the act in their states, and what their legal and professional responsibilities are accordingly.

■ Are the state dental association and the state board of examiners parts of the same organization?

No. The dental association within a state is the professional organization that represents dentists and their interests, just as the state dental assistant organization represents dental assistants. Neither organization has political status.

The board of examiners is an agency of the state government. It functions as a legal entity of the state with authority from the legislature to regulate the profession of dentistry in the public interest.

■ What is the responsibility of dentist employers for acts of the auxiliary employees functioning under their direction and supervision?

According to the law of principle and agent, the principle of *respondeat superior,* "let the higher one answer," places the dentist employer in a position of responsibility for the acts of the auxiliary employee when such acts are performed within the scope of employment. Support for this principle is based on the rationale that as the employer has control and direction over the acts performed, responsibility for any consequences of these acts must also be assumed. Also the employer has placed the employee in a position that might cause harm, and therefore the employer must be responsible, should such harm occur. It must be stated, however, that *this does not automatically relieve the auxiliary employee of individual responsibility for the harmful act or resultant injury to a third party, that is, a patient.*

■ **Can dental assistants be held personally responsible for performing functions delegated to them legally or illegally?**

Yes, under the law persons are accountable for their own actions. Each state practice act determines what constitutes the practice of dentistry. If the duties are legally delegated, the dental assistant is expected to perform competently to that standard of skill and care required of other dental assistants legally performing those same functions. Any unqualified person performing functions that constitute dental services for a patient may be found guilty of practicing dentistry without a license and may be prosecuted for a criminal act. Any action brought against the employer dentist would be a *separate* action from the illegal practice of dentistry.

■ **Should dental assistants carry their own liability insurance even though covered through the office of employment?**

Yes. The dental assistant *as an individual is not covered* through the office of employment. Although lawsuits against dental assistants have been few, court actions in general are increasing. As additional functions are delegated to dental assistants, it seems only reasonable to suppose that lawsuits will be more frequent in dental assisting as well. A little known *fact* that is often misunderstood is that an office liability insurance policy carried by the dentist protects the *dentist* if an auxiliary employee is sued for negligence or malpractice. The office policy *does not protect the dental assistant as an in-*

dividual. For example, if a dentist and the dental assistant are *both* sued for negligence, the dental assistant *will not have protection* unless a separate liability insurance policy is carried by that assistant.

■ **Will liability insurance cover the performance of illegal duties?**

No. Policies are written only to cover those duties that can be legally delegated to a person legally qualified to perform them.

■ **In the dentist-patient relationship, what legal responsibilities does the dentist have?**

To establish a legal relationship the patient must first seek dental services, and the dentist must accept the individual as a patient. Once the dentist has accepted the patient, there are responsibilities imposed by law as a part of the contractual relationship, and there are those responsibilities implied as part of a professional relationship and established in common law. Following is an outline of these duties.

Imposed by the contractual relationship:
— Attend to all the needs of a patient or to those needs agreed on until completion of treatment.
— Protect and respect the patient's property and privacy.
— Do only those things to which the patient has consented.
— Satisfy the patient, but only if satisfaction has been promised or guaranteed.

Implied by the professional relationship and established in common law:
— Charge a reasonable fee for treatment when one has not been agreed on in advance.
— Exercise reasonable care in treatment.
— Adhere to the "duty of care," which refers to:
   Duty to possess the skill and learning established as necessary for a licensed practitioner
   Duty to exercise the acceptable standard of skill and care

A dentist who fails to recognize or abide by these imposed and implied duties may be held liable for breach of contract or negligence.

■ **Is an agreement between a dentist and a patient for the completion of a determined treatment considered a legal and binding contract, although it may not be written?**

Yes. A contract is defined as an agreement between two or more competent parties covering a specific lawful act for a consideration. To be binding, such an agreement must have legally competent persons making the agreement, the agreed on service or act cannot be against the law, and there must be some form of payment for the service. A contract may be either expressed or implied. An expressed contract may be an oral or written agreement; an implied contract may exist when there has been no discussion of fees or terms. In any case if the three factors listed before are met, the contract is considered legal and binding. A violation of such an agreement by either the patient or the dentist is called a "breach of contract," and damages may be sought.

■ **In the dentist-patient relationship, what legal responsibilities does the patient have?**

The patient is responsible for two aspects of this relationship. The first is to follow instructions both during and after treatment. Proof of failure to do this could constitute contributory negligence, and the patient would then be unable to collect damages in a suit alleging malpractice or breach of contract. The patient has a duty to cooperate in the treatment agreed on. Second is the responsibility of the patient to pay a reasonable fee for treatment. To avoid misunderstanding, a fee that is agreed on prior to treatment is best; however, the patient is still responsible for paying a fee for services rendered, whether discussed or not.

■ **When a dentist determines that a particular treatment is necessary, is it always important to obtain permission from the patient before proceeding with that treatment?**

Yes, *always*. Each individual has the legal right not to be touched by another without consent. Legal action brought against a dentist may charge that the dentist, whether intentionally or inadvertently, performed services not authorized by the patient. Even if the service has been of benefit to the patient, the dentist may be liable for technical assault. It has been established that a patient, seated in the dental chair, has thereby given implied consent to an examination, diagnosis, and consultation. At that point, however, it is for the patient to determine what treatment, if any, is to be performed.

Not all patients are considered competent to give legal consent for treatment. A minor is one example of such a patient. It would be necessary, then, to obtain permission from the parent or legal guardian before proceeding.

■ **What determines the standard of skill and care that a practitioner must possess to provide patient services?**

The standard of skill and care is determined by the following factors. The practitioner must meet the standard of practice of other practitioners in that same locale or community under similar conditions or circumstances. An evaluation or judgment of that skill and care must be made by the practitioner's peers. This applies to all practitioners, whether dentists, dental assistants, or dental hygienists. An extreme example might be a general dentist who makes a house call in the town to a bedridden patient and removes a tooth. An evaluation of the conditions would include the probable poor light source, no opportunity for an x-ray film, limited instruments available, and limited or no assistance with the procedure. The evaluation would be done by other general dentists in that town or area who must consider performing the service under those same conditions. A specialist in this situation, for example, an oral surgeon, would be judged by other oral surgeons, not by general dentists or specialists in other areas.

■ **Must a dentist accept all patients that express a need for treatment or that make an appointment?**

Legally, a dentist is not obligated to see or treat any new patient, even in an emergency situation. For a legal relationship to exist, the patient must seek dental services, and the dentist must accept the patient. The fact that a receptionist accepts a new patient for an appointment does not constitute a legal contract until the *dentist* accepts the patient. In an emergency situation the dentist may have an ethical obligation to accept the patient, depending on the circumstances, but there is no legal obligation. It should be noted, however, that civil rights laws and participation in federally or state-funded dental programs prohibit dentists from refusing treatment to patients based on race, creed, color, national origin, etc.

■ **Can a dentist refuse to continue treatment or care of a patient without the patient's consent?**

Not very easily. Treatment may be terminated by the dentist only under very specific conditions and with certain risks. The dentist wishing to discontinue treatment must notify the patient in writing of this intent, with a minimum of 30 days advance notice of the effective date, specifying the need for and consequences of not receiving further treatment. The letter should be sent by registered or certified mail with a return receipt requested. The letter and receipt should be placed in the patient file. Even when the conditions are strictly met, the dentist may be relieved only from liability for malpractice. He may still be held liable for breach of contract.

■ **How does liability differ between negligence and malpractice?**

First let us establish the definition of each term. *Negligence* is defined as either failing to do something that a reasonable person would do, or doing something that a reasonable person would not do. *Malpractice* has been defined as any professional misconduct or any unreasonable lack of skill or fidelity in performance of professional duties, practice contrary to established rules. These two terms are often used interchangeably, but there is a distinction between them. When a dentist is negligent and when this negligence results in harm or injury to a patient during treatment, it is usually called malpractice. One example might be failing to inform a patient that a root tip has been left in

his jaw following an extraction. Necessary removal of the root tip some time later may result in a malpractice suit. A dentist may, however, be negligent with regard to a patient without dental treatment being involved. An example would be a patient injuring his head on the unit light as he is dismissed from the dental chair. Although either case could be very damaging to a professional reputation, a suit of negligence might be the least damaging, depending on the circumstances.

■ **How can the dental assistant help to prevent a lawsuit?**

Unfortunately, there is no one answer to this question but there are some key points that can be emphasized.
   —Remain courteous, regardless of the situation or circumstance.
   —Keep accurate patient records including medical, dental, and financial information.
   —Remain in the treatment room with the dentist and patient at all times.
   —In the event that an accident occurs, *say nothing*. A statement made by the dental assistant may be quoted in court. Reassuring the patient is often helpful, but no comment on the work should be made.
   —Maintain an unquestionable standard of sterilization and cleanliness procedures.
   —Maintain the integrity and confidence of the patients and office staff by not discussing patient and office business with persons outside the dental office.

■ **What can dental assistants do if a lawsuit is threatened against their employers or themselves?**

The dental assistant should maintain absolute silence on matters relating to the case. The insurance company and/or an attorney should be notified *immediately*.

■ **When a patient files a suit for malpractice against a dentist, is the patient held responsible for proving the allegation?**

Yes, the burden of proof is with the patient. There are four factors the patient should consider before taking such action. It must be clearly demonstrated that (1) a legal duty was owed the patient by the dentist in question, (2) the duty was breached by the dentist, (3) the patient suffered harm or damage as a result of the breach of this legal duty, and (4) the harm or damage was caused directly as a result of the dentist's breach of duty. If any *one* of these factors cannot be established, the dentist cannot be held liable for malpractice.

■ What does statute of limitations mean?

This term refers to the time allowed a person who feels a wrong has been committed to file a civil suit for damages. Generally, when the question is one of negligence or malpractice, the time limit is 2 years from the date the alleged wrong was committed or from the time the patient became aware of the problem. *The action must be filed within that time limit,* not necessarily resolved. In matters concerning breach of contract, the time limit is usually 6 years.

Since state laws differ in this matter, dentists and their staffs should be familiar with the law in their respective states.

MULTIPLE-CHOICE QUESTIONS

1. _____ established the science of dentistry and is regarded as the "father of dentistry."
   a. S. P. Hullihen
   b. John W. Riggs
   c. Pierre Fauchard

2. The man responsible for the standardized system of cavity classification, preparation, and design still taught in dental schools today is:
   a. G. V. Black
   b. Chapin Harris
   c. Sir John Tomes

3. The first known woman dental assistant was employed in New Orleans by:
   a. Dr. T. G. Morton
   b. Dr. C. Edmund Kells
   c. Dr. Horace Hayden

4. Dr. C. Edmund Kells may best be remembered for his introduction and use of _____ in America.
   a. Sterile surgical procedures
   b. X radiation
   c. Anesthetics

5. The founder of the first dental assistant organization was:
   a. Annette Stoker
   b. Lucy Hobbs
   c. Juliette Southard

6. The certified dental assistant and the edu-cational requirement to qualify were formally recognized by the American Dental Association in:
   a. 1960
   b. 1948
   c. 1969

7. The Certifying Board of the ADAA was established for the primary purpose of:
   a. Preparing educational courses for dental assistants
   b. Credentialing qualified dental assistants
   c. Accrediting dental assisting programs

8. The central office of the American Dental Assistants Association is located in:
   a. La Porte, Indiana
   b. New Orleans, Louisiana
   c. Chicago, Illinois

9. A registered dental assistant is defined as one who:
   a. Is qualified by work experience
   b. Is a certified dental assistant also
   c. Meets the criteria set by the dental practice act in that person's individual state

10. Personal decisions based on what conduct may be morally right or wrong are questions of:
    a. Law
    b. Ethics
    c. Judicial decision

11. Laws dealing with the rights and duties of

people toward one another and the violations of these rights and duties are referred to as _____ laws.
a. Tort
b. Constitutional
c. Contract

12. A state law that regulates and controls the practice of dentistry within that state is *most correctly* termed the:
a. Civil law
b. Dental law
c. Dental practice act

13. The agency within state government designated to administer and enforce the dental practices act is the board of:
a. The dental association
b. Dental legislators
c. Dental examiners

14. Performing dental treatment without the consent of the patient makes the dentist liable for:
a. Technical assault
b. Breach of contract
c. Invasion of privacy

15. Total patient satisfaction with dental treatment is not always required if it can be shown that the dentist:

a. Had good intentions
b. Was assisted by competent auxiliaries
c. Maintained an acceptable standard of skill and care

16. The dental assistant should purchase an individual liability insurance policy because:
a. The protection is good when performing illegal duties.
b. An office policy does not cover the individual assistant who is sued for negligence.
c. Patients are suing dentists and dental assistants more frequently than ever before.

SUGGESTED READINGS

Bremner, M. D. K.: The story of dentistry, ed 3, Brooklyn, N.Y., 1964, Dental Items of Interest Publishing Co., Inc.

Ehrlich, A.: Ethics and jurisprudence, Champaign, Ill., 1976, The Colwell Co.

Miller, S. L.: Legal aspects of dentistry, New York, 1970, G. P. Putnam's Sons.

Motley, W. E.: Ethics, jurisprudence, and history, ed. 2, Philadelphia, 1976, Lea & Febiger.

Sarner, H.: Dental jurisprudence, Tampa, Fla., 1963, W. P. Poe Associates, Inc.

Torres, H. O., and Ehrlich, A.: Modern dental assisting, Philadelphia, 1976, W. B. Saunders Co.

CHAPTER 3

The dental business office

BETTY A. LADLEY and JERRY CROWE PATT

■ **The object of a letter of application is to make your reader interested enough in your skills and abilities to grant you an interview. How can this objective be accomplished?**

The letter of application must be attractive and typed in the correct format, using correct spelling, grammar, and good quality stationery.

The letter of application states the applicant's qualifications. The first paragraph should state the objective for writing the letter and for applying for a specific position. The second paragraph informs the reader about the applicant and the applicant's qualifications. This paragraph should have positive and accurate statements about the applicant's ability. The concluding paragraph should ask for an interview and give the phone number and hours when you can be reached, making it convenient for the reader to respond.

■ **List the parts of a business letter.**

Heading
Inside address
Salutation
Body of the letter
Complimentary closing
Typewritten signature
Reference initials

■ **Identify three methods of filing.**

Alphabetic: a system whereby names appear in an alphabetic sequence.

Geographic: a filing system that uses location as a factor of reference. With geographic filing, entries are arranged alphabetically by a territorial division such as a state, city, and street rather than by name.

Numeric: a method of assigning numbers to patients or accounts.

■ **Define the two methods of transferring business records in the dental office.**

Two common methods of transferring business records are:

Perpetual: a method that provides for the constant transfer of materials from active to inactive files

Periodic: a method that provides for the transfer of records from active to inactive files at stated intervals

■ **List the duties of the business assistant when functioning in the role of receptionist.**

Acknowledge patients in a friendly manner as they enter the office.
Keep the reception room neat.
Provide current reading material that has a wide variety of interest.
Inform patients of delays.
Manage properly the patient who talks too much and upsets other patients.
Remind the patient when the patient is leaving the office (1) that treatment is complete, (2) of the next appointment, or (3) of the scheduled recall.

■ **Explain the purpose of an appointment matrix.**

The appointment matrix is a framework around which appointments are made. The matrix is completed prior to beginning a new appointment book and includes special events in the office, such as holidays, professional meetings, and staff meetings.

■ **What vital information should be included in the appointment book entry?**

The following information should be included in the appointment book entry:
— Patient's full name, with cross-reference in case of duplication of names
— Home and business phone numbers
— Treatment to be given
— Length of the appointment indicated with an arrow
— Special notations, that is, new patient, premedication, laboratory case

■ **Identify the functions of a clinical record.**

It serves as a guide to the medical and dental history of the patient and includes notes on past and future treatment of that patient.
It aids in identification of bodies.
It may be used as evidence in a malpractice suit.
It provides verification of treatment rendered for internal revenue purposes.
In third party payment plans, it can be reviewed by dental consultants to determine if services have been rendered.

■ **Describe the function of an office policy.**

The office policy is a written communication designed to establish a better understanding between the patient and the dental staff. The policy should include information about the dentist's philosophy, office hours, appointment control, payment methods, recall procedures, auxiliary duties, and office location and phone numbers.

■ **State the reasons for maintenance of a financial record.**

Financial records provide (1) protection for the dentist and patient, (2) information to be used for tax purposes, and (3) data for business analysis.

■ **What systems of bookkeeping are commonly used in dental offices?**

Three basic systems of bookkeeping may be used in a dental business office:
The log system: a method that requires separate entries in the journal, ledger cards, and receipts and is rapidly being phased out of the business office.

The pegboard: a "write it once" system that provides entry on a daily journal sheet, ledger card, receipt, and in some instances, an insurance claim form or statement.
The computerized system: this system is rapidly gaining acceptance in dentistry and may be used for common bookkeeping procedures plus a variety of other business activities.

■ **Define third party payment.**

The term *third party payment* refers to dental insurance coverage. Altogether there are four persons involved in dental insurance: the patient, the group, the carrier or insurance agency, and the dentist. Four basic types of coverage exist in dentistry: (1) usual, customary, and reasonable fee, (2) fixed, (3) closed panel, and (4) table of allowances.

■ **Explain coordination of benefits.**

When a patient is covered by more than one insurance plan, it is necessary to coordinate the two plans to assure that the patient receives maximum coverage not in excess of 100%. Coordination of benefits occurs when (1) the patient is covered by two or more plans, (2) the patient is covered by a state plan and a commercial plan, or (3) the patient is covered by two commercial plans. Many variables exist in individual policies, and the business assistant should be aware of the common procedures of the various carriers.

■ **List the procedures for reconciling a bank statement.**

Verify the amount of the cancelled checks with the amounts on the bank statement. (The cancelled checks are usually returned in the order listed on the statement.)
Arrange the cancelled checks numerically.
Compare the amounts on the cancelled checks and deposits with the amounts written in the checkbook register.
List the outstanding checks with the check number and the amount. Total the outstanding checks.
Add deposits to the bank statement balance if they do not appear on the bank statement. Add deposits before subtracting outstanding checks.
Look for charges, other than checks, listed

on the bank statement that have been deducted from the account, for example, service charge (SC), debit memo (DM), and overdraft (OD). These charges must be subtracted from the checkbook register.

■ **List equipment common to an efficiently run business office and explain the design of a dental business office, including the desk, typing table, reception window, and counter heights.**

An efficient dental business office is well designed to include arrangement of equipment that will reduce stress and maximize productivity. Equipment will include a typewriter (dual pitch gives the option of selecting pica or elite type), calculator, postage meter, Rolodex file, lateral or vertical files, telephone with multiple lines, copier, intercom, clock, music system controls, fireproof safe, chairs, and a variety of organizational trays and/or baskets.

Following are criteria for an efficient business office arrangement:

— Two desk heights are required. The typing level should be approximately 66 to 68.5 cm (26 to 27 inches), and the writing level should be about 73.7 to 76.2 cm (29 to 30 inches). The counter depth need not exceed 50.8 cm (20 inches). A counter for patients to write on will be about 112 cm (44 inches) high.
— The business assistant should face the reception room.

— Adequate storage should be provided for stationery supplies.
— All cabinet drawers should have full suspension to allow maximum use.
— A small private area should be adjacent to the business office for private calls.

■ **List six suggestions for success with the dental team in a new job.**

Learn the names of staff members.
Use a notebook and calendar for important information.
Observe office hours.
Use good judgment when working overtime and when taking breaks.
Prove your ability through your work rather than by flaunting your education and abilities.
Review the office policy and adhere to it.
Be yourself.

■ **List factors to consider when asking for a raise.**

Have you performed your duties well enough to deserve a raise?
Have you improved or advanced your assisting skills since beginning the job?
Have you been cooperative with other members of the dental team?
Has the dentist's productivity increased because of your assistance?
Do economic factors within the practice, as well as the national economy, make a raise warranted?

MULTIPLE-CHOICE QUESTIONS

1. The most important person(s) in the dental practice is/are the:
   a. Dentist
   b. Dental assistant
   c. Dental hygienist
   d. Laboratory technician
   e. Patient

2. A staff meeting should (1) be held regularly, (2) review accomplishments, (3) be a gripe session, (4) be a time to establish future goals, and/or (5) be held only when a crisis arises.

a. All of the above
b. 1, 2, 3, and 4
c. 2, 4, and 5
d. 1, 2, and 4

3. To be *phonogenic,* you must (1) develop a pleasant telephone voice, (2) speak loudly because people are hard-of-hearing, (3) answer the telephone promptly, (4) attempt to terminate a call to allow other incoming calls to be received, and/or (5) be cordial and responsive to the caller.
   a. 1, 2, and 3

b. 1, 3, and 4

c. 1, 3, and 5

d. 3, 4, and 5

4. Which of the following telephone services would be used in the dental office that would enable the dental assistant to make calls within a specified service area at a monthly rate, rather than on a per-call basis:

a. Conference call

b. Centrex system

c. Touch-a-matic

d. Wide area telephone service (WATS)

5. Which of the following rules apply to dental office correspondence: (1) conciseness, (2) curtness, (3) correctness, and/or (4) courtesy?

a. 1, 2, and 3

b. 1, 3, and 4

c. 2, 3, and 4

d. 1, 2, and 4

6. Mail can be classified as: (1) First class—letters, postcards, business reply mail, and bills; (2) Second class—books, circulars, catalogs, or miscellaneous printed material weighing less than 16 ounces; (3) Third class—newspapers and published periodicals; and/or (4) Fourth class—parcel post, and printed material and packages weighing over 16 ounces.

a. 1 and 2

b. 2 and 3

c. 1 and 4

d. 3 and 4

7. When selecting a copying machine for a dental office, the following features should be considered: (1) quality of copy, (2) paper size for reports, ledger cards, and letters, (3) ability to make microfilms, (4) ability to reproduce from colored original or colored ink, and/or (5) speed and output of copy reproduction.

a. 1, 2, 4, and 5

b. 1, 2, 3, and 4

c. 2, 3, 4, and 5

d. 1, 3, 4, and 5

8. Computers can be used in a dental office to (1) expedite the processing of insurance claim forms, (2) file radiographs, (3) process accounting statements, (4) process the daily schedule of patients, and/or (5) process day sheets that list receivables.

a. 1, 2, 3, and 4

b. 1, 3, 4, and 5

c. 2, 3, 4, and 5

d. 1, 2, 3, and 5

9. Rules for efficient appointment management require that (1) one person be in charge of the appointment book, (2) a treatment plan for the patient be well-defined, (3) all patients be scheduled for short appointments, (4) the patient's needs be accommodated while control of the appointment book is maintained, and/or (5) entries are made in ink.

a. 1, 2, and 4

b. 2, 4, and 5

c. 1, 2, 4, and 5

d. 3, 4, and 5

10. A young child is being scheduled for an appointment. It is wise to schedule an appointment that (1) avoids nap time, (2) is of long duration, (3) is of short duration, (4) is in the early morning, and/or (5) is shortly after lunch.

a. 1, 2, and 4

b. 1, 3, and 4

c. 2 and 5

d. 2 and 4

11. A patient calls the office with an emergency caused by an unexpected accident. You should:

a. Schedule him for the earliest appointment next week.

b. Tell him you are "all booked up" and that perhaps he should call someone else.

c. Tell him to come in during your first available time in the day at which time you will treat the emergency and schedule another treatment if you are unable to complete treatment today.

d. Express your sympathy, and tell him the dentist will phone in a prescription to the pharmacist.

12. When a patient calls the office and states that he has an emergency, which of the following questions should be asked: (1) "How long have you had the discomfort?" (2) "When was your last prophylaxis?"

(3) "What type of discomfort are you experiencing?" and/or (4) "Is it sensitive to hot, cold, or pressure?"
a. 1, 2, and 3
b. 2, 3, and 4
c. 1, 3, and 4
d. 1, 2, and 4

13. A patient requires a series of appointments for treatment over several weeks. The best appointment scheduling for the patient would be:
a. A variety of days and times
b. The same day and time each week
c. Alternate days—Monday the first week, Tuesday the second week, etc.

14. A patient cancels an appointment on short notice. You should:
a. Announce a staff break
b. Seek to fill the appointment with a patient who is readily available
c. Consider this time as a buffer period for the day
d. Quickly announce a staff meeting

15. An enamel hatchet is an example of a/an:
a. Expendable supply
b. Nonexpendable supply
c. Capital item

16. A listing of the stock and equipment in the dental office is referred to as a/an:
a. Accounts receivable
b. Accounts payable
c. Inventory system
d. Total assets

17. Overhead refers to:
a. Gross income
b. Net income
c. Operational costs
d. Liabilities

18. A statement listing services rendered, date of services, and an itemization of the fees is a:
a. Claim form
b. Certificate of eligibility
c. Purchase order
d. Table of allowances

19. Failure to maintain a recall system will result in:
a. Neglect of the patient's oral health
b. Diminished activity in the appointment book

c. Decreased accounts receivable
d. All of the above

20. A disadvantage of the advanced appointment system for recall is:
a. Simplicity
b. Amount of time required of the assistant
c. Lack of knowledge of future commitments

21. The success of a recall system depends on:
a. Dental health education
b. Motivation
c. Consistent follow-up
d. All of the above

22. The term *accounts receivable* refers to:
a. Total charges of the day
b. Total of all outstanding accounts
c. Total of payments received for the day
d. Total of all payments received to date for the year

23. Management of financial arrangements for a patient should (1) represent sound business concepts, (2) provide options for the patient, (3) consider the patient's convenience only, (4) conform to community standards, and/or (5) be presented in a written form to the patient.
a. 1, 2, 4, and 5
b. 1, 3, 4, and 5
c. 2, 3, 4, and 5
d. 1, 2, 3, and 4

24. A patient is seen for treatment for a total fee of $84. The previous balance on the account was $225. The patient pays $60. The new balance is:
a. $301
b. $239
c. $249
d. cr $49

25. A patient has a previous balance of $150. The fee today is $125, and he pays $500. The new balance is:
a. $225
b. $275
c. cr $225
d. cr $275

26. Which of the following groups is a correct computation of totals for the columns given on p. 22?
a. Col A = $420   Col C = $1050
   Col B = $240   Col D = $1020

b. Col A = $420   Col C = $900
   Col B = $240   Col D = $720
   Col C = $975   d. Col A = $410
   Col D = $870   Col B = $140
c. Col A = $420   Col C = $900
   Col B = $240   Col D = $720

	A	B	C	D
	Charge	Credit	New balance	Previous balance
	$75	—	cr $75	cr $150
	$120	—	$400	$280
	$175	$150	$525	$500
	$50	$90	$50	$90
TOTALS				

27. The formula used in pegboard bookkeeping to determine the proof of posting is:
    a. Previous balance + credits − charges = New balance
    b. Previous balance + charges − credits = New balance
    c. New balance − charges + credits = Previous balance
    d. Previous balance + charges − cash received − insurance charges = New balance

28. The employee's earnings record should provide the following information: (1) name of employee, address, social security number, and rate of pay; (2) withholding status, marital status, and special reductions, such as credit unions, bonds, etc.; (3) regular and overtime earnings; and/or (4) quarterly and annual totals.
    a. 1 and 2

b. 1 and 3
c. 2 and 3
d. 3 and 4
e. All of the above
f. None of the above

29. A check that is the bank's own order to make payment out of the bank fund is a:
    a. Certified check
    b. Cashier's check
    c. Money order
    d. Voucher check
    e. Bank draft

30. A credit bureau:
    a. Lends money
    b. Denies credit
    c. Reports information about a person's payment habits
    d. Collects money

31. Using standard-sized stationery (8½ × 11 in), the following procedures would be true: (1) with paper guide at zero, scale reads 0 to 85 for a pica machine; (2) with paper guide at zero, scale reads 1 to 102 for an elite machine; (3) a pica machine has 12 spaces per horizontal inch; and/or (4) an elite machine has 10 spaces per horizontal inch.
    a. 1 and 3
    b. 2 and 4
    c. 1 and 2
    d. 2 and 3

SUGGESTED READINGS

Ehrlich, A. B., and Ehrlich, S. F.: Dental practice management: the teamwork approach, Philadelphia, 1969, W. B. Saunders Co.
Ladley, B. A., and Patt, J. C.: Office procedures for the dental team, St. Louis, 1977, The C. V. Mosby Co.
Miller, S. L.: Legal aspects of dentistry: a programmed course in dental jurisprudence, New York, 1970, G. P. Putnam's Sons.

CHAPTER 4

Oral diagnosis and charting

ELIZABETH OCHOA

■ **What is oral diagnosis?**

Oral diagnosis is recording and evaluating the results of an oral examination and recommending dental treatment to a patient.

■ **What is the responsibility of a dental assistant during oral diagnosis?**

The dental assistant's responsibility is first, to observe the physical condition of the patient, that is, the use of a cane, a limp, the presence of a hearing aid, skin coloring, etc. The dental assistant may be given the responsibility of obtaining a complete health and personal history. It will also be the duty of the dental assistant to accurately record all intraoral and extraoral findings.

■ **Why is a complete medical/dental history vital for an accurate oral diagnosis?**

A complete medical/dental history is vital for determining a patient's current health status. The past dental treatment, history of systemic diseases, medications, existing conditions, and symptoms are contributing factors in diagnosis and treatment planning procedures.

■ **What are vital signs, and why should these findings be recorded?**

The vital signs are blood pressure, pulse rate, temperature, and respiration.

Blood pressure. Blood pressure is the pressure of the blood on the walls of the arteries, and this pressure is dependent on energy of the heart action, elasticity of the walls of the arteries, resistance in the capillaries, and volume and viscosity of the blood.

The two types of blood pressure recorded are *systolic* and *diastolic*. Systolic pressure is the greatest pressure exerted on the circulatory system by the contraction of the left ventricle. The contraction of this ventricle forces blood out into the aorta, which is the largest blood vessel in the circulatory system. The blood then passes into the large arteries, arterioles, and capillaries and then into the tissue. Diastolic pressure refers to the lowest pressure of the circulatory system that occurs when the heart muscle rests prior to the next contraction.

The normal range for blood pressure is 100 to 140/160 systolic and 60 to 90/95 diastolic.

Pulse rate. Pulse rate is the expansion and contraction of an artery, and this can be felt with the finger. The pulse is usually felt on the radial artery at the wrist, or it may be felt at the carotid, temporal, femoral, or other arteries. The normal number of pulsations per minute varies from 70 to 72 in males and from 78 to 82 in females.

Temperature. Normal temperature is 98.6° F or 37° C.

Respiration. The act by which air is drawn in and expelled from the lungs, inspiration and expiration, is referred to as respiration. The normal pattern of respiration is 17 to 20 breaths per minute.

In oral diagnosis it is important that these vital signs be recorded. Any deviation from the normal may indicate a medical or dental problem.

■ **What are the objectives of dental charting?**

To establish accurate records for future reference or legal purposes

To identify existing conditions in the oral cavity

To maintain records for identification of a body in case of death

To establish a permanent record of oral conditions from the time of the initial visit

■ What are the four methods of naming and coding teeth?

The common methods used in dental charting include (1) Name, (2) Universal, (3) Palmer Notation System, and (4) FDI (Federation Dentaire Internationale).

Name. When identifying a specific tooth list the dentition, arch, quadrant, and tooth name in that order. For example, a permanent maxillary right first premolar instead of right first premolar maxillary permanent.

Universal. This system uses the arabic numerals 1 to 32 to identify the permanent dentition. For primary dentition, the letters A to T are used. The number designation begins by assigning the number 1 to the permanent maxillary right third molar. The numbers proceed to the permanent maxillary left third molar, 16, descending to the permanent mandibular third molar, 17, and terminating on the permanent mandibular right third molar, 32. In a similar manner, the A to T nomenclature is applied to the primary dentition with A being assigned to the primary maxillary right second molar and T to the primary mandibular right second molar.

Palmer. In the Palmer Notation System the arch is divided in brackets.

MAXILLARY RIGHT	MAXILLARY LEFT
8 7 6 5 4 3 2 1	1 2 3 4 5 6 7 8
8 7 6 5 4 3 2 1	1 2 3 4 5 6 7 8
MANDIBULAR RIGHT	MANDIBULAR LEFT

In the Palmer Notation System the lowest number is closest to the midline; therefore all teeth designated 1 are central incisors. If a separate tooth is to be designated, as is often the case, the following symbol would be used to denote the permanent mandibular left first molar ‾| 6.

To indicate the primary dentition using the Palmer Notation System the letters A to E are used in the same manner.

MAXILLARY RIGHT	MAXILLARY LEFT
E D C B A	A B C D E
E D C B A	A B C D E
MANDIBULAR RIGHT	MANDIBULAR LEFT

FDI. This system is a simple numerical method that designates each tooth by two digits, facilitating communication between dentists and satisfying the need for data processing. The first digit identifies quadrants and dentitions, and the second digit denotes individual teeth. The numbers 1 to 8 are used in the first digit as follows:

1—maxillary right permanent
2—maxillary left permanent
3—mandibular left permanent
4—mandibular right permanent
5—maxillary right primary
6—maxillary left primary
7—mandibular left primary
8—mandibular right primary

Moving clockwise, the sequence begins with the upper right quadrant and ends with the lower right quadrant.

For the second digit the numerals 1 to 8 are also used as follows:

1—permanent or primary central incisor
2—permanent or primary lateral incisor
3—permanent or primary cuspid
4—first premolar or primary first molar
5—second premolar or primary second molar
6—permanent first molar
7—permanent second molar
8—permanent third molar

The following charts indicate the application of these digits.

PERMANENT DENTITION

MAXILLARY RIGHT	MAXILLARY LEFT
18 17 16 15 14 13 12 11	21 22 23 24 25 26 27 28
48 47 46 45 44 43 42 41	31 32 33 34 35 36 37 38
MANDIBULAR RIGHT	MANDIBULAR LEFT

PRIMARY DENTITION

MAXILLARY RIGHT	MAXILLARY LEFT
55 54 53 52 51	61 62 63 64 65
85 84 83 82 81	71 72 73 74 75
MANDIBULAR RIGHT	MANDIBULAR LEFT

■ **List guidelines the dental assistant should follow when charting an oral examination.**

Use a No 2 black lead pencil, *not* a pen.

Be familiar with the codes and symbols the dentist uses; do *not* use longhand.

Use colored pencils to differentiate between restorations and caries, that is, *blue* to designate amalgam restorations, *yellow* for gold restorations, *red* for caries, *blue* diagonal lines to denote porcelain jacket crowns, etc.

Make accurate entries.

Make entries neatly and avoid smudges.

■ **What aids are used for a complete and accurate diagnosis?**

A dentist will use a variety of materials and techniques to aid in the diagnosis of a patient's condition.

Clinical examination. This examination includes a visual inspection and palpation to reveal any abnormal conditions of intraoral hard and soft tissues or extraoral structures.

Radiographs. These films are valuable aids for detecting what the eye does not see, that is, bone loss, proximal caries, cysts, and pulp stones.

Study models. These reproductions of a patient's dentition provide information on teeth and their occlusion and the shape and contour of soft tissues.

Pulp tests. These tests indicate the vitality of a specific tooth or teeth. The tests include the use of an electric vitalometer or a thermal test using ice or heated gutta-percha.

Plaque disclosure. Disclosing solutions are applied to the patient's teeth to reveal the presence of plaque.

Photographs. Photographs offer an opportunity to consult with other dentists, provide an accurate record of treatment progress, and provide a vivid record of the before and after status of the patient.

Bacterial analysis. This procedure is often used on a patient with rampant caries to determine the presence and quantity of the lactobacillus organisms.

Medical tests. These tests are becoming more routine in a dental practice to aid complete and accurate diagnosis and include blood pressure measurement, a variety of blood and urine studies, and a vitamin C test.

■ **Using your customary method of charting, record the following conditions on chart A.**

a. Maxillary right third molar is to be extracted.

b. Maxillary right second molar has bucco-occlusal caries.

c. Maxillary right first premolar has mesio-occlusal caries.

d. Maxillary right lateral incisor has a mesial composite restoration.

e. Maxillary left cuspid has a porcelain veneer crown and is a mesial abutment for a fixed bridge.

f. Maxillary left first premolar is missing.

g. Maxillary left second premolar has a three-quarter gold crown as a distal abutment to the fixed bridge replacing the first premolar.

h. Maxillary left second molar has a mesio-occlusodistal amalgam restoration.

i. Maxillary left second molar has a buccal pit amalgam restoration.

j. Maxillary left third molar is missing.

k. Mandibular left third molar is to be extracted.

l. Mandibular left second molar has a full gold crown and root canal therapy.

m. Mandibular left first molar is missing.

n. Mandibular left second premolar is missing.

o. Mandibular left first premolar has a mesio-occlusal gold inlay.

p. Mandibular left cuspid has a distal amalgam restoration.

q. Mandibular left central incisor has a mesial composite restoration.

r. Mandibular right central incisor has distal caries.

s. Mandibular right lateral incisor has a mesial composite restoration.

t. Mandibular right lateral incisor has a distal composite restoration.

u. Mandibular right first premolar has a mesio-occlusodistal gold inlay.

Chart A

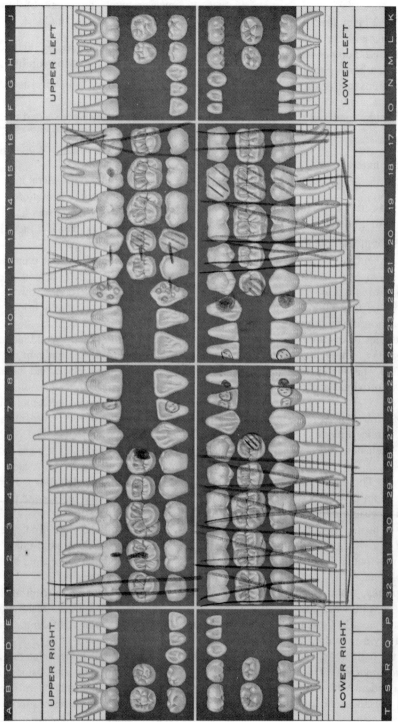

From Professional Publishers, P.O. Box 10113, Palo Alto, Calif. 94303. Reprinted by permission.

Chart B

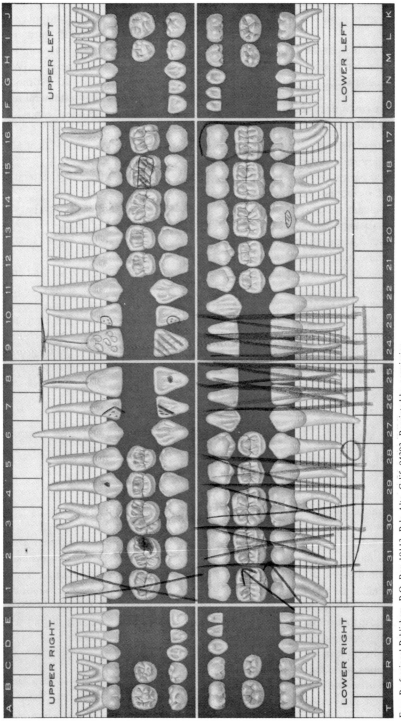

From Professional Publishers, P.O. Box 10113, Palo Alto, Calif. 94303. Reprinted by permission.

v. Mandibular right second premolar is missing.

w. Mandibular right first molar is missing.

x. Mandibular right second molar is missing.

y. Mandibular right third molar is missing.

z. A partial denture is replacing all missing mandibular teeth.

■ **Using your customary method of charting, record the following conditions on chart B.**

a. Maxillary right third molar is missing.

b. Maxillary right second molar has mesio-occlusal caries.

c. Maxillary second premolar has a buccal pit amalgam restoration.

d. Maxillary right lateral incisor has a class IV distal composite restoration.

e. Maxillary right central incisor has root canal therapy and a lingual pit amalgam restoration.

f. Maxillary left central incisor has root canal therapy and a porcelain veneer crown.

g. Maxillary left lateral incisor has a mesial class III composite restoration.

h. Maxillary left first premolar needs a porcelain veneer crown.

i. Maxillary left second molar has a mesio-occlusodistal gold inlay.

j. Mandibular left third molar is partially erupted and pericoronitis is present.

k. There is a buccal class V gold foil on the mandibular left first molar.

l. Mandibular left lateral incisor is missing.

m. Mandibular left central incisor is missing.

n. Mandibular right central incisor is missing.

o. Mandibular right lateral incisor is missing.

p. Mandibular right first premolar has a periapical abscess.

q. Mandibular right second premolar is missing.

r. Mandibular right first molar is missing.

s. Mandibular right second molar is missing.

t. Mandibular right third molar has drifted mesially into the second molar position.

u. There is a mandibular partial denture replacing all missing mandibular teeth.

MULTIPLE-CHOICE QUESTIONS

1. The _____ have no distal teeth.
   a. Central incisors
   b. Cuspids
   c. First molars
   d. Third molars
2. First premolars have _____ to the mesial aspect and _____ to distal aspect.
   a. Laterals; second premolars
   b. Cuspids; first molars
   c. Cuspids; second premolars
   d. Laterals; first molars
3. Radiographs are vital in the diagnosis of (1) tooth vitality, (2) supportive tissue, (3) faulty restorations, (4) tooth mobility, and/ or (5) restorative material.
   a. 2 and 4
   b. 1 and 4

   c. 2 and 3
   d. 3 and 5
   e. 1 and 3
4. The role of the dental assistant in oral diagnosis is to (1) evaluate the patient's physical condition, (2) observe any outward sign of abnormalities, (3) transcribe the dictation of the dentist accurately, and/ or (4) serve as a second set of eyes in general observation.
   a. 1 and 2
   b. 2 and 4
   c. 1 and 4
   d. All of the above
5. The average temperature of an adult male is:
   a. 98.6° F/42° C

b. 86.9° F/39° C

c. 98.6° F/37° C

d. 9.68° F/40° C

6. The average pulse rate of an adult female is:
   a. 60 per minute
   b. 20 per second
   c. 10 per second
   d. 80 per minute

7. The average blood pressure of an adult is:
   a. 100/50 mm Hg
   b. 80/120 mm Hg
   c. 50/100 mm Hg
   d. 120/80 mm Hg

8. Hypertension is the condition known as:
   a. Hypergloxinia
   b. Hyperlymphatic
   c. High blood pressure
   d. High blood urea level

9. During the recording of a medical history the patient states the presence of a renal condition. This information is vital for safe dental treatment because:
   a. The patient cannot receive a local anesthetic.
   b. If a local anesthetic is administered, there will be inflammation of the kidneys.
   c. Slow healing will occur because of excess glucose in the kidneys.
   d. The kidneys serve as a filter of impurities, and therefore a renal condition could hinder the healing process.

10. The first objective in oral diagnosis is:
    a. Secure x-ray films of the patient immediately and evaluate the underlying tissue.
    b. Take and record vital signs to determine the physical status of the patient.
    c. Observe patients initially as they are ushered to the operatory (dental chair).
    d. Record a complete medical history prior to the beginning of treatment.

11. Vital signs are (1) blood pressure and pulse, (2) temperature and respiration, (3) blood pressure and nerve reaction to sharp instruments, and/or (4) pulse and temperature.
    a. 1 and 3
    b. 2 and 4

c. 2 and 3

d. 1 and 2

12. The *primary* purpose of oral diagnosis is to:
    a. Determine treatment needed
    b. Detect abnormalities
    c. Warn the patient of physical health hazards
    d. Prevent caries

13. The blood disease that is contracted only by members of the Negroid race is:
    a. Dextrodeficiency
    b. Plasma impurity
    c. Sickle cell anemia
    d. Neurotic anemia

14. Accurate charting is required for (1) legal purposes, (2) death identification, (3) public knowledge, and/or (4) diagnosis.
    a. 1, 2, and 4
    b. 1, 2, and 3
    c. 2, 3, and 4
    d. 1, 3, and 4

15. The armamentarium required for a visual oral examination is:
    a. Medical history and radiographs
    b. Measurement of vital signs and blood test
    c. Vitalometer and periodontal probe
    d. Mirror, explorer, and periodontal probe
    e. All of the above
    f. None of the above

16. The vitalometer measures:
    a. Pulp mobility
    b. Reaction
    c. Tissue depth
    d. Vital signs
    e. None of the above
    f. All of the above

17. The dental patient's complete record requires accurate notation because (1) records are required should there be a legal action brought against the dentist, (2) records detail past and current treatment, (3) records are necessary in forensic identification, and/or (4) records indicate a patient's physical condition.
    a. 1 and 3
    b. 3 and 4
    c. 2 and 3
    d. 2 and 4

e. All of the above

f. None of the above

Use the Universal System of tooth coding to answer questions 18 to 26.

18. The permanent maxillary right first molar is tooth:

a. 1

b. 14

c. 3

d. 6

19. The permanent mandibular right second molar is tooth:

a. 31

b. 18

c. 15

d. 3

20. The permanent third molars are teeth:

a. 1, 16, 17, and 32

b. 3, 6, 22, and 27

c. 1, 18, 32, and 16

d. 3, 14, 17, and 30

21. The permanent mandibular left second premolar is tooth:

a. 21

b. 13

c. 28

d. 20

22. Tooth 6 is the:

a. Maxillary right cuspid

b. Maxillary right first molar

c. Mandibular left cuspid

d. Mandibular right first molar

23. Tooth 8 is the:

a. Maxillary right central incisor

b. Maxillary right lateral

c. Maxillary right third molar

d. Maxillary left third molar

24. Tooth 21 is the:

a. Mandibular left second premolar

b. Mandibular right first premolar

c. Mandibular left first premolar

d. Maxillary left first premolar

25. Teeth 24 and 25:

a. Contact on the distal surface

b. Contact on the labial surface

c. Contact on the mesial surface

d. Are in different arches

26. The primary mandibular right cuspid is:

a. M

b. C

c. R

d. Q

Use the Palmer Notation System of tooth coding to answer questions 27 to 29.

27. $\overline{3|}$ is the:

a. Permanent mandibular left first premolar

b. Permanent mandibular right first premolar

c. Permanent maxillary right cuspid

d. Permanent mandibular right cuspid

28. The permanent maxillary right first molar is:

a. $\overline{6|}$

b. $\underline{6|}$

c. $\overline{|6}$

d. $\underline{|6}$

e. None of the above

29. Which tooth is represented by $\underline{|E}$?

a. The primary maxillary right central incisor

b. The primary maxillary left central incisor

c. The primary maxillary right second molar

d. The primary maxillary left second molar

30. Which tooth is represented by $\overline{B|}$?

a. The primary maxillary right cuspid

b. The primary mandibular right cuspid

c. The primary mandibular right lateral incisor

d. The primary mandibular left lateral incisor

Use the completed chart A on p. 26 to answer questions 31 to 37.

31. Which teeth have total coverage?

a. Mandibular left second molar and maxillary left cuspid

b. Mandibular left first bicuspid and mandibular left first bicuspid

c. Mandibular left second molar and mandibular right first bicuspid

d. Mandibular left cuspid and mandibular left first bicuspid

32. How many surfaces of amalgam are present?

a. 12
b. 3
c. 5
d. 15

33. How many posterior teeth have caries?
a. 2
b. 1
c. 3
d. 4

34. Which tooth is nonvital?
a. Mandibular left cuspid
b. Mandibular right central
c. Mandibular left third molar
d. Mandibular left second molar

35. What type partial denture does the patient have?
a. Bilateral
b. Unilateral
c. Free end
d. Complex
e. Labial bar

36. How many teeth are missing?
a. 12
b. 6
c. 8
d. 10

37. The mesial abutments of the partial denture are:
a. Mandibular left second molar and mandibular right second bicuspid
b. Mandibular right second bicuspid and mandibular right third molar
c. Mandibular left first bicuspid and mandibular right first bicuspid
d. Mandibular right first bicuspid and mandibular left second molar

Use the completed chart B on p. 27 to answer questions 38 to 42.

38. There is inflammation around the crown of the:
a. Maxillary right central incisor
b. Maxillary left central incisor
c. Mandibular left third molar
d. Mandibular right third molar

39. Which tooth has periapical involvement?
a. 30
b. 28
c. 21
d. 19

40. Endodontic treatment has been completed on teeth:
a. 24 and 25
b. 9 and 11
c. 7 and 8
d. 8 and 9

41. There is a cervical cohesive gold restoration on tooth:
a. 16
b. 36
c. 26
d. 46

42. A composite involving the distoincisal angle has been placed on tooth:
a. 12
b. 21
c. 32
d. 43

SUGGESTED READINGS

Brand, R. W., and Isselhard, D. E.: Anatomy of orofacial structures, St. Louis, 1977, The C. V. Mosby Co.

Chasteen, J. E.: Essentials of clinical dental assisting, St. Louis, 1975, The C. V. Mosby Co.

Ehrlich, A.: Fundamentals for dental auxiliaries; introduction to recording dental charting, Champaign, Ill., 1974, The Colwell Co.

Ladley, B. A., and Patt, J. C.: Office procedures for the dental team, St. Louis, 1977, The C. V. Mosby Co.

CHAPTER 5

Dental instruments

ANN EHRLICH

■ **Describe G. V. Black's instrument formula, and state the criteria that determine when the three-number or the four-number formula should be used.**

G. V. Black developed the universal instrument formula that bears his name as a means of precisely describing an instrument with reference to its shaft, blade, and cutting edge. If the cutting edge of an instrument forms a right angle with the blade of that instrument, a three-unit formula is used. If the cutting edge forms anything other than a right angle with the blade, a four-unit formula is used.

Enamel hatchets and chisels exemplify instruments fitting the criteria of the three-unit formula, whereas gingival margin trimmers and angle formers are typical of instruments meeting the criteria of the four-unit formula.

■ **Identify the parts of a hand instrument.**

A hand instrument's components include the handle or shaft, shank, and nib or blade. In hand cutting instruments the blade terminates in a bevel and cutting edge, whereas in other hand instruments the working end is referred to as a nib.

■ **Identify instruments that have right and left ends from instruments that have standard and reverse bevels.**

Hatchets, angle formers, and gingival margin trimmers possess right and left ends, whereas chisels and hoes possess standard and reverse bevels. Manufacturers often denote left from right and mesial from distal by an indented ring.

■ **What is the primary use of the enamel hatchet?**

The enamel hatchet is used primarily to plane cavity walls and cervical floors to remove any roughness created by burs during cavity preparation. It is used to sharpen line and point angles in the cavity preparation.

■ **What is a spoon excavator?**

The spoon excavator is a double-planed instrument designed to remove debris and caries from an extensively damaged tooth.

■ **Describe the primary function of a dental hoe and the type of motion required in its use.**

A hoe is used to smooth and finish the walls and floor of the cavity preparation. This instrument is similar in design to a garden hoe and is used with a pull motion.

■ **Describe the primary use of a finishing file and the type of motion required in its use.**

A finishing file is used to trim away excess restorative material. The blade is very thin, and the teeth of the blade are designed so that the file may be used as either a push or a pull instrument.

■ **Describe the design and primary function of the gingival margin trimmer.**

The gingival margin trimmer is a modified hatchet with a curved blade. This curvature aids in the efficiency of the instrument when it is used in a lateral scraping motion. It is used primarily to place a bevel along the cervical cavosurface margin in amalgam and inlay preparations.

■ **What is a periodontal probe, and how does it differ from an explorer?**

A periodontal probe is an instrument with millimeter gradations and is used to measure the depth of bone resorption in a periodontal pocket. An explorer has a fine sharp tip; the tip of a probe is gently rounded.

■ **Describe a matrix and how it is used?**

A matrix is a flexible, adaptive metal or plastic strip designed to supply the form of the missing tooth wall in the placement and condensation steps of a tooth restoration. Matrices may be held in place by hand, with a clip, or by a holder such as a Tofflemire retainer.

■ **Describe the design and use of an amalgam condenser.**

An amalgam condenser is a metal hand instrument designed to pack and condense plastic-type material, such as amalgam, within a cavity preparation. The nib of the condenser may be smooth or serrated. The shank and nib can be placed at various angles to the shaft for use in different areas of the mouth.

■ **Name and describe the function of the three instruments that are used in most standard dental procedures.**

Mouth mirror. This instrument is used for an indirect view of the operating field, to reflect light, to retract the tongue and cheek, and to protect tissues from injury during the procedure.

Explorer. The explorer is commonly used to probe the less accessible areas of the teeth to detect discrepancies on tooth surfaces.

Pliers. Pliers (commonly referred to as cotton pliers and/or forceps) are used to pick up and transfer cotton rolls, pellets, and medicaments into the oral cavity without contamination.

■ **Describe the primary function of the ultra high-speed and conventional speed handpieces in cavity preparation.**

The ultra high-speed handpiece is used for gaining entry into the tooth, for rapid cutting of tooth structure, and for removal of bulk tooth structure. The conventional handpiece is used for removal of caries and refinement of the preparation.

■ **Describe how the friction-grip and latch-type contra-angles hold burs in position.**

Friction-grip contra-angles hold the instrument with a friction chuck that grasps the entire shaft in the head of the contra-angle. A latch-type contra-angle holds the end of the cutting instrument by mechanically grasping a small groove on the end of the bur shaft.

■ **What is the primary difference in use between carbide burs and plain steel burs?**

The carbide steel bur operates most efficiently at high speeds. It is able to retain its sharp cutting capability during repeated use and is generally favored in operative dentistry. Plain steel burs are effective in cutting at low speed on dense, hard tissue. Frequently, the plain steel bur at low speed will generate heat in the tissues of the tooth, causing discomfort to the patient.

MULTIPLE-CHOICE QUESTIONS*

1. In Black's instrument formula that uses a three-digit number, the _____ number indicates the length of the blade in millimeters.
   a. First
   b. Second
   c. Third
   d. Fourth

2. The _____ of an instrument connects the blade or nib with the shaft. In some instruments this is _____ to bring the working edge of the instrument within 2 mm of the long axis of the handle.
   a. Connector; slanted
   b. Neck; angled
   c. Shank; binangled
   d. Shank; contra-angled

3. Plastic instruments are so named because they are:
   a. Made of plastic material
   b. Used only with nonmetallic materials such as composites
   c. Used to move and pack materials while they are still soft and easily changed in shape
   d. a and b above
   e. None of the above

4. A _____ is used in a push motion to cut along the lines of the enamel rods and accessible margins of a cavity preparation. Instrument _____ is an example of this type of instrument.
   a. Carver; F
   b. Chisel; B
   c. Hatchet; I
   d. Hoe; J

5. Ultra high-speed handpieces have very little torque. This means:
   a. The operator must apply pressure to make it work
   b. It is best suited for finishing a cavity preparation
   c. The handpiece must be used with a very light touch
   d. a and b above

6. An example of a hand cutting instrument with a three-number formula is a/an:
   a. Binangle chisel
   b. Explorer
   c. Gingival margin trimmer
   d. Angle former

7. A _____ is a hand cutting instrument with the blade at right angles to the long axis of the instrument shaft. It is used with a pull motion. Instrument _____ is an example of this type of instrument.
   a. Chisel; B
   b. Chisel; J
   c. Hatchet; H
   d. Hoe; H

8. Which of the following instruments do *not* have sharp knifelike edges?
   a. Carvers
   b. Chisels
   c. Excavators
   d. Hatchets
   e. Hoes

9. Instrument _____ is a modified enamel hatchet. It is called a _____.
   a. D; Wedelstaedt hatchet
   b. F; Black angle former
   c. H; Hollenback hatchet
   d. J; gingival margin trimmer

10. A _____ is used to reproduce tooth anatomy in amalgam or wax. Instrument _____ is an example of this.
    a. Burnisher; E
    b. Carver; F
    c. Condensor; A
    d. Plastic instrument; G
    e. Gingival margin trimmer; I

11. Nonmetallic instruments are used with composite restorations because:
    a. Metal instruments may leave marks on the restoration.
    b. Metal retards the set of the material.
    c. Metallic instruments set up galvanic action.
    d. Nonmetal instruments will not stick to the material.

12. Which of the following is/are example(s) of burnishers?
    a. Beaver-tail
    b. Egg

---

*Refer to Figs. A to R on pp. 37-39 when responding to those questions that require you to identify instruments according to a letter of the alphabet.

c. Football
d. Round
e. All of the above

13. A ''red imp'' (dental stone) is used to:
    a. Contour an amalgam restoration
    b. Place holes in a custom impression tray
    c. Polish amalgam restorations
    d. Sharpen instruments
    e. Take a ''quickie'' impression

14. A finishing file is used with a _____ motion.
    a. Pull
    b. Push
    c. Lateral
    d. Rotating
    e. a and b

15. The operator wants to use a handpiece to remove the remaining carious dentin. For this purpose a/an _____ bur and a _____ handpiece are indicated.
    a. Inverted cone; low-speed
    b. Inverted cone; high-speed
    c. Tapered fissure; high-speed
    d. Round; high-speed
    e. Round; low-speed

16. When the operator asks for a right-angle handpiece, the procedure is likely to be:
    a. Cutting a crown preparation
    b. Opening a carious lesion
    c. Polishing the teeth or restoration
    d. Preparing for pin retention
    e. Toileting the cavity

17. You are preparing to mix zinc phosphate cement. For this you would use instrument _____.
    a. F
    b. K
    c. L
    d. Not shown

18. The operator asks for a 33½ bur. This is a _____ bur and is shown in Fig. _____.
    a. Large crosscut tapered fissure; P
    b. Large inverted cone; Q
    c. Large round; M
    d. Medium pear; R
    e. Small inverted cone; N

19. A cleoid-discoid instrument can be used to:
    a. Carve the occlusal detail in a posterior restoration
    b. Contour the matrix band
    c. Finish the cavity preparation

d. Smooth and finish a composite restoration
e. All of the above

20. An instrument that represents Black's four-number instrument formula is the:
    a. Angle former
    b. Black's wax and amalgam carver
    c. Hoe
    d. Spoon excavator
    e. None of the above

21. An Arkansas stone is used to:
    a. Finish composite restorations
    b. Polish amalgam restorations
    c. Smooth and finish custom trays
    d. Sharpen hand instruments
    e. Trim dentures

22. Instrument _____ may have a serrated working end. It is used to condense amalgam.
    a. A
    b. C
    c. F
    d. G
    e. J

23. A Wedelstaedt file is a finishing instrument modified by a/an _____ in the shank.
    a. Angle
    b. Contra-angle
    c. Right-angle
    d. Slight curve

24. The operator is working in a hard-to-reach area of a posterior tooth. You are asked for a binangle chisel. This is instrument _____.
    a. B
    b. D
    c. F
    d. H
    e. I

25. _____ is/are impregnated into metal to form a bur or wheel that is used as a rotary cutting instrument to reduce tooth structure.
    a. Carbide silicon
    b. Dentates
    c. Diamonds
    d. Stainless steel chips

26. The operator is ready to use a hand instrument to remove any remaining decay. You have instrument _____ ready to pass.
    a. A
    b. C

c. H
d. I
e. J

27. The operator is ready to use a hand instrument to condense the amalgam. The instrument of choice is instrument _____.
a. A
b. E
c. F
d. G
e. I

28. A _____ is a mounting device used to hold abrasive disks in the handpiece.
a. Friction grip
b. Garnet
c. Latch key
d. Mandrel
e. Spindle

29. The amalgam restoration has a slight overhang on the interproximal gingival margin. The operator may use instrument _____ to correct this.
a. B
b. D
c. F
d. I
e. J

30. The _____ handpiece is most effective for polishing or refining a cavity preparation.
a. low-speed (6000 to 7000 rpm)
b. high-speed (6000 to 100,000 rpm)
c. ultrasonic (30,000 to 400,000 rpm)
d. ultra high-speed (100,000 to 800,000 rpm)

31. The operator is ready to carve the anatomy in an amalgam restoration. You pass instrument _____.
a. A
b. E
c. F
d. G
e. Correct instrument not shown

32. To open a carious lesion and to begin the cavity preparation, the operator may request a _____ handpiece and instrument _____.
a. high-speed; M

b. high-speed; N
c. low-speed; Q
d. low-speed; R

33. Instrument _____ has the angle of the cutting edge at right angles to the axis of the blade. It is designed to cut enamel along the lines of the enamel rods.
a. B
b. D
c. H
d. I
e. None of the above

34. The operator is using a direct technique to prepare an inlay pattern. Instrument _____ will be used to shape the occlusal contours of the wax pattern.
a. A
b. C
c. E
d. F
e. G

35. Instrument _____ is a tapered fissure crosscut bur.
a. N
b. O
c. P
d. R

36. Instrument _____ is a plain straight fissure bur. It is called plain because _____.
a. N; the top is not curved
b. O; it is not crosscut
c. Q; it is not tapered
d. R; it is not diamond impregnated

37. Instrument _____ is a bur in the series numbered from ¼ to 8.
a. M
b. O
c. P
d. Q
e. R

SUGGESTED READINGS

Chasteen, J. E.: Essentials of clinical dental assisting, St. Louis, 1975, The C. V. Mosby Co.

Ehrlich, A.: Dental hand instrument study cards, Champaign, Ill., 1974, The Colwell Co.

Torres, H. O., and Ehrlich, A.: Modern dental assisting, Philadelphia, 1976, W. B. Saunders Co.

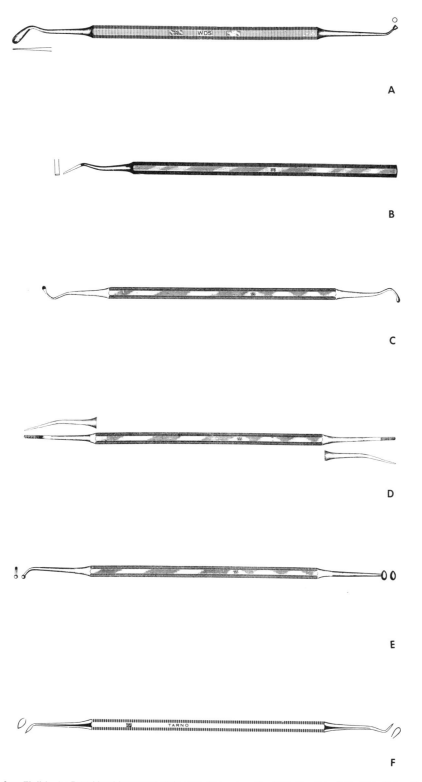

A

B

C

D

E

F

A to **L** from Ehrlich, A.: Dental hand instrument study cards, Champaign, Ill., 1974, The Colwell Co. **M** to **R** from Torres, H. O., and Ehrlich, A.: Modern dental assisting, Philadelphia, 1976, W. B. Saunders Co.

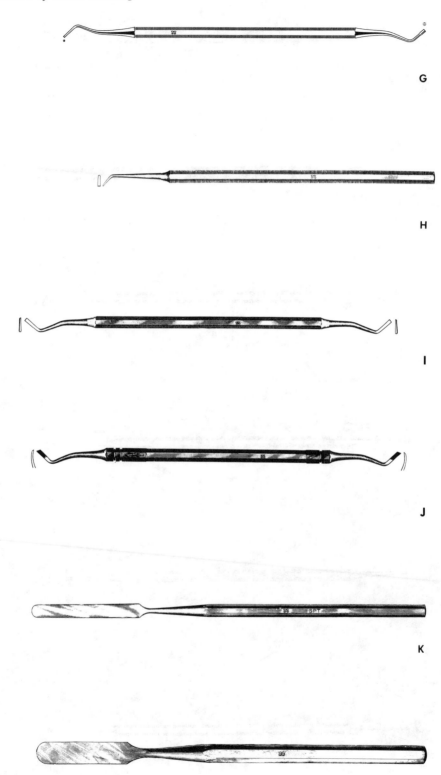

G

H

I

J

K

L

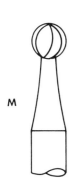

M

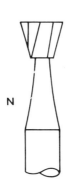

N

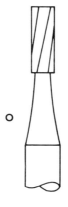

O

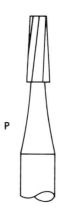

P

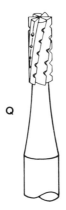

Q

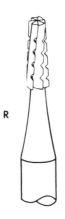

R

CHAPTER 6

Office emergencies

JOHN P. GOBETTI

■ **What is an office emergency?**

The term *office emergency* refers to a medical emergency that occurs in the dental office. An emergency in medicine is a sudden, unexpected change in a person's health status that calls for immediate action. The major concept in this definition is that *immediate action* is necessary.

■ **Why is it necessary to prepare for an office emergency?**

Through the amazing progress of modern medical, pharmacologic, and surgical techniques, more persons are surviving in spite of their diseases. Approximately 60% of all persons over 60 years of age suffer from some chronic disease, and cardiac and circulatory diseases are the cause of 54% of all deaths in this age group. Perks confirms the potential risks involved during dental treatments with his data; 31.8% of the dental patients surveyed had a medical disorder. Included in the figure were 7.5% who had a "major" medical disorder. Barclay found that 21.2% of dental patients were receiving pharmacologic agents, and 40% of those patients were taking two or more medications concurrently. There is a tendency especially for senior citizen patients to be receiving multiple drug therapy. The large percentage of patients receiving drug therapy increases the potential of possible side effects and drug interactions during dental procedures. The greater number of patients who are receiving treatment for medical problems produces a greater risk in the practice of modern dentistry, which uses pharmacologic agents administered orally, intramuscularly, intravascularly, or by inhalation.

Patient population, advances in medicine, drug therapy, and new dental procedures must all be considered when preparing for an office emergency.

■ **What is the first step in preparing for an office emergency?**

Prevention! The best preparation is prevention. Many potential emergency situations can be minimized or totally avoided if they are anticipated. Therefore, the best preventive measure is a thorough history to alert the dental professional to potential problems.

■ **What composes a thorough history?**

An adequate and thorough history must be composed of several sections: medical history, drug history, dental history, review of systems, and personal and social factors. When used to avoid an office emergency, the major functions of a history are to elicit information about *known* and *unknown* systemic diseases and problems. Questions help the patient remember known diseases (angina pectoris, diabetes mellitus, etc.). Diseases that are undiagnosed may be suspected by correlation of positive answers to questions about signs and symptoms. (Do you experience chest pains?) The best method of history procurement is a questionnaire to be filled out in ink by the patient, combined with an oral interview.

■ **How should the medical history be recorded?**

The information obtained from the history is seldom explored in depth for pertinent details. A history of angina pectoris is only the most superficial information. Additional questions must be answered to evaluate the process. How long has the person had angina? What are the frequency and severity of the attacks? How does the patient's angina attack manifest itself? The medical history should record the precipitating factors, location of pain, quality of pain, modifying features (such as shortness of breath), duration of the attack, response to drug therapy, and physician's instructions to the patient in the event of an attack. The recorded information enables the dental personnel to rapidly recognize and comprehend the signs and symptoms for a specific appraisal of the patient's medical condition.

■ **How should the drug history be recorded?**

Side effects or the primary therapeutic effect of medications in combination with dental therapy and stress may precipitate a crisis. All medications, over-the-counter and prescription, should be evaluated. Basic drug information, drug name and dosage, should be obtained from the patient, from the prescription container, from the dispensing pharmacist, or from the patient's physician. The drug information should be recorded as single words or short phrases. Minimal information would be (1) name of reference book where drug is described, (2) page in that reference book, (3) names of therapeutic agent, both brand and generic, (4) components of the agent, (5) indications, (6) actions, (7) contraindications and drug interactions, (8) side effects, (9) normal dosage, and (10) patient's dosage. The accessibility of this detailed review of a drug saves precious time during an emergency. The drug history may help prevent an emergency, since rational changes in the dental treatment may be made to avoid future problems or exacerbating existing conditions.

■ **How are problems of interpretation of the history resolved?**

Any patient with a dubious history, questionable medical condition, poorly controlled disease, or complex drug regimen should have a *written consultation* from the physician before proceeding with dental treatment.

■ **Is any other patient data necessary before beginning treatment?**

Yes. The history serves as a guide for a limited physical examination. It is mandatory to record baseline physiologic information. A "normal" blood pressure reading is an important reference necessary for comparison with blood pressure changes during an emergency. The blood pressure should be taken at the end of the initial dental appointment to avoid patient anxiety being a biologic variable in the recording. It is important to update the blood pressure determination at recall appointments. If there is a history of hypertension, a recording of the blood pressure should be entered in the patient notes at the beginning of each dental appointment. When indicated by the history, securing the pulse and respiration rates provides valuable background information that should be noted in the patient record.

■ **Is there anything else that can be done to prevent an office emergency?**

Yes. Routine office procedures should be altered as indicated by the patient's history and limited physical examination. Appointment times can be arranged to coincide with specific medical requirements. Patients with a history of cardiac disease (congestive heart failure, angina pectoris, hypertension, etc.) and respiratory diseases (asthma, emphysema, etc.) tolerate dental procedures much better in the morning when they are rested and not stressed. Diabetic patients and others with a strict mealtime regimen should be scheduled after meals. Patients who require premedication before dental treatment (sedation for emotional problems and anxiety) should have increased length and decreased number of appointments to reduce the exposure risk of precipitating an untoward event from the stress of dental procedures or drug interactions. Persons taking diuretics should be given frequent breaks during lengthy procedures.

Correct chair positioning of a dental patient can alleviate or eliminate potential problems. Patients with a history of cardiac or respiratory disease are more comfortable and experience less physical and mental stress (fear of suffocation in patients with some respiratory diseases) if placed in an upright or slightly reclining position. The same position is best for pregnant patients in the last trimester who must have dental therapy. Most procedures on pregnant patients should be planned during the second trimester or wait until after delivery.

Compromising the airway during dental procedures in a healthy individual is a minor inconvenience but could cause a crisis for some patients. The patients with this potential for problems include not only cardiac and respiratory patients, but also persons with allergies, sinus conditions, and nasal obstruction. They become anxious and stressed with rubber dam placement, impressions, radiographic techniques, and some restorative procedures. Also a hyperactive gag reflex demands special attention and appropriate modifications in technique.

Proper patient dismissal procedures may prevent an emergency. Each step in the dismissal process allows sufficient time for the cardiovascular system to adjust to the new positions. The first step is to bring the patient to a sitting position. After a time interval, the patient swings his legs to one side and sits with the feet on the floor. Then, the patient stands next to the dental chair and proceeds slowly from the operatory. If the patient has been sedated or for any reason requires constant attention, accompany the patient to the waiting room and deliver the patient to a responsible adult who will take the patient home.

■ **Prevention is the first step. What is the next step in managing a potential office emergency?**

Recognition. The potential problem must be recognized to be appreciated, diagnosed, and managed. Early recognition permits prompt action and possible interruption of the sequence of events. Constantly observe the patient for any signs or symptoms that might indicate stress or difficulty. Specific signs and symptoms may be anticipated by scrutiny of the patient's history for known problems. Notice the patient's eyes, facial expressions, and hands for any signs of distress. Be aware of patient movements, actions, reactions to specific treatments, and changes in body position. Listen for departures from normal patterns of respiration. Look

for anything that might signify the development of an emergency.

■ **Once the problem is recognized, what actions should be taken?**

Position the patient immediately. All conscious patients with cardiac or respiratory difficulty or a history of cardiac or respiratory problems must be placed with the back of the chair in the upright position. All *unconscious* patients are placed in the Trendelenburg position (horizontal with head slightly lower than feet). An exception is the unconscious pregnant patient who is placed on her left side. Patients who do not fit these general categories are placed in the most comfortable position for them. After a tentative diagnosis is made, the patient may be repositioned. The whole chair is lowered close to the floor to facilitate other emergency procedures.

■ **What is the next step after positioning the patient?**

Rapidly proceed with the ABCs of basic life support.

A for is airway. Many dental chairs with headrests that support the occipital part of the skull can cause the airway to be closed off in unconscious patients. The occipital headrest pushes the chin down on the chest when the neck muscles relax in the state of unconsciousness. Therefore, as the patient is being placed in the Trendelenburg position, the headrest must be released and lowered to extend the neck. Extending the neck opens the airway mechanically by keeping the tongue from blocking the oropharynx.

B is for breathing. *Look, listen,* and *feel* for breathing in an unconscious patient. *Look* at both the abdomen and chest for a rise and fall of respiratory movements. Place your ear close to the patient's mouth to *listen* for the sounds of breathing while looking at the chest and abdomen. At the same time, *feel* for exhaled air. If there are no signs of respiration, begin artificial respiration.

C is for circulation. Rapidly determine the presence or absence of a pulse in an unconscious patient. The carotid pulse is evaluated by placing the tips of the index and middle fingers on the laryngeal prominence (Adam's apple) and sliding the fingers laterally to the carotid artery located anterior to the sternocleidomastoid muscle. The carotid body, or pressure-sensing structure, lies in the anatomic area of palpation for the pulse. If the carotid body is compressed vigorously, physiologic responses occur that may have a deleterious effect on the heart of an unconscious patient. Use gentle fingertip pressure to avoid the carotid body response. If there is no pulse, begin artificial circulation.

Cardiopulmonary resuscitation (CPR) will not be discussed in detail because I feel strongly that it is a motor skill best learned with mannequin practice. Excellent participation courses are offered by the American Red Cross and local chapters of the American Heart Association. Both programs offer certification on successful completion of the basic life-support course. *All* office personnel should be certified in CPR.

■ **What procedure should be followed if something is in the mouth and the patient develops a respiratory problem?**

Proceed with *A,* airway. Ensure an open airway for the patient by removing all potentially obstructive material from the mouth. Cotton rolls, saliva ejectors, rubber dam, dentures, or anything else removable should be taken out of the mouth. Sometimes judgment is necessary, and impressions that have not set up are left in place until they can be easily removed. While clearing the mouth, make sure all restrictive clothing about the neck is loosened and opened.

■ **How do you evaluate the breathing of a conscious patient?**

In a conscious patient the character of respirations reveals a tremendous amount of information about the cardiac and respiratory systems. The rate, rhythm, depth, and effort of breathing are informative diagnostic signs. Precise data facilitate differentiation of emergency states, such as a cardiac condition from an allergy problem.

■ **What criteria are used to evaluate circulation in the conscious patient?**

The circulation must be appraised and appre-ciated to have any diagnostic significance. The pulse rate, rhythm, regularity, and force are minimum necessary data. A pulse rate of over 100 beats per minute is tachycardia. Under 60 beats per minute is bradycardia. To fully appraise the circulatory system, a blood pressure determination must accompany pulse data. A patient's blood pressure is subject to many biologic variables and, to be properly interpreted, must be compared with a baseline or "normal" blood pressure recording. The normal range is 100 to 140/160 systolic pressure and 60 to 90/95 diastolic pressure.

■ **Should any additional observations be made and recorded?**

Yes. Carefully observe the patient's exposed skin surfaces for diagnostic clues. The skin discloses the degree of oxygenation (cyanotic or blue indicating poor oxygenation), the condition of the autonomic nervous system (perspiration, temperature changes, etc.), and allergic conditions (pruritus, urticaria, and rashes). Visually inspect the nail beds, hands, and lips to correlate these observations with findings obtained from palpation of the skin.

The degree of dilation or constriction of the pupils is an index of severity of cerebral hypoxia. Pupil reactivity to light (constricting when a bright light is directed at the pupil) aids in determination of the patient's cerebral status. Nonreactive pupils indicate biologic death of the cerebral tissue. This is most important to determine in an unconscious patient.

The evaluative process should include a consideration of the mental state of the patient. How does the patient respond to simple commands? Is the patient oriented? What is the level of consciousness? What is the emotional status and level of anxiety? With these questions answered the mental status of the patient can be rapidly assessed, a necessary determination for epileptic seizures and other central nervous system emergencies.

■ **How can the dental office personnel prepare for an emergency?**

An office emergency plan should be developed. This is an organized, detailed plan for managing and treating *any* emergency that might occur in the dental office. The office emergency plan eliminates wasted motion by distributing responsibilities in advance to *all* office personnel. Many factors must be considered when developing an emergency plan: the type of dental practice (general or specialized), locale of practice with nearby resources and medical facilities considered, the presence or absence of associates in the practice, office personnel, and number of staff available. The most important factor is the dentist's personality, training, and ability.

■ What are the duties of the dentist in an office emergency plan?

The dentist has primary responsibility for the patient's welfare. He initiates and directs the emergency system. It should be implemented as unobtrusively as possible so as not to alarm the patient or other patients in the office. The dentist monitors the patient and administers any indicated emergency drugs.

■ What are the duties of the chairside assistant?

The chairside assistant's duties vary depending on the nature of the emergency. She quietly and unexcitedly alerts the other office staff members. Then she gathers the necessary emergency equipment: drug kit, portable oxygen tank, Ambu bag, blankets, backboard (to be placed behind the patient's back if cardiopulmonary resuscitation is necessary), etc. She obtains and prepares emergency drugs for the dentist to administer. She assists in monitoring the patient's responses and reactions. The chairside assistant performs any function demanded by the emergency situation and the involvement of the dentist.

■ What are the responsibilities of a second assistant or the hygienist?

Another assistant or the hygienist should record details of the event on the emergency record sheet that is kept in the emergency kit. Various headings are listed on the emergency record sheet so that important data will not be omitted. Specific factual data are recorded: the patient's name, age, and sex; the date and time; the events preceding the emergency; signs; symptoms; drugs used before and during the emergency; dosages; routes of administration; and outcome of the emergency treatment. If possible the patient's vital signs and condition should be recorded at 5-minute intervals. The emergency record is a valuable source of information and should have attached carbon copies. If removal of the patient to a hospital becomes necessary, a copy of the emergency record should accompany the patient. The recorder's other duties are dictated by the emergency.

■ What are the duties of the receptionist in an office emergency?

The receptionist manages crowd control and keeps the other patients away from the emergency area. This member of the staff may have to clear the waiting room if transportation of the victim is necessary. The receptionist keeps the telephone lines open for use during the emergency and makes all the necessary telephone calls to prearranged and predetermined numbers: local emergency number, fire department rescue squad, ambulance, police, hospital emergency room (either for instructions or to inform them about the patient being brought to them), and a nearby physician who has agreed to offer assistance during an emergency. The dentist may ask the receptionist to call the patient's family physician to seek advice and assistance. This staff member must be ready to rotate duties in any manner required.

■ How are all the duties coordinated?

Each person in the office *must* know everyone else's responsibilities so they can fill in during someone's absence and so the team actions will be coordinated. For maximum efficiency and effectiveness, frequent practice and review are essential. At 3-month intervals, the entire staff should sit down at an office meeting and review the total emergency office plan, their responsibilities, and emergency procedures. A planned "simulated" emergency permits unforeseen contingencies to be corrected before an actual emergency. The major concern should be to maintain a high level of preparation by frequent updating of information, continuing education, practice, and review.

MULTIPLE-CHOICE QUESTIONS

1. The major concept in the definition of an emergency is:
   a. Sudden onset
   b. Unexpected change
   c. Immediate action

2. What percentage of patients over 60 years of age suffer from a chronic disease?
   a. 20%
   b. 40%
   c. 60%
   d. 80%

3. The first step in prevention of an office emergency is a thorough history because:
   a. The history screens for known systemic diseases and problems.
   b. The history permits rational changes in the treatment plan.
   c. The history helps by anticipating potential problems.
   d. The history enables a rapid recognition and comprehension of the patient's medical condition.
   e. All of the above.

4. Basic drug information recorded should include:
   a. Page in the reference source
   b. Components of the agent
   c. Actions of the drug
   d. Normal dosage
   e. All of the above

5. When should the blood pressure be taken during the initial dental appointment?
   a. At the beginning of the appointment
   b. At the end of the appointment

6. Patients with a history of cardiac disease should have:
   a. Morning appointments
   b. Appointments after meals
   c. Short, but frequent appointments
   d. All of the above

7. Varying office procedures can prevent emergencies. Easily modified procedures include:
   a. Correct chair position
   b. Airway maintenance
   c. Patient dismissal procedures
   d. Preoperative sedation
   e. All of the above

8. All unconscious patients are placed in the Trendelenburg position except for:
   a. Patients with a history of cardiac problems
   b. Patients with a history of respiratory problems
   c. Patients with a history of allergy problems
   d. Pregnant patients
   e. All of the above

9. To evaluate the circulatory system in a conscious patient, the following information is necessary:
   a. Pulse rhythm
   b. Pulse regularity
   c. Pulse force
   d. Blood pressure determination
   e. All of the above

10. Patient distress may be manifested by the:
    a. Eyes
    b. Hands
    c. Facial expression
    d. Changes in body position
    e. All of the above

11. Factors to be considered when establishing an office emergency plan are:
    a. Type of dental practice
    b. Location of dental practice
    c. Whether it is a group or single practice
    d. Dentist's personality, training, and abilities
    e. All of the above

12. The duties of the chairside dental assistant in an office emergency are:
    a. To alert the other office staff members
    b. To gather the necessary emergency equipment
    c. To perform CPR if necessary
    d. To monitor the patient's responses and reactions
    e. All of the above

13. Required on the emergency record sheet is information about:
    a. Events preceding the emergency
    b. Signs and symptoms
    c. Patient's vital signs
    d. Outcome of the emergency treatment
    e. All of the above

14. The receptionist's duties include:
    a. Crowd control
    b. Calling the emergency numbers
    c. Calling the patient's family physician
    d. Performing CPR if necessary
    e. All of the above

15. A conscious patient starts to have difficulty breathing. The first thing to be done is to:
    a. Position the patient
    b. Count the respirations
    c. Check the blood pressure
    d. Extend the neck

16. A conscious patient starts to perspire and feels ill. How do you position this patient?
    a. In an upright position
    b. In the Trendelenburg position
    c. In any comfortable position

17. An unconscious patient's pupils are dilated. This means:
    a. A lack of oxygen to the brain
    b. That patient will regain consciousness soon
    c. A lack of oxygen to the heart
    d. All of the above

18. The carotid body may be stimulated when checking the patient's:
    a. Breathing
    b. Pulse
    c. Blood pressure
    d. Pupils

19. To maintain peak proficiency as a dental assistant, it is necessary to:
    a. Frequently review emergency procedures
    b. Practice
    c. Take continuing education courses
    d. Maintain certification in CPR
    e. All of the above

20. What is the rate of breathing for an adult when respiration has stopped?
    a. Once every second
    b. Once every 3 seconds
    c. Once every 5 seconds
    d. Once every 15 seconds

21. What is the rate of chest compressions for one-rescuer CPR on an adult victim?
    a. 12 per minute
    b. 60 per minute
    c. 80 per minute
    d. 100 per minute

22. How are the fingers held when one is performing chest compressions on an adult?
    a. Hold the fingers off the chest.
    b. Push lightly with the fingers.
    c. Push firmly with the fingers.
    d. It does not matter.

23. What is the ratio of breaths to compressions in two-rescuer CPR for an adult?
    a. 1 breath to 5 compressions
    b. 1 breath to 15 compressions
    c. 2 breaths to 5 compressions
    d. 2 breaths to 15 compressions

24. To allow time for a breath in two-rescuer CPR for an adult, the person given chest compressions should:
    a. Stop giving compressions.
    b. Slow down the compressions.
    c. Keep the same speed of compressions.
    d. It does not matter.

25. Where are chest compressions performed on a small child or baby?
    a. Over the left nipple
    b. Over the xiphoid process
    c. At the middle of the sternum
    d. At the top half of the sternum

SUGGESTED READINGS

Ballinger, C. M.: Sudden death in the dental office: preparing for the inevitable will save lives, American Institute of Oral Biology, Proceedings of the Thirty-first Annual Meeting, Oct. 25-29, 1974, pp. 48-70.

Bell, W. H.: Emergencies in and out of the dental office: a pilot study in the state of Texas, J. Am. Dent. Assoc. **74:**778, 1967.

Blair, K. P.: Editorial—C.P.R., J. Can. Dent. Assoc. **6:**8, 1978.

Capello, J., and Wheatley, F.: Medical emergencies: the dental team approach, Dent. Survey **53:**24, 1977.

Council on Dental Therapeutics: Emergency kits, J. Am. Dent. Assoc. **87:**909, 1973.

Donaldson, D., and Wood, W. W.: Recognition and control of emergencies in the dental office, J. Can. Dent. Assoc. **41:**228, 1975.

Freeman, N. S., et al.: Office emergencies: an outline of causes, symptoms, and treatment, J. Am. Dent. Assoc. **94:**91, 1977.

Malamed, S. F.: Handbook of medical emergencies in the dental office, St. Louis, 1978, The C. V. Mosby Co.

Schijatschky, M. M.: Life-threatening emergencies in the dental office, Chicago, 1975, Quintessenz.

Tomme, C.: C.P.R.: A trend in modern dentistry, J. Am. Dent. Assoc. **95:**900, 1977.

CHAPTER 7

Oral and maxillofacial surgery

PAMELA M. PETERS

■ **Define the dental specialty of oral and maxillofacial surgery.**

The American Dental Association defines the specialty of oral and maxillofacial surgery as "the diagnosis, the surgical and adjunctive treatment of the diseases, injuries and defects of the human jaws and associated structures, within the limits of the professional qualifications and training of the individual practitioner, and within the limits of agreements made at the local level by those concerned with the total health care of the patient."

■ **What are the educational requirements for an oral and maxillofacial surgeon?**

To become an oral and maxillofacial surgeon one must obtain a Doctor of Dental Science (DDS) degree or Doctor of Dental Medicine (DMD) degree and complete an oral surgery training program. The training programs are 3 to 5 years long. Individuals graduating from 5-year programs receive a Doctor of Medicine (MD) degree in addition to their oral surgery credential. Those who wish to remain in an academic career may also receive a Masters of Science (MS) degree or a Doctor of Philosophy (PhD) degree.

■ **Define exodontia.**

Exodontia is a term that describes the procedure for removing or extracting teeth. This procedure may range from the removal of one tooth to the extraction of multiple teeth.

■ **What is meant by the term "impacted tooth?"**

An impacted tooth is one that is unable to erupt because of its location beneath or within tissue, bone, or other teeth. The effects of the impacted tooth on the health of the oral cavity will determine whether or not it needs to be extracted.

■ **Briefly describe the procedures to remove an erupted tooth and to remove an impacted tooth.**

If there are no unforeseen difficulties, the extraction of an erupted tooth involves severing the periodontium with a surgical curet, expanding the size of the alveolus using a periosteal elevator, and using a rocking or luxating motion with forceps to remove the tooth from its socket.

The procedure for removing an impacted tooth is somewhat more complicated than that for removing an erupted tooth. Initially, an incision with a scalpel must be made to gain access to the tooth. If the tooth is impacted in bone, either a surgical bur or mallet and chisel must be employed additionally. An elevator is then used to either luxate and extract the tooth or prepare the tooth to be removed with forceps. In certain situations a tooth cannot be removed from the alveolus in one piece. In these circumstances the tooth must be sectioned with a surgical bur or a mallet and chisel.

■ **What is the purpose of performing an alveolectomy?**

The reason for performing an alveolectomy is to remove rough or sharp areas of bone from the maxilla or mandible. These projections may be the result of single or multiple extractions or irregularities in the ridges from wear or disease.

■ **Define the term "tori" and describe the indications or contraindications for the removal of tori.**

Tori are bony projections (exostoses) found most often on the palate of the maxilla, in the lingual area of the mandible, or in both areas. These bony growths are present in approximately 25% of the population. Unless the tori are preventing proper fit of a removable prosthetic device or causing undue discomfort to the patient, removal is not indicated.

■ **What is a biopsy?**

The appearance of various types of lesions is not totally uncommon in the oral cavity. To make sure that these growths are not placing the patient's health in jeopardy, a sample of tissue is removed and examined for abnormalities. This procedure, called a *biopsy,* can be accomplished using several different techniques.

■ **Explain the difference between excisional, incisional, exfoliative cytologic, and exploratory biopsy procedures.**

Excisional. Excisional biopsies are performed when the lesion is rather small. Because of limited tissue involvement, the entire lesion can be removed and examined. So that the pathologist can compare the lesion with the patient's normal tissue, a piece of adjacent tissue is excised along with the specimen.

Incisional. When the lesion is large, only a sample of normal and abnormal tissue is incised for examination. The rationale for this action is that the final diagnosis will determine whether or not there is a malignancy and will thus dictate the extent of surgery required.

Exfoliative cytologic. An exfoliative cytologic biopsy is a nonsurgical procedure in which sample cells are scraped from the surface of the lesion. This procedure is not as predictable or conclusive as the incisional and excisional biopsies. However, it is sometimes helpful when performed in conjunction with other types of biopsies.

Exploratory. An exploratory biopsy is a technique used when the abnormal tissue is deeply positioned. The sample to be examined is obtained by making an extensive incision into the tissue. After the diagnosis is made, the lesion is removed if necessary.

■ **Why is maxillofacial surgery performed?**

Maxillofacial surgery is performed for a variety of reasons, such as, to reduce fractures of the mandible or maxilla caused by accidents, to correct occlusal or facial abnormalities, to render a patient in a better oral condition for dentures, or to reconstruct the jaws after trauma or tumor surgery. Normally these procedures will not be performed by the general practitioner; rather, they are done by an oral and maxillofacial surgeon.

■ **Discuss the dental assistant's role in presurgical preparation.**

The dental assistant has many responsibilities in preparing the patient and operatory for surgery. First, the assistant should carefully and thoroughly review the patient's medical and dental history for information pertaining to premedication needs, anesthetic preferences and tolerances, and health considerations in light of the proposed procedure. The importance and thoroughness of this procedure cannot be overemphasized. Second, it is the auxiliary's duty to accurately take and record the patient's vital signs. Third, the dental assistant is delegated the task of establishing an aseptic surgical environment. This includes disinfecting the dental equipment, securing a sterile instrument tray setup, dressing in the appropriate attire, draping the patient, and scrubbing for surgery. In addition to these responsibilities, the auxiliary must attempt to allay any fears expressed by the patient through psychologic support.

■ **Describe the dental assistant's presurgical role in establishing an aseptic environment in a dental office.**

The goal of establishing an aseptic environment is to eliminate the possibility of introducing the patient to disease-producing microorganisms. Thus every precaution must be taken by the dental team to prevent cross contamination. Following is a summary of the dental assistant's responsibility in this procedure:

Wipe the dental chair, unit, light, and equipment with a disinfectant solution.

Secure a sterile surgical tray setup.

Prepare the patient by removing glasses and other obstacles that may interfere with surgery. Additionally, provide the patient with a drape to protect clothing.

Scrub hands and obtain appropriate attire. "Appropriate attire" may or may not include a sterile gown and cap. However, surgical gloves and masks should be the minimum required.

Lay a sterile covering on the patient's chest to prevent the auxiliary or operator from touching unsterile areas.

Unwrap, assemble, and arrange instruments on the tray.

■ **Briefly discuss the role of the dental assistant during a surgical procedure.**

The dental assistant's responsibility in oral surgery, as in any other area of dentistry, is to facilitate an efficient and effective procedure. In oral surgery, specifically, the assistant must transfer instruments and materials, maintain a clear field of operation, monitor the patient's responses, and retract the cheek and tongue. The ease and efficiency with which these procedures are performed demonstrate the expertise of the auxiliary.

■ **Define and describe the treatment for alveolitis (dry socket).**

Alveolitis is a condition that occurs when a blood clot does not form in the alveolus of an extracted tooth. The classic symptoms include severe pain and a foul odor and are manifested from 2 to 5 days after the surgery. The treatment for alveolitis is to irrigate the socket with hydrogen peroxide or a saline solution, apply a sedative dressing, and prescribe an analgesic for the pain. This treatment is repeated in 24 hours and then as often as is necessary.

■ **What is the treatment for excessive and prolonged surgical hemorrhaging?**

The treatment for prolonged and excessive bleeding varies with the amount of hemorrhaging and the length of time that has elapsed since the surgery. However, a typical treatment for postoperative extraction complications would include having the patient apply pressure to gauze compresses placed on the site of extraction for a period of time. If this does not alleviate the situation, the patient would be asked to return to the office. At this time, an absorbable material that controls hemorrhage would be packed into the alveolus.

■ **Describe the symptoms and treatment for postsurgical infection.**

The symptoms of postsurgical infection include swelling, pain, and the accumulation of exudate in the area of the face over the surgical site. Initial treatment would include rinsing the oral cavity with warm saline solution and lancing the tissue once the infection has been localized. Antibiotics and analgesics are prescribed as needed.

■ **Describe the characteristics and function of the following surgical instruments:**

Forceps. Forceps are instruments used to grasp and remove a tooth from its alveolus. These instruments, resembling pliers in appearance, are available in a variety of designs. Forceps differ in design according to the area of the oral cavity in which they will be used.

Elevator. There are several types of surgical elevators. Examples include the periosteal, straight, and apical elevators. The periosteal elevator has a long handle with a single broad or thin working end or a double end containing both. Periosteal elevators are used to reflect the attached gingiva or mucoperiosteum from the bone, which slightly separates the alveolar bone from the tooth's root. Additionally, this instrument is used to deflect a tissue flap during a surgical procedure.

Straight elevators have rather short bulbous handles with nibs of varying designs. Their function is to loosen the tooth within its alveolus. Often this action alone will remove a tooth.

Apical elevators are used to gain access to small root tips that may have broken away from the tooth and remain in the socket. The handles of these instruments are thin or bulbous in appearance, whereas their shanks and working ends have differing angulations and forms.

Scalpel. The scalpel is composed of a handle and varying interchangeable blades. It is used to make incisions into the soft tissue. The blades are disposable to ensure sharpness and sterility.

Surgical curet. A surgical curet can be used in several different ways during a surgical procedure. It releases the epithelial attachment of the gingiva surrounding the tooth during the early stages of an extraction and removes necrotic tissue, bone, or root fragments following the tooth's removal. The curet has a long thin handle with either large or small spoon-shaped nibs.

Hemostat. The hemostat is used to clamp blood vessels and to grasp and remove small pieces of tissue, roots, or bone chips from the surgical site. It resembles a pair of scissors with varying types of beaks and ratchet-type locks on the handles.

Needle holder. The function of a needle holder is to grasp and manipulate the needle and thread during placement of the sutures. This instrument is similar in appearance to a hemostat. The major differences are that the beaks are finer and the serrations are in patterns arranged to secure the needle.

Suture and needle. Extensive incisions into the soft tissue must be sutured to facilitate healing. The materials required to perform this procedure include the needle, the suture material, and the needle holder that was previously described. Needles are available with or without an eye and in many shapes and sizes. The suture material, produced in a variety of thicknesses, is manufactured in gut, silk, and various man-made materials such as nylon.

Mallet and chisel. Mallets and chisels serve to remove or to reshape bone and to resect teeth. The mallet, resembling a hammer in appearance, is used to strike the chisel that in turn chips the bone or sections the tooth. Chisels are either single or bibeveled and have varying styles of handles.

Rongeur forceps. A rongeur forceps is a type of forceps used to produce a cutting or nipping action. Most often these instruments serve to trim and reshape bone after a multiple extraction. Rongeur forceps are produced in several styles; blunt-nose and side-cutting are examples of two common types.

Bone file. A bone file is used to smooth sharp edges of bone following multiple extractions. The handle is long and thin, and the working ends are composed of sharp elevations.

Surgical scissors. There are many types of surgical scissors with various characteristics. Scissors can be curved or straight with serrated or smooth blades and with long or short handles. The sharp blades of surgical scissors are used to cut tissue and sutures.

Tissue forceps. The purpose of using tissue forceps is to grasp soft tissue either during suturing or excisional procedures. The serrated beaks provide a positive hold on the tissue without undue pressure. This instrument is produced in a number of styles. Some tissue forceps resemble cotton pliers; others are similar in design to a hemostat.

Suction tip. The surgical suction tip is similar to those used in restorative dentistry. The main difference is that the surgical suction tip is much thinner in appearance, and the opening is small. This instrument removes blood, saliva, and small debris from the oral cavity during a surgical procedure.

Surgical burs. Surgical burs are used to section teeth and remove bone. The most common cutting surfaces are the round and crosscut fissure. Surgical burs are available for use in both high-speed and slow-speed handpieces.

Mouth props. Mouth props are produced in two basic designs. One is a rubber block available in small, medium, and large sizes. The second is a scissorslike, adjustable lock-handled instrument with small rubber pads on the ends. These instruments are positioned within the oral cavity to keep the mouth open during a surgical procedure. Mouth props are often used with children and patients who are under general anesthesia.

Tongue, cheek, and tissue retractors. So that the surgical site is clearly visible, instruments that retract the cheek, tongue, or mucosa may be required. Tongue and cheek retractors made of pieces of plastic or metal with bends or hooks on their ends are used for this purpose. Tissue retractors have long flat metal handles with large scoop-shaped ends.

MULTIPLE-CHOICE QUESTIONS

Use the letters assigned to the instruments in Fig. 7-1 to answer questions 1 to 6.

1. The doctor informs you that he will be removing and smoothing the sharp projections of bone on a patient's mandibular ridge. Which of the following groups of instruments should be included in the tray setup?
   a. K, B, G, A, and I
   b. K, G, and I
   c. B, A, and I
   d. K, B, G, and A
2. The doctor is preparing to remove an impacted tooth with a surrounding cyst. You are presented with the following instruments for this procedure: B, A, D, C, and H. In which of the following groups are these instruments placed in the correct sequence of use?
   a. B, D, A, H, C
   b. D, B, A, C, H
   c. A, D, H, C, B
   d. C, D, A, B, H
3. You are preparing a tray setup for a single erupted tooth extraction procedure. Instruments that would be included are in which of the following groups?
   a. K, D, and A
   b. B, K, R, and D
   c. R, K, and B
   d. B, A, and R
4. The instrument used to keep the oral cavity open during a surgical procedure is:
   a. L
   b. Q
   c. K
   d. M
5. The patient is having a horizontally impacted third molar extracted. The procedure to be used requires that the tooth be sectioned. Which of the following groups of instruments would the operator most likely use to perform this procedure?
   a. F, C, and K
   b. F, G, and P
   c. C, G, and K
   d. F, G, P, and K
6. Which of the following armamentarium

would be required during the placement of sutures?
   a. H, J, and L
   b. H and J
   c. K and D
   d. K, H, D, and L
7. One of the presurgical responsibilities of the dental assistant is to take and record the patient's vital signs. Which of the following statistics would this include?
   a. Blood pressure, temperature, pulse, and respiration
   b. Blood pressure and temperature
   c. Blood pressure, pulse, and respiration
   d. Blood pressure, temperature, and pulse
8. The dental auxiliary's major function during the administration of a general anesthetic is to:
   a. Administer the anesthetic
   b. Monitor the patient's responses
   c. Provide the patient with psychologic support
   d. Retract the tongue and cheek

With the following information in mind, respond to the next three questions. A female patient has come to your office to have an erupted maxillary second molar extracted. After reviewing her chart, you note the following facts: (1) she is not allergic to any medication, (2) her blood pressure is a little high, and (3) she is not an apprehensive or nervous patient. It is your responsibility to prepare the operatory and to prepare the patient for treatment.

9. A desirable local anesthetic solution would be one:
   a. With a vasoconstrictor, of slow onset, and of long duration
   b. With a vasoconstrictor, of rapid onset, and of short duration
   c. Without a vasoconstrictor, of rapid onset, and of short duration
   d. Without a vasoconstrictor, of slow onset, and of long duration
10. What is the minimum amount of time that you should spend scrubbing your hands, nails, and forearms before the first surgery of the day?

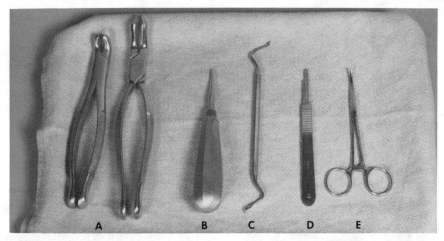

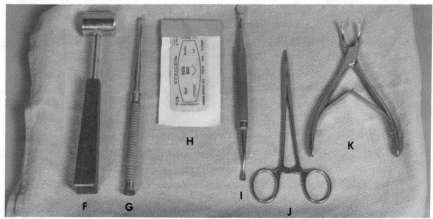

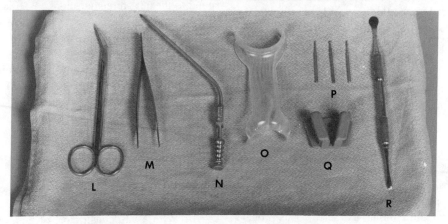

Fig. 7-1. Instruments used in oral and maxillofacial surgery.

A. Forceps
B. Elevator (straight)
C. Curet
D. Scalpel
E. Hemostat
F. Mallet
G. Chisel
H. Suture and needle
I. Bone file

J. Needle holder
K. Rongeur forceps
L. Surgical scissors
M. Tissue forceps
N. Suction tip
O. Retractors
P. Surgical burs
Q. Mouth prop
R. Periosteal elevator

a. 1 minute
b. 6 minutes
c. 10 minutes
d. 3 minutes

11. Which of the following groups of instruments should be included on the tray setup?
    a. Scalpel and rongeur forceps
    b. Forceps, periosteal elevator, and straight elevator
    c. Forceps, scalpel, and periosteal elevator
    d. Forceps, scalpel, rongeur forceps, periosteal elevator, and straight elevator

12. What method of instrument transfer should the dental team use when exchanging forceps?
    a. Two-handed palm grasp
    b. Two-handed pen grasp
    c. One-handed palm grasp
    d. One-handed pen grasp

13. Following a single surgical extraction, which of the following postoperative instructions should be given to the patient?
    a. Use a straw for consuming liquids, apply cold packs immediately after surgery, and maintain pressure on a square of gauze for at least 30 minutes.
    b. Use a straw for consuming liquids, and rinse the oral cavity with a saline solution shortly after surgery.
    c. Rinse the oral cavity with a saline solution shortly after surgery, and maintain pressure on a square of gauze for at least 30 minutes.
    d. Apply cold packs immediately after surgery, and maintain pressure on a square of gauze for at least 30 minutes.

14. Prior to dismissing a patient following surgery, the dental team must make sure that the patient is not:
    a. In pain, hemorrhaging excessively, or dizzy
    b. In pain or experiencing swelling
    c. Hemorrhaging excessively or dizzy
    d. In pain, hemorrhaging excessively, dizzy, or experiencing swelling

SUGGESTED READINGS

Chasteen, E.: Essentials of clinical dental assisting, St. Louis, 1975, The C. V. Mosby Co.

Dunn, M. J., Booth, D. F., and Clancy, M.: Pharmacology—pain control—sterile techniques—oral surgery, Baltimore, 1975, The Williams & Wilkins Co.

Emmitt, C. R., and White, R.: Fundamentals of oral surgery, Philadelphia, 1971, W. B. Saunders Co.

Richardson, R. E., and Barton, R. E.: The dental assistant, ed. 5, New York, 1978, McGraw-Hill Book Co.

Torres, H. O., and Ehrlich, A.: Modern dental assisting, Philadelphia, 1976, W. B. Saunders Co.

CHAPTER 8

Pedodontics

ROSLYN M. CIDADO

■ **What is pedodontics?**

Pedodontics is the branch of dentistry that deals with treatment of the child patient.

■ **What is the main objective of pedodontics?**

The overall objective of the pedodontist is to show concern for the total well-being, both physical and emotional, of the child patient. This is accomplished by prevention of oral diseases and abnormal development, early treatment when these occur, and relief of discomfort and suffering if present.

■ **What are some developmental considerations for the pedodontic patient?**

The developmental considerations for the pedodontic patient are physical and psychologic. In considering physical development, it is necessary to be aware of the normal development of dentition as it compares to various hereditary and developmental anomalies. From the embryonic stages of bud, cap, and bell through the eruption patterns to their eventual exfoliation, the primary teeth may be subjected to a variety of internal or external disturbances that could produce marked effects on the child patient.

■ **What are some common problems associated with the eruption and exfoliation of primary teeth?**

The eruption of the primary dentition covers the period from 6 months to 3 years. During this time a child may have many minor illnesses that appear suddenly, remain briefly, and leave rapidly. Disturbances of this nature are likely to be attributed by mothers and physicians to the teething process. While irritability, exces-sive drooling, and mild localized facial swelling are symptoms often connected with this process, it is important to know that the more severe symptoms warrant expert medical advice. The "cyst of eruption" that refers to the swelling of the mucosa covering the unerupted tooth is a common disturbance associated with eruption. Left untreated, this condition is often resolved with the eruption of the tooth.

Exfoliation, or the shedding of primary teeth, may cause the child patient varying degrees of discomfort. If the tooth remains attached to a thin piece of root, the surrounding soft tissue may become red and swollen. Children should be encouraged to remove the tooth themselves.

■ **How does the premature loss of primary teeth affect the child patient?**

Primary teeth reserve space for 20 teeth of the permanent dentition, assist in the development of the jaw through function, and are essential in the development of speech. Premature loss of these teeth may result in the improper positioning of secondary teeth, difficulty in learning the pronunciation of certain words, and feelings of self-consciousness, especially with the premature loss of anterior teeth.

■ **What are various signs of psychologic development in the pedodontic patient?**

During the course of dental treatment the normal child will undergo definite mental growth as well as physical growth. This is apparent as one observes the child constantly acquiring, shedding, or modifying habits. This may also be the reason that a child's reaction to the dental office may vary from one appointment to the next. Because no two children share the same rhythm and style of growth, we can observe the individuality of their personalities.

■ **How do the child's psychologic characteristics differ from birth through adolescence?**

Birth. The infant learns from varied experiences and is nurtured by environmental occurrences. Although children within the same age groups vary considerably in growth patterns, there are certain similarities in their behavior that are predictable.

Age two. Dental appointments should be initiated when the child reaches 2 years of age. There are considerable differences among children in vocabulary development. Work can be successfully completed for some, but with others there is limited cooperation. The child is too young to be reached by words but should be allowed to handle and touch objects used as part of his treatment. Separation from his parents, especially where there are unfamiliar people and surroundings, arouses fear in the 2-year-old child. For this reason the child should be accompanied by the parents to the treatment room.

Age three. This child is usually eager to communicate and is receptive to positive rather than negative reinforcement. The 3-year-old patients will often do things they are instructed not to do. These children are also insecure when separated from their parents.

Age four. The 4-year-old child is a good listener and responds to verbal communication. A child at this age has an active mind, talks freely, and has a tendency to exaggerate in conversation. Although the 4-year-old child may become defiant, the child who has had a normal amount of parental discipline and training will generally be a cooperative patient.

Age five. The 5-year-old child displays more independence than a younger child. As the ego develops, the child engages in more group activities and social relationships. With proper preparation from his parents, fear of visits to the dental office becomes minimal. The 5-year-old child may use the imaginative process to deal with the discomfort encountered during a dental procedure.

Ages six, seven, and eight. The 6-, 7-, or 8-year-old child depends less on family for security and relies more on friends for support. Children in this age group exhibit a variety of characteristics, from anxiety during the transition period to becoming an active member of the dental team during treatment. The ability to reason and to accept directives increases with the 7- and 8-year-old child. An important facet of their personality and self-appraisal is their concern for bigness and smallness of size.

Ages nine, ten, and eleven. Being with children of the same sex and age is important to the 9-, 10-, and 11-year-old child. Children at this age are characterized by a need to be viewed as being in control of self and events affecting them. For this reason, the preadolescent patient accepts and adjusts well to dental treatment.

Age twelve. At age twelve the child's personality and physiology begin to undergo an enormous change that continues through the adolescent years. During this hypersensitive period a bond is formed between the child and the peer group. This patient is in control of his emotions, displays self-discipline during dental treatment, and appreciates direct and honest communication from the dentist and auxiliaries.

■ **What are the four most common reactions to the dental experience?**

The four most common reactions to the dental experience are fear, anxiety, resistance, and timidity. The child will usually present a combination of these reactions, creating a complicated management task for the dentist and the auxiliaries.

Fear. Fear is an emotion frequently observed when treating the child. It can be the result of insecurity, acquired by imitating one who is afraid, or directly related to a previous unpleasant experience.

Anxiety. Anxiety is closely related to fear. An anxious child is unable to develop necessary assurance and remains insecure long after he should have outgrown such feelings.

Resistance. Resistance is observed when a child rebels against the environment. It can be an outlet for anxiety and insecurity. Home training and previous experiences will dictate the extent to which the child will be resistant.

Timidity. Timidity is usual when a child visits the dental office. Because of a lack of social experiences, the child who is timid will need to go through a warming-up period.

■ **How is the "normal" child managed in the dental office?**

The term "normal" refers to the patient who exhibits no apparent mental or physical handicaps. The management of this patient will depend on the ability of the dentist and auxiliaries to convey a positive and friendly manner. A child patient's bad habits should be rejected or overcome at the outset; his good habits should be encouraged with praise. Through kindness, firmness, and a sincere enthusiasm for the child's total well-being, the dentist and assistants gain the child's confidence while establishing a successful doctor-patient relationship.

■ **How does the management of the mentally and/or physically handicapped child vary from the management of the "normal" child?**

Oral needs vary considerably for mentally and/or physically handicapped children, and these children must be examined and their needs evaluated on an individual basis. Although there may not be specific dental problems, the child's mental or physical handicap may complicate dental treatment. If the child is mentally handicapped and the customary behavior management techniques are ineffective, it may be necessary to employ restraints or physical control. In this case every effort should be made to carry out the procedure quickly, with as little discomfort to the patient as possible. The child with a physical or mental handicap may require special preoperative or postoperative medications, assistance to and from the waiting area, and physical assistance during the dental procedure.

■ **What are the various types of parental behavior?**

The four most common types of parental behavior seen by the pedodontist are *overindulgence, rejection of the child, overanxiety, and domineering behavior.* Each of these has a dramatic effect on the behavior of the child patient.

The child of an overindulgent parent will display unlimited methods for gaining attention. When this type of behavior is evident, it is necessary for the dentist and assistants to respond with an attitude of discipline.

The child who is rejected by parents will appear quiet and unsure of himself and may eventually become aggressive and disobedient. If approached with a friendly and understanding manner, the child will realize that obedience will result in a quicker, more comfortable dental procedure.

The overanxious parent creates an atmosphere of constant concern with the child's health and well-being, causing the child to become shy and fearful. If the dentist and staff members indicate their confidence in the child as a dental patient, the child should present few management problems during treatment.

The domineering parent places excessive responsibilities on the child, and at the same time nags and criticizes the child into a state of submission. The dentist and staff can avoid perpetuating the child's feelings of inadequacy in the dental office by treating the child with respect and understanding.

■ **Outline the concepts of four-handed dentistry in the restorative phases of pedodontics.**

Operative or restorative procedures for the child patient are very similar technically to those performed on the adult patient. The chairside role of the dental assistant during these procedures varies slightly. Because of the short attention span of the child, it is imperative to provide the maximum amount of dental service in the minimum amount of time. One of the assistant's chief responsibilities in a pedodontic practice is the thorough preparation of the operatory prior to seating the child. The longer the child has to sit in the patient chair, the less cooperative he will be toward the end of the procedure.

Following is an outline of the usual restorative process followed by a pedodontist and his assistant(s).

The patient's records and armamentarium required during this procedure are set out prior to seating the patient.

Once the patient is brought from the reception area and seated, the assistant remains beside the child.

After reviewing the anticipated procedure, the dentist anesthetizes the child patient. A local anesthetic is routinely administered to avoid the possibility of pain associated with the removal of deep carious lesions. Premedication of the child is usually indicated only in cases presenting severe management problems or for the very young child. Learning to handle stress-related situations is part of the normal child's maturation process.

After administration of the anesthetic, the rubber dam should be placed. In addition to the advantages of its use in general dentistry, the rubber dam is helpful in the management of the child, especially to exclude the child's tongue from the working area.

During the preparation of the tooth, proper coolants and evacuation techniques are employed. Following its completion, the preparation is cleaned and dried. The dentist then may choose to insert a sedative base and cavity liner.

The matrix band, usually of the spot-welded or T-band variety, is placed around the tooth and properly wedged to reproduce the tooth's contour.

Amalgam is used extensively for restoring the posterior teeth of the child patient. For use as esthetic restorative materials, the composite resins have dramatically increased in popularity over the silicate restorative materials. Because of the exfoliation of primary teeth, amalgam may be indicated as the restorative material of choice for some anterior restorations.

After the amalgam is mixed, it is placed and condensed into the cavity preparation using the methods of four-handed dentistry.

Following condensation, the excess restorative material is removed, and the dentist proceeds to carve and recontour the tooth to its proper proportion. During this stage of the procedure the assistant's responsibility is to maintain a clear working field while transferring the appropriate instruments.

The rubber dam is removed at the completion of the restoration. The occlusion is checked with articulating paper for high spots in its contour and adjusted if necessary.

■ **Discuss the three basic techniques employed in pulpal management of primary and immature permanent teeth.**

Direct pulp capping. This is the protection of a small exposure in a healthy pulp by the application of a medicament to stimulate the odontoblast cells to produce secondary dentin. An indirect pulp capping is the result of a medicament, such as calcium hydroxide, being applied to the last remaining layer of carious dentin to prevent an exposure and encourage the growth of secondary dentin.

Pulpotomy. This procedure is the removal of the coronal portion of the pulp because of an exposure resulting from the excavation of deep caries or exposure resulting from a fractured tooth. It is the treatment most widely used in the management of primary pulpal degeneration. Once the coronal pulp is removed, a cotton pellet moistened with formocresol is placed in the chamber and left for 5 minutes. At the end of this time, the pellet is removed. If the bleeding from the root pulp is well controlled, a layer of fast-setting zinc oxide–eugenol is placed in the pulpal chamber, and the tooth is covered with a stainless steel crown or an amalgam restoration. If the bleeding is difficult to control or if there is active infection in the root pulp, the pellet with formocresol is sealed in the tooth with a suitable temporary cement.

Pulpectomy. This is the complete extirpation or removal of pulpal tissue from both the crown and the root portion of the tooth. Pulpectomy in the primary teeth is usually limited to the single-rooted anterior teeth. It is not a widely employed technique because the configuration of the primary root canals make hermetic sealing of the canals difficult.

■ **Explain the function of a chrome or stainless steel crown in pedodontics.**

The chrome or stainless steel crown used in

pedodontics is a very durable type of restoration. It has played a decisive role in preventing premature loss of primary teeth. Following are the indications for use of the chrome or stainless steel crown: (1) following removal of extensive carious lesions on three or more surfaces, (2) following a pulpotomy, (3) as a transitional crown on a permanent tooth prior to the complete development of occlusal relationships, (4) in temporary retention of malformed teeth, (5) in restoring teeth for the handicapped child, and (6) as an abutment for space maintainers and habit appliances.

■ **Why are interceptive orthodontic procedures necessary for the pedodontic patient?**

By maintaining good alignment of the primary teeth, malalignment of the permanent teeth may be prevented. This is the theory in interceptive or preventive orthodontics. A fixed or removable space maintainer is used when there is premature loss of a primary tooth. Some of these appliances are designed to regain, as well as maintain, space. The type of space maintainer employed depends on the child's age, oral hygiene, and stage of development of permanent dentition.

An acrylic bite plane is an appliance designed to rotate the lingual position of an incisor facially to free it from a locked-in position. As the anterior tooth in question gently strikes the bite plane, it is guided outward. This type of apparatus is cemented onto the opposing

anteriors and is easily removed when treatment is completed.

Various oral habits of the child, such as thumb-sucking, tongue thrusting, nail biting, or bruxism may be the chief causes of the malpositioning of teeth. Prior to treatment these habits must be broken. The dentist and the assistant should provide instruction and encouragement to the child and the parents to aid the child in overcoming the problem.

■ **When is hospital dentistry for the pedodontic patient indicated?**

Although most dental procedures are best performed in the dental office, there are occasions when hospitalization of the child patient is necessary. Indications for hospitalization are systemic complications, major surgical procedures, or operations requiring prolonged general anesthesia. It is the responsibility of the dentist and the assistant to know hospital rules and regulations, the hospital code of conduct, operating room decorum, and the hospital's record-keeping system. The dentist, with the help of the assistant, can ensure an organized treatment of the hospitalized child if the following responsibilities are executed: (1) coordination and scheduling of admission and operating times, (2) proper ordering of laboratory tests and medications, (3) scheduling of examinations and consultations, and (4) dictation of operative and discharge notes.

MULTIPLE-CHOICE QUESTIONS

1. The procedure that involves removal of the coronal portion of the pulp is referred to as:
   a. Pulpectomy
   b. Direct pulp capping
   c. Indirect pulp capping
   d. Pulpotomy
2. The type of parent who produces a shy and fearful child by constantly being concerned about his health and well-being is termed:
   a. Overanxious
   b. Domineering

   c. Rejective
   d. Stable
3. At this age the child is in control of his emotions, is disciplined during dental treatment, and hypersensitive in his relationships with others:
   a. 8 years old
   b. 12 years old
   c. 3 years old
   d. 5 years old
4. This reaction to the dental experience is

usually associated with the first appointment and caused by the child's lack of social experiences.

   a. Anxiety
   b. Fear
   c. Resistance
   d. Timidity

5. The type of anterior fracture that is the most extensive and involves the enamel, dentin, and pulp is classified as:
   a. Class I
   b. Class II
   c. Class III
   d. Class IV

6. Factors used to determine the type of space maintainer to be constructed are all but which one of the following?
   a. Age of the child
   b. Cost of the appliance
   c. Patient's oral hygiene
   d. Development of the permanent dentition

7. All but which one of the following would be considered a preventive procedure in the pedodontic office?
   a. Fluoride therapy
   b. Treatment of fractures
   c. A plaque control program
   d. Nutritional counseling

8. Put the following stages in restorative dentistry in the correct sequence.
   a. Administration of a local anesthetic
   b. Placement and contouring of matrix
   c. Seating of the patient
   d. Preparation of instruments and patient's records
   e. Completion of the cavity preparation
   f. Carving and contouring of the restoration
   g. Application of the rubber dam
   h. Condensation and placement of restorative material

9. All but which one of the following would be indications for the hospitalization of the child patient:
   a. General restorations
   b. Major surgical procedures
   c. Operations requiring prolonged anesthesia
   d. Systemic complications

10. The diagnostic aids that assist the dentist in visualizing the relationship of the arches as well as the various stages of the growth process are:
   a. Study casts
   b. Blood tests
   c. Bite-wing radiographs
   d. Medical history

11. All but which one of the following are symptoms often associated with the teething process:
   a. Irritability
   b. Mild localized facial swelling
   c. Intense headaches
   d. Excessive drooling

12. Dental appointments should be initiated when the child is:
   a. 2 years old
   b. 4 years old
   c. 5 years old
   d. 6 months old

SUGGESTED READINGS

Costano, F. A., and Alden, B. A.: Handbook of expanded dental auxiliary practice, Philadelphia, 1973, J. B. Lippincott Co.

Gershen, J. A.: Maternal influence on the behavior patterns of children in the dental situation, J. Am. Dent. Assistants Assoc. **46:**17, 1977.

Holloway, P. J., and Swallow, J. N.: Child dental health, ed. 2, Bristol, 1975, John Wright & Sons, Ltd.

Meyers, A.: Injuries to anterior teeth, J. Am. Dent. Assistants Assoc. **47:**24, 1978.

McDonald, R. E., and Avery, D. R.: Dentistry for the child and adolescent, ed. 3, St. Louis, 1978, The C. V. Mosby Co.

Richardson, R. E., Barton, R. E., and Brauer, J. C.: The dental assistant, ed. 4, New York, 1974, McGraw-Hill Book Co.

Steinberg, A. D.: The role of dental auxiliary personnel in dentistry for the handicapped, J. Am. Dent. Assistants Assoc. **47:**20, 1978.

Torres, H. O., and Ehrlich, A.: Modern dental assisting, Philadelphia, 1976, W. B. Saunders Co.

CHAPTER 9

Orthodontics

DANIEL R. BALBACH

■ **What is orthodontics?**

Orthodontics is the branch of dentistry concerned with growth of the craniofacial complex, development of occlusion, and treatment of irregularities and imbalances in the teeth, the facial skeleton, and the orofacial musculature. Orthodontics is the largest dental specialty, and it derives its name from two Greek words, *orthos* meaning straight and *odontos* meaning tooth. An orthodontist is a dentist who has had 2 years of advanced training in treating malocclusions. Membership in the American Association of Orthodontists indicates that the orthodontist has met certain standards of training, education, and experience.

■ **How does the craniofacial skeleton change from childhood to adulthood?**

The growth of the craniofacial skeleton is extremely complex. A number of growth centers are involved with each one growing at different rates and at different times. For example, the cranium (the brain case) often reaches its adult size by 7 years of age, whereas the maxillary complex (upper face and jaw) continues to grow until a person is 15 to 16 years old. The mandible (lower jaw) often shows evidence of growth until a person is 20 to 25 years old. These varying growth rates produce the changes we all observe in the facial profile of children as they mature.

■ **Why is an understanding of facial growth so important in orthodontics?**

Certain orthodontic appliances are designed to be used during a particular phase of the patient's facial growth. Consequently, knowledge of facial growth is crucial in the *timing of treatment*. Orthodontic appliances also may have a significant impact on the direction and rate of growth of various areas within the face. A knowledge of the relationships between parts of the face is essential when choosing the amount and direction of force to be applied to the patient's craniofacial skeleton. Severe aberrations in the development of the face such as a cleft lip and/or palate usually require the knowledge and efforts of a team of health care specialists of which the orthodontist is a member.

■ **What is malocclusion?**

The term *malocclusion* refers to crooked or irregularly positioned teeth ("mal" meaning bad and "occlusion" meaning how well the teeth are aligned and how well they close together). In reality most malocclusions result from imbalances or irregularities not only in the position of the teeth, but also in the bony structures of the face and musculature of the face and oral cavity.

■ **How are malocclusion and malpositions of teeth classified and described?**

The most commonly used classification is the Angle system (Fig. 9-1). This classification is based primarily on the anteroposterior relationship of the upper first molar to its lower counterpart, and the divisions are based on the position of the incisors. The basic classes are as follows:

CLASS I—a normal molar relationship with the mesiobuccal cusp of the upper molar seated over the buccal groove of the lower molar.

CLASS II—the upper arch is positioned mesially or

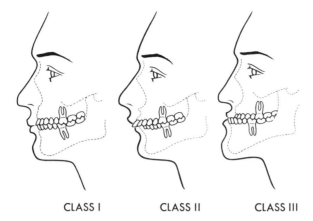

CLASS I   CLASS II   CLASS III

Fig. 9-1. Angle classification of occlusion. (Courtesy Rocky Mountain Data Systems, Inc., Encino, Calif.)

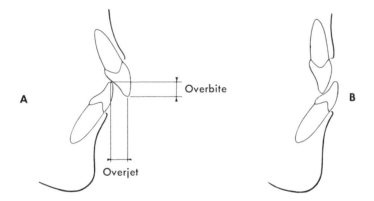

Fig. 9-2. A, Overbite and overjet relationships. **B,** Negative overjet/anterior crossbite. (Courtesy Rocky Mountain/Orthodontics, Denver.)

forward. The mesiobuccal cusp of the upper molar is seated over the embrasure between the lower first molar and second premolar.

DIVISION 1—all the upper incisors are tipped forward.

DIVISION 2—the central incisors are usually upright or tipped backward, and the lateral incisors are often flared.

CLASS III—the lower arch is positioned forward with the mesiobuccal cusp of the upper molar occluding distally to the buccal groove of the lower molar.

Following are additional terms that describe the position of groups of teeth.

Overjet. This term describes the horizontal relationship of the upper incisors to the lower incisors. Ideally the upper incisors should ex-tend 2 to 3 mm ahead of the lower incisors. The school yard term "buck teeth" can be described in the kinder and more correct term "an excessive overjet." When the lower incisors are ahead of the upper incisors, the relationship is described as a negative overjet and is a characteristic of a class III malocclusion (Fig. 9-2).

Overbite. Overbite describes the extent to which the upper incisors overlap the lower incisors in a vertical direction. Ideally, when the posterior teeth are in occlusion, only the upper to middle one third of the lower incisors should be covered, and there should be tooth-to-tooth contact. In some patients the lower incisors impinge on the soft palatal tissue; such an *impinging overbite* is functionally unhealthy (Fig.

9-3). The opposite of the deep, impinging overbite occurs when there is no vertical overlap of the front teeth. This relationship is called an anterior *open bite* and frequently is associated with a thumb or finger habit or with abnormal tongue function (Fig. 9-4). Posterior open bites occur less frequently.

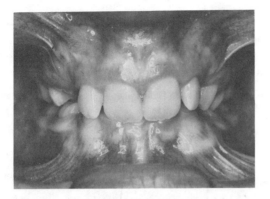

Fig. 9-3. Impinging overbite.

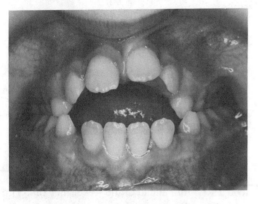

Fig. 9-4. Anterior open bite due to a thumb habit. Note posterior crossbite.

Crossbite. This term is used to indicate an abnormal buccolingual (labiolingual) relationship of the teeth. The most common crossbite is that of the buccal cusps of the maxillary molars occluding lingually to the buccal cusps of the lower teeth. An *anterior crossbite* is present when one or more maxillary incisors are lingual to the lower incisors. A *posterior crossbite* is present when one or more posterior teeth are locked in an abnormal buccal or lingual relationship (Fig. 9-5).

■ What is the etiology of malocclusion?

Heredity is the major causative factor in malocclusion. Most malocclusions that require orthodontic treatment result either from imbalances between the sizes of the jaws and the sizes of the teeth or from disharmony between the various parts of the facial skeleton. Essentially, both of these conditions are genetically determined. However, other factors may cause malocclusion. Early or late loss of primary teeth can produce alignment problems in the permanent dentition. Environmental factors such as a thumb-sucking or finger-sucking habit, abnormal swallowing, mouth breathing, or tongue and lip habits can produce significant irregularities of the teeth. If such habits are causative factors of the malocclusion, then they must be eliminated before treatment can be conducted successfully. Injury to the face and various systemic and local diseases may also cause some orthodontic problems.

The causative factors mentioned before may act on various tissue systems, namely, the *neuromuscular system* (the muscles of mastication and facial expression and the tongue), *the bone*

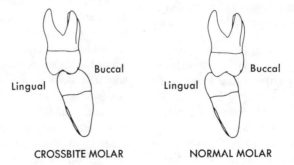

Fig. 9-5. Posterior crossbite. (Courtesy Rocky Mountain/Orthodontics, Denver.)

(maxilla, mandible, and other bones of the craniofacial complex), *the teeth* (primary and permanent), and *the soft tissues* (periodontal membrane, mucosa, skin, and connective tissues). It should be evident that the evaluation and treatment of a malocclusion require broad knowledge of all the tissue systems of the face.

■ How does a thumb-sucking or finger-sucking habit affect the teeth?

Frequently, the upper incisors are moved forward, and the lower incisors are moved backward; this movement produces an excessive overjet (Fig. 9-6). In addition the normal position of the upper and lower lip and the general profile of the child are affected. Failure to break such a habit at a reasonable age can result in improper development and positioning of the teeth and jaws.

■ What is tongue thrusting, and how does it affect the teeth?

Tongue thrusting consists of pushing the tongue against or between the teeth when swallowing or of posturing the tongue between the teeth when the mouth is closed (Fig. 9-7). In some cases its cause may be linked to heredity. In others cases tongue thrusting may be a maturational failure of the child to grow out of the swallowing pattern of infancy. Occasionally a tongue thrust remains after a broken thumb sucking habit. Most often an openbite is a sign of a tongue thrust.

■ Why should a malocclusion be treated?

A malocclusion may cause tooth decay, loss of teeth, diseased gums, bone destruction, and joint problems. It also affects a person's appearance. Although some people are not bothered by their malocclusion, others become self-conscious about it and even depressed as a result of it. The treatment of a malocclusion not only may improve the health of the teeth and gums and improve the functional relationships of the teeth but also may strengthen the patient's self-esteem.

■ When should treatment for a malocclusion be started?

Orthodontists can improve most malocclusions at any age, but there is usually a maximum age in terms of improvement that can be achieved, the type of treatment that can be employed, and the cost required. This age is determined by the character of the malocclusion, the age that the child's teeth come in, and the extent of the treatment needed. The American Dental Association has recommended that the proper age for a first visit to the family dentist is when the child is 2 to 3 years old. Likewise, the American Association of Orthodontists has recommended that the proper age for a first visit to the orthodontist is when the child is 7 years old. Early examinations can reveal existing or potential conditions that may respond to interceptive orthodontic treatment. The family dentist can usually determine if orthodontic help is needed and can then refer the patient to an orthodontist.

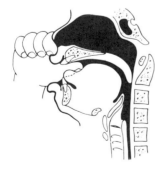

Fig. 9-6. Effect of thumb-sucking on teeth, tongue, mandible, and the circumoral musculature. (Courtesy Rocky Mountain/Orthodontics, Denver.)

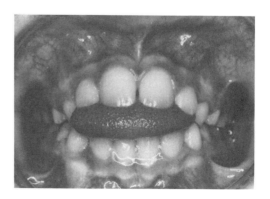

Fig. 9-7. Anterior tongue thrust.

■ **In what sequence does an orthodontic treatment proceed?**

An orthodontic treatment begins with a clinical *examination* of the patient. At this time a decision is made either to initiate treatment or to observe the patient while additional dental development is taking place.

If treatment is to begin immediately, a detailed study of *orthodontic records* and a *treatment plan* are made and presented to the parties involved. Orthodontic appliances are then fabricated and placed. The patient has thus begun the *active phase of treatment* and is usually seen once every 4 to 6 weeks for adjustments and changes in the appliances. Most malocclusions require about 2 years of active treatment; however, some malocclusions may take from a few weeks to a few months, whereas the more complicated conditions may take from 4 to 5 years. Once the functional and esthetic goals of treatment have been achieved, the fixed appliances are removed and the retentive phase of treatment begins. During this phase retainers are used to allow further stabilization of the teeth, bone, and oral musculature. The patient is often monitored during the retentive phase for approximately the same period of time as the active phase of treatment covered; however, appointments are much less frequent.

■ **What diagnostic aids are used in planning and monitoring an orthodontic treatment?**

When an orthodontist evaluates a patient's problem, he must consider not only the alignment and functional relationships of the teeth, but he must also evaluate the patient's facial skeleton and neuromuscular system (lip, tongue, swallowing pattern, cheek musculature, mouth breathing) that surround the teeth. In making this evaluation the following diagnostic aids are typically used: a thorough clinical examination, plaster study models, full face and profile photographs, full mouth periapical or panoramic radiographs, and standardized radiographs of the head (cephalograms) (Fig. 9-8). Using these materials, the orthodontist is able to identify areas of disharmony, quantitate the amount of disharmony, project future growth of the face, and determine the treatment necessary to correct the problems.

These records also serve as reference points throughout treatment and are the means by which the progress of treatment is closely monitored.

■ **What is an orthodontic appliance?**

An orthodontic appliance is a mechanism for the application of force to the teeth and their supporting tissues to produce changes in the relationship of the teeth and the related osseous structures. The term "appliance" is used in preference to "brace," since the latter implies a rigid immobile contrivance rather than a device that can be manipulated to tip, move bodily, and rotate the teeth. A wide variety of fixed (cemented) and removable appliances are used by orthodontists.

■ **What are fixed orthodontic appliances?**

Fixed appliances are cemented to the teeth (Fig. 9-9). They often consist of individual *bands* that fit around each tooth and are cemented onto the tooth. On the cheek or lip surface of the band is a bracket with one of a variety of configurations depending on the biomechanical system used by the orthodontist.

The *bracket* may also be bonded directly to the enamel by use of the acid-etch technique with various polymeric resins. The bracket is the means by which forces are applied to the teeth. *Arch wires* that may be round, square, or rectangular extend around the dental arch and are attached to the teeth by means of the bracket. Frequently a wire is found resting on the lingual aspect (tongue side) of the teeth or across part of the palate. This type of appliance is called a *lingual wire* (Fig. 9-10). Small rubber bands or latex elastics often are seen running from a hook on one part of the appliances to another. These elastics are used to move teeth by the pitting of one group of teeth against another. The elastics usually are worn all the time, although the length of time varies with the specific treatment objectives. The elastics are replaced by the patient daily or when they break.

■ **What is a removable appliance?**

Any orthodontic appliance that the patient is able to insert and remove from the mouth is a

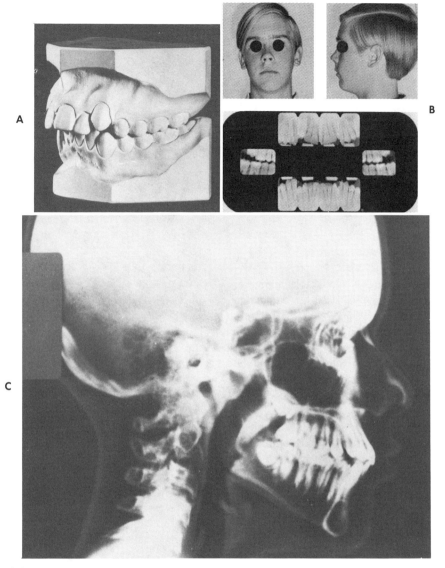

Fig. 9-8. A, Study models. **B,** Extraoral photographs and periapical radiographs. **C,** Lateral cephalogram. (Courtesy Rocky Mountain Data Systems, Inc., Encino, Calif.)

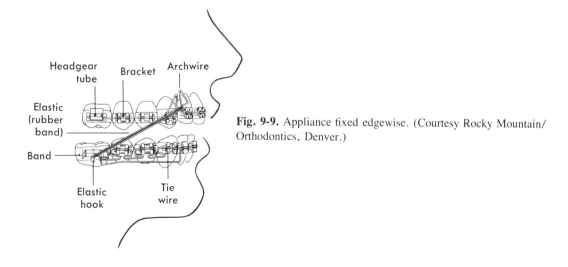

Headgear tube Bracket Archwire

Elastic (rubber band)

Band

Elastic hook   Tie wire

Fig. 9-9. Appliance fixed edgewise. (Courtesy Rocky Mountain/ Orthodontics, Denver.)

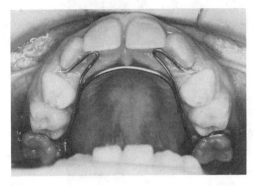

Fig. 9-10. Lingual wire with auxiliary springs to move the lateral incisors labially.

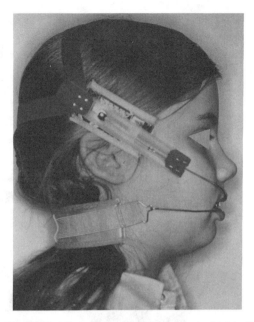

Fig. 9-11. A face-bow and neck strap and a high pull headcap. These extraoral appliances are removable.

removable appliance. A removable appliance called a *headgear* is often used in conjunction with fixed appliances (Fig. 9-11). There are a variety of headgear designs, but all use the head and/or neck as a point of resistance for forces that then are applied to the teeth and the jaws. This type of appliance is usually worn for 12 to 16 hours a day or as instructed by the orthodontist.

A *retainer* is another removable appliance that is generally used after the fixed appliances are removed (Fig. 9-12). The retainers allow further stabilization of the teeth, bone, and oral musculature. Retainers are usually worn full time for several months, and then the wearing time is gradually reduced to periods determined by the orthodontist.

■ **How do orthodontic appliances move the teeth?**

The capability of the appliances described previously to move teeth within bone is due to the biologic property of bone that causes it to resorb or dissolve under pressure and to deposit new bone under tension. The efficiency of these tooth movements depends on the following factors: (1) the magnitude of the force, (2) the duration of the force, (3) the direction of the force, and (4) the age of the patient. These factors must be considered when the orthodontist selects the size of the arch wires, the strength of the elastics, the type of headgear, and the amount of time the various appliances are to be worn.

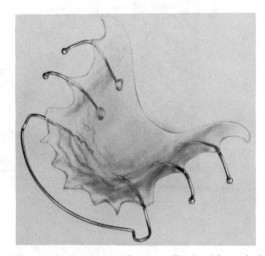

Fig. 9-12. Retainer. (Courtesy Rocky Mountain/ Orthodontics, Denver.)

■ **Will there be discomfort with orthodontic appliances?**

Following placement of orthodontic appliances the new additions to the oral cavity often will be annoying to the patient temporarily. The projections of the brackets and wires may be annoying to the mucosa of the lips, cheeks, and tongue. The added bulk of a retainer or lingual appliance may interfere with certain consonant and vowel sounds. The teeth may be sore and sensitive to biting forces. Fortunately, these annoyances should decrease rapidly over the ensuing 2 to 3 days. Soft wax is usually provided to cover any offending projections, and aspirin will help reduce soreness of the teeth. Occasionally, wires break or become distorted, causing pricking or scratching of the mucosa. In such instances the soft wax should be used to cover the point of irritation, and the orthodontist should be contacted immediately. Likewise if a band or a bracket becomes loose, the patient should save the band or any other appliance, call the office for an appointment, and bring all parts back to the office.

■ **Should orthodontic patients alter their diet?**

There are three adverse effects from poor eating habits: (1) loose bands and brackets, (2) distorted arch wires, and (3) caries on the exposed parts of the teeth. To avoid these problems the patient must avoid hard foods that can bend the wires and break the brackets and bands. Biting ice cubes, pencils, and the unpopped kernels of popcorn must be avoided. Fresh fruits and vegetables should be cut in small thin pieces before eating. Sticky foods can also bend the wires and pull loose the bands. Taffy apples, caramels, and bubble gum must also be avoided. Foods with a high sugar content increase the danger of cavities and must obviously be eliminated as much as is possible.

■ **Does toothbrushing have to be modified while orthodontic appliances are in place?**

There are many more nooks and crannies in which food can collect when appliances are in place, and thorough toothbrushing is a major responsibility of the orthodontic patient. One of the most commonly expressed fears concerning orthodontics is that the bands may cause decay. Actually the parts of the teeth that are covered by the bands are protected from caries as long as the cement seal is present. The result of brushing is more important than the method. Every office may teach a slightly different brushing technique, but without exception toothbrushing and good oral hygiene are emphasized in orthodontic offices. Many orthodontists recommend the regular use of fluoride toothpastes, fluoride mouth rinses, and pulsating irrigating devices as part of their oral hygiene program.

The areas that present the most trouble and in turn require the greatest attention are (1) the area between the band and the gingival tissue, (2) the space behind the arch wires and loops, (3) the teeth that are blocked out, and (4) newly erupted molars. Patients should brush within 5 minutes after eating, morning and night, and when in school they should swish and rinse vigorously with water after lunch. Proper brushing should result in bands that look clean and shiny, the small half-moon area of the tooth between the band and gingiva should be free from plaque, and the gingiva should be firm and light pink in color.

MULTIPLE-CHOICE QUESTIONS

1. Orthodontics is the branch of dentistry concerned with all of the following areas except:
   a. Development of occlusion
   b. Growth of the face
   c. Treatment of crowded teeth
   d. Filling of a root canal
2. Which of the following statements regarding the growth of the craniofacial skeleton is false:
   a. It is a very complex process.
   b. The mandible generally ceases growth before the maxilla.
   c. There is evidence that some parts of the craniofacial skeleton continue growing until 20 to 25 years of age.

d. The cranium often reaches its adult size by age 7 years.

3. The orthodontist must understand facial growth to:
   a. Always avoid orthodontic treatment until all growth has occurred
   b. Choose the proper time for treatment
   c. Correct a deviated nasal septum
   d. Impress the patient

4. The mean age for eruption of the first deciduous tooth is:
   a. 5 months
   b. 1½ years
   c. 7½ months
   d. 12 months

5. The sequence of eruption of deciduous teeth is usually characterized by:
   a. The upper teeth erupting before their lower counterparts
   b. The teeth erupting in sequence from back to front
   c. The lower teeth erupting before their upper counterparts with the exception of the lateral incisors
   d. A complete deciduous dentition by 1½ years of age

6. The mean age for eruption of the first permanent tooth is:
   a. 5 years
   b. 5½ years
   c. 6 years
   d. 6½ years

7. The first permanent tooth to erupt is usually:
   a. The upper central incisor
   b. The lower first permanent molar
   c. The lower central incisor
   d. The upper first permanent molar

8. Which of the following statements regarding the sequence of eruption of the permanent dentition is true?
   a. The upper arch sequence begins with the first molars and then proceeds from front to back.
   b. The lower arch sequence begins with the first molar and then proceeds from front to back.
   c. The upper teeth generally erupt before their lower counterparts.

d. The permanent teeth of males tend to erupt 5 months earlier than those of females.

9. Which of the following statements regarding the mixed dentition period is false?
   a. The mixed dentition period is generally from 6 to 12 years of age.
   b. Since so many changes in occlusion are occurring, orthodontic treatment is never initiated during this period.
   c. This period is characterized by the presence of both primary and permanent teeth.
   d. Critical adaptive changes in the occlusion occur during the transition from the deciduous to the permanent dentition.

10. Which statement regarding ankylosis of teeth is false?
   a. The frequency of ankylosed teeth is greatest in the primary dentition.
   b. Upper teeth are involved more frequently than lower teeth.
   c. Ankylosed teeth may contribute to an open bite.
   d. Ankylosed primary teeth may interfere with normal eruption of the underlying permanent teeth.

11. With the exception of third molars the most frequently congenitally missing teeth are:
   a. The lower second bicuspids
   b. The upper lateral incisors
   c. The upper second bicuspids
   d. The upper first bicuspids

12. Supernumerary teeth are:
   a. More often found in the mandible than the maxilla
   b. Found in about 10% of the population
   c. Often found in the area of the maxillary central and lateral incisors
   d. A result of trauma

13. The Angle classification of occlusal relationships is based primarily on:
   a. The presence of crossbites
   b. The size of the overjet
   c. The number of rotated teeth
   d. The relationship of the upper first molar with the lower first molar

14. The Angle classification system:

a. Has five major classes
b. Has divisions that are based on the position of the cuspids
c. Primarily describes lateral relationships
d. Is the most commonly used classification system

15. An overjet:
a. Describes the vertical relationship between the upper and lower incisors
b. Is considered normal when the upper incisors are 5 to 7 mm ahead of the lower incisors
c. Is often a characteristic of class II malocclusions when it is negative
d. Is negative when the lower incisors are ahead of the upper incisors

16. An overbite:
a. Is impinging when the lower incisors contact the palatal tissue lingual to the upper incisors
b. Describes the horizontal relationship between the upper and lower incisors
c. Is cause for esthetic concern when it is impinging but functionally is not a problem
d. Is evaluated when the posterior teeth are apart and the jaws are in a rest position

17. Which of the following statements about an open bite are false?
a. It is often associated with a thumb or finger habit.
b. It is often associated with a tongue thrust.
c. It is the opposite of an impinging overbite.
d. It is most frequently found in the buccal segments.

18. Which of the following statements about a crossbite are false?
a. It is an abnormal anteroposterior relationship of the posterior teeth.
b. It indicates an abnormal buccolingual (labiolingual) relationship of the teeth.
c. It is a malocclusion.
d. It often involves groups of anterior and posterior teeth.

19. The major etiologic factor in malocclusions is:

a. Tongue habits
b. Early loss of deciduous teeth
c. Injury to the face
d. Heredity

20. Environmental factors causing malocclusion may be all the following except:
a. Large teeth
b. Thumb-sucking
c. Abnormal swallowing
d. Mouth breathing

21. The orthodontist must consider the impact that an etiologic factor has on:
a. The thumb habit
b. Only the teeth and the jawbones
c. The teeth, bone, soft tissue, and neuromuscular system
d. Heredity

22. The results of a thumb-sucking or finger-sucking habit may be all of the following except:
a. An excessive overjet
b. An anterior open bite
c. Large teeth
d. Tipping of the upper and lower incisors

23. An untreated malocclusion may make a patient prone to all of the following except:
a. Tooth decay
b. Periodontal problems
c. Temporomandibular joint problems
d. A cleft palate

24. The American Association of Orthodontists has recommended that the proper age for a child's first visit to the orthodontist is when the child is:
a. 2 to 3 years old
b. 7 years old
c. 11 years old
d. 16 years old

25. During the active phase of orthodontic treatment the patient:
a. Is seen infrequently
b. Is seen every 4 to 6 weeks
c. Usually wears retainers
d. Is awaiting final stabilization of the teeth, bone, and oral musculature

26. An orthodontic bracket is not:
a. The means by which forces are applied to the teeth
b. Part of a removable appliance

    c. Held on the tooth by bands or by direct bonding

    d. Used to attach the arch wires to the tooth

27. A retainer:

    a. Is used during the active phase of treatment to align the teeth

    b. Is commonly used before fixed appliances are placed

    c. Is usually worn full time for several months, and then wearing time is gradually reduced

    d. Is an example of a fixed appliance

28. A headgear:

    a. Is a removable appliance

    b. Uses the muscles of mastication to produce force

    c. Can only be inserted and removed by the orthodontist

    d. Should be worn no more than 4 to 6 hours per day

29. Orthodontic appliances move teeth because:

    a. Bone is elastic

    b. Roots dissolve

    c. Bone resorbs under tension

    d. New bone forms under tension and dissolves under pressure

30. The efficiency of tooth movement is affected by all of the following factors except:

    a. The magnitude of the force

    b. The duration and direction of the force

    c. The age of the patient

    d. The type of orthodontic cement

31. An orthodontic patient should contact the orthodontist immediately if:

    a. The teeth are sore to pressure for 2 to 3 days following the initial placement of appliances

    b. A band or bracket comes loose or an arch wire breaks

    c. Teeth are sore to pressure for 2 to 3 days following a change in arch wires

    d. Molars are sore following the initial use of a headgear

32. Which of the following statements regarding an orthodontic patient's eating habits is false:

    a. Poor eating habits can cause loose bands.

    b. Poor eating habits can cause distorted arch wires.

    c. Extremely hard foods and sticky foods must be avoided.

    d. High sugar content foods are not of concern, since the bands cover much of the teeth.

33. Which of the following statements regarding toothbrushing is false:

    a. The orthodontic patient must concentrate on the area between the band and the gum tissue.

    b. Orthodontic bands and wires will become dull and tarnished from the oral fluids and dull and tarnished bands and wires are not indicative of poor toothbrushing.

    c. Teeth that are blocked out and rotated require special attention when brushing.

    d. If patients are unable to brush after eating, they should rinse vigorously with water.

SUGGESTED READINGS

Graber, T. M.: Orthodontics—principles and practice, ed. 3, Philadelphia, 1973, W. B. Saunders Co.

Horowtiz, S. L., and Hixon, E. H.: The nature of orthodontic diagnosis, St. Louis, 1966, The C. V. Mosby Co.

Moyers, R. E.: Handbook of orthodontics, ed. 3, Chicago, 1973, Year Book Medical Publishers, Inc.

Reynolds, J. M., and Arai, H. Y.: Welcome to the world of orthodontics, Lubbock, Tex., 1973, Zulauf, Inc.

CHAPTER 10

Endodontics

ELIZABETH GORMAN ALLEN

■ **Define the specialty of endodontics.**

Endodontics is that branch of dentistry that deals with the prevention, diagnosis, and treatment of diseases and injuries of the pulp and periapical tissues.

■ **What is the purpose of endodontics?**

The purpose of endodontics is to restore the diseased tooth to a healthy status, resulting in a tooth that is free of disease and functional.

■ **Identify the five causes of a nonvital tooth.**

A tooth may become nonvital because of bacterial invasion, chemical irritation, mechanical exposure, thermal change, and trauma.

■ **Define the diseases of the pulp.**

Hyperemia. This term refers to excess blood in any body part. As it applies to endodontics, hyperemia occurs when there has been an injury to the pulp and the arterioles within the pulp become engorged with blood and dilate.

Pulpitis. Pulpitis is an inflammation of the dental pulp.

Necrosis. Necrosis refers to the death of a cell or group of cells. Pulpal necrosis occurs as a result of pulpitis.

Apical periodontitis. This is an inflammatory reaction of the tissues surrounding the apex of the root of a tooth.

Periapical abscess. This is a severe inflammation at the apex of the tooth that results from untreated apical periodontitis. Symptoms include acute pain, edema, dilated blood vessels, and pressure caused by invasion of white blood cells, resulting in *pus* formation.

Periapical granuloma. This is a tumorlike mass made up of granulation tissue that occurs

as a result of resorption of the bone it replaces. The tissue has good repair potential and converts to normal periapical tissue when the irritant is removed from the root canal.

Periapical cyst. A periapical cyst is a fluid-filled sac lined with epithelial cells located in the bone at the apex of a pulpless tooth. These cysts may increase in size and create pressure than can result in significant bone loss and tooth mobility.

■ **What is a pulp stone?**

Pulp stones (denticles) are calcified substances occurring in the coronal portion of the pulp. Depending on their structure, they are classified as true or false denticles. *True* denticles consist of irregular dentin, whereas *false* denticles are made up of concentric layers of degenerated or calcified tissue. These calcifications may be attached to the pulpal wall or free of any attachment. They are generally harmless concretions, although occasionally may cause pain as a result of their impingement on nerve fibers. *Diffuse calcification* occurs in the form of multiple calcified bodies in the root portion of the pulp. This calcification is significant in clinical endodontics, since it may complicate a procedure.

■ **Describe the role of the dental assistant in the evaluative procedures prior to endodontic treatment.**

The dental assistant should obtain a complete medical/dental history, chart the findings during a clinical examination, obtain the necessary radiographs, and ask key questions such as, "Which tooth is causing discomfort? When did the pain begin? How long does it last? Is the pain becoming increasingly worse? What gives you relief?'' The dental assistant records responses in the patient's record.

■ **Identify the diagnostic aids used in endodontics.**

There are several aids used in endodontic diagnosis.

Palpation. Finger pressure on the soft tissue area, buccolingually, will identify the site of inflammation or edema.

Percussion. The handle of a mouth mirror is often used to tap the incisal surface to stimulate pain. If the patient reacts, it can be noted as periapical inflammation.

Radiograph. A bite-wing radiograph will indicate caries and periodontal disease, whereas a periapical radiograph will indicate the presence of periapical disease or an abnormality in the pulp canal.

Thermal pulp testing. A *cold* pulp test may be accomplished by directly applying a cone of ice to the tooth. A severe response from the patient indicates an abnormal condition. It should also be noted that no response may indicate either a normal or an abnormal condition. A *heat* pulp test may be accomplished by the direct application of hot gutta-percha sticks to the tooth. A hot instrument or a rubber rotary instrument may also be used to stimulate a pulpal reaction. A severe response indicates an abnormal condition. No response may indicate a normal or abnormal condition. A severe reaction from the patient will require an immediate application of ice or cold water to the site.

Probing. The use of a periodontal probe into the sulcus will aid in determining the periodontal status and/or presence of an endodontic lesion.

Electric pulp testing. A vitalometer probe, with gradations of electric current, is placed on a dried tooth to stimulate a response from the pulp.

Other diagnostic aids may include a bite test, selective anesthesia, or even the removal of dentin. No one test can determine the vitality of a tooth, and it is often necessary to perform several tests before the final diagnosis is made.

■ **Explain the use of a vitalometer.**

The vitalometer is an electric pulp tester used to determine tooth vitality. The following steps are common to the use of most vitalometers:

Explain the use of the device to the patient and assure him that you will remove the probe from the tooth as soon as he reacts positively.

Isolate the teeth to be tested with cotton rolls or rubber dam and dry with air.

Set the dial at zero.

Place the probe of the pulp tester into toothpaste or a pumice mixture.

The probe should be placed on a normal adjacent tooth prior to testing the suspected tooth, so the patient may have a contrast of sensations.

Place the probe onto the cervical portion of the tooth to be tested. Avoid placing the probe near the gingiva or on metallic restorations.

Slowly advance the dial until the patient responds. More than one reading should be taken, and the results should be averaged and recorded.

■ **Describe the various types of intracanal instruments or devices.**

There are several instruments for intracanal usage.

Broach. This instrument is designed for removing pulp tissue, paper points, and cotton pellets, but *not* for enlarging the canal. The barbs on this instrument are notched out of the shaft; this presents a weakened point and a possible site for breakage if torque is applied (Fig. 10-1).

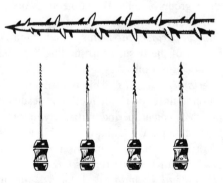

Fig. 10-1. Endodontic barbed broach.

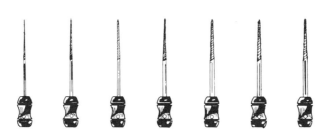

Fig. 10-2. K-files.

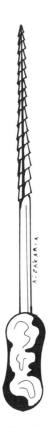

Fig. 10-3. Hedstrom file. (From Bence, R.: Handbook of clinical endodontics, St. Louis, 1976, The C. V. Mosby Co.)

K-file. This instrument is designed for enlarging and removing hard tissue from the canals. The instrument is made from carbon or stainless steel square rods twisted in a series of cutting flutes. K-files are color coded according to the instrument's diameter (Fig. 10-2).

Hedstrom file. This file consists of a series of sharp cone-shaped cutting segments that are similar to wood screws. The disadvantage of this instrument is that it is weakened where gouged during the manufacturing process and may break at that point if binding occurs during rotation in the canal (Fig. 10-3).

Reamer. The reamer is designed to cleanse and enlarge the canals. It is constructed from a triangular piece of carbon or stainless steel rod that is twisted into a tapered instrument with gradual spirals (Fig. 10-4).

Instrument stops. These small metal, rubber, or silicone rings are placed on files to mark the measured length of the root canal. This eliminates overextension of the file into the apical space.

■ **Which instruments are placed on the standard tray setup for root canal preparation?** (See Figs. 10-5 and 10-6.)

The following items are required on a standard tray setup:

Mouth mirror

Endodontic explorer

Endodontic excavator

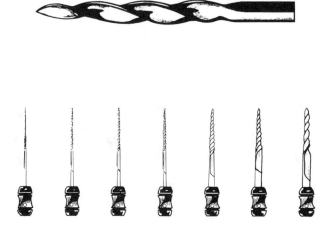

Fig. 10-4. Reamers.

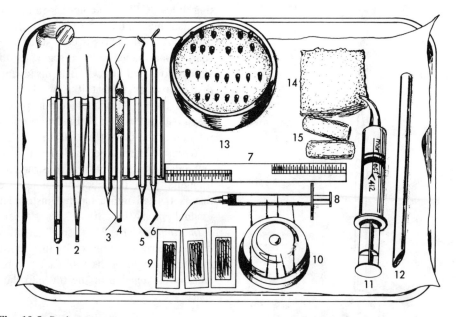

Fig. 10-5. Basic tray setup.

1. Mirror
2. Cotton pliers
3. Endodontic explorer
4. Periodontal probe
5. Spoon excavator
6. Plastic instrument
7. Ruler
8. Disposable irrigating syringe
9. Paper points
10. Bur holder with burs
11. Large disposable syringe containing rc-prep
12. Suction tip
13. Assorted files
14. Gauze sponges
15. Cotton rolls

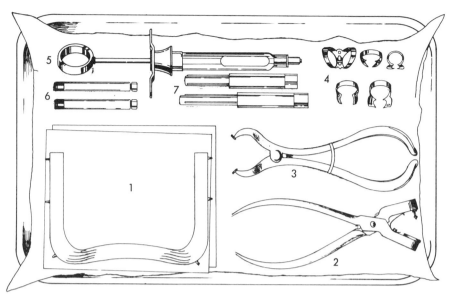

Fig. 10-6. Rubber dam and anesthetic tray.

1. Rubber dam material and frame
2. Rubber dam punch
3. Rubber dam clamp holder
4. Assorted clamps
5. Anesthetic syringe (aspirating type)
6. Anesthetic solution cartridges
7. Sterile needles in plastic capsules (1 inch and 1⅝ inches in length for infiltration or block anesthetic)

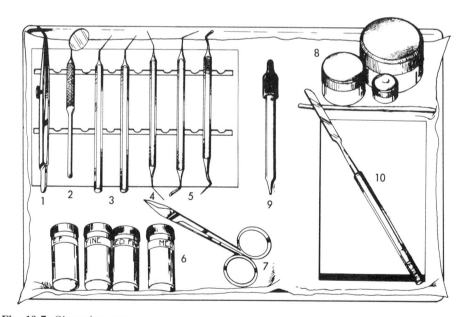

Fig. 10-7. Obturation tray.

1. Endodontic locking pliers
2. Mouth mirror
3. Endodontic pluggers of various diameters
4. Endodontic spreader
5. Plastic instruments
6. Assorted gutta-percha points
7. Scissors
8. Root canal sealer
9. Dropper
10. Sterile glass slab and spatula

Endodontic cotton pliers
Periodontal probe
Plastic instrument
Endodontic ruler (metal)
Endodontic syringe filled with sodium hypochlorite solution
Assorted files
Rubber dam frame
Rubber dam forceps
Assorted rubber dam clamps
Rubber dam
Disinfectant and cotton applicator
Contra-angle and burs (No 2, 4, 6, 557, and 701)
Gauze sponges and cotton pellets
Absorbent paper points
Anesthetic syringe
X-ray film and film holder

The additional instruments necessary for root canal filling include the following (see Fig. 10-7):

Endodontic spreader
Root canal plugger
Heat source
Absorbent paper points
Gutta-percha cones
Root canal sealer
Glass slab and spatula

■ What special considerations should be given to rubber dam application in endodontic therapy?

The same armamentarium used in rubber dam application in operative dentistry is used in endodontics. Several special considerations exist, however:

A radiolucent rubber dam frame eliminates the problems of radiographic procedures being cumbersome and anatomic structures being obscured.

A single hole is punched for endodontic treatment. Multiple holes are punched only if more than one tooth is involved endodontically.

The isolated tooth and adjacent dam are swabbed with tincture of nitromersol (Metaphen) or other disinfectant.

Care should be taken to avoid potential seepage by using a clamp that fits the tooth

snugly, by replacing a torn dam, and by not punching a hole that is too large.

■ Discuss the phases of root canal preparation.

The phases of root canal preparation include biomechanical preparation, chemical preparation, disinfection, culturing, and obturation.

During biomechanical preparation, once access to the pulp has been achieved, the pulp is extirpated with a barbed broach. Then enlargement and débridement of the canal is accomplished with files and reamers of assorted sizes.

Chemicals may be used to dissolve dentin or pulp tissue debris. The canal is disinfected, and cultures may be taken at the option of the operator.

The purpose of the root canal filling (obturation) is to seal the canal to prevent entry of bacteria to the periapical tissue.

■ Describe the steps to be followed in measuring length of the tooth accurately.

The shadow of a tooth is measured on a good preoperative x-ray film. The reverse or unsterile end of the endodontic ruler is placed on x-ray films.

Subtract 2 mm to allow for image distortion or measuring error.

Place the endodontic ruler at this measurement and adjust the rubber stop on the file at that site.

Insert the file into the canal until the rubber stop is at the specific point of measurement unless pain is felt; in which instance, the file is left at that point, and the rubber stop is readjusted to this new point of reference.

Expose and develop another x-ray film.

Measure the difference between the end of the instrument and the site where the canal leaves the root. Add this figure to the original measured length of the instrument extended into the tooth. If the file has perforated the apex, subtract this difference.

Using the adjusted length of tooth, subtract 0.5 mm as a safety factor to conform with the apical termination of the root canal at the cementodentinal junction.

Set the endodontic ruler at this corrected

length, and readjust the rubber stop on the file. Take another x-ray film to confirm the adjusted length.

Reset the endodontic ruler at this measurement, and record this figure and the occlusal reference point on the patient's record.

■ **What is a chelating agent?**

A chelating agent is a chemical placed into a canal during the enlarging process that softens sclerotic areas of dentin so that the dentin may be easily removed.

■ **Discuss the purpose and method of irrigating the canal.**

The primary purpose of irrigating the canal is to wash out organic debris, microorganisms, and pieces of dentin. The best method of irrigation is to use alternating solutions of hydrogen peroxide and sodium hypochlorite. It has been recommended that sodium hypochlorite solution should be used following the hydrogen peroxide irrigation because of the release of oxygen from the hydrogen peroxide which will cause pressure and, ultimately, pain if left in the canal.

■ **Describe the procedure of drying a canal.**

On completion of canal irrigation, thorough drying of the canal is necessary. Excess irrigating solution may be withdrawn from the canal slowly with the irrigating syringe. Large sterile absorbent points are inserted to contact the canal walls. Then absorbent points narrower than the canal are inserted and extended to the apical constriction to ensure that the apical portion is dry. If the point perforates the apical constriction, it will appear tinged with blood or wet with tissue fluids. It is important to note that compressed air should *never* be used to dry the canal.

■ **Describe the procedure for obtaining a trial point.**

Either a gutta-percha point or silver point is selected and disinfected. Gutta-percha is placed in a germicide. A silver point is heated in a Bunsen burner, and overheating is avoided. The point is placed in a germicide to cool it and anneal it. The selected point is measured and then placed into the canal. The point is tested visually, tactilely, and radiographically to assure correct placement.

■ **Which agents are used as intracanal medicaments?**

Although the philosophy of using intracanal medicaments has been replaced with emphasis on débridement, many practitioners continue to use drugs as interim treatment dressings. The drugs used include the following:

Beechwood creosote: a clear yellow oily liquid with a highly pungent odor. It is considered less toxic and irritating than phenol.

Camphorated parachlorophenol (CPCP): an oily light-amber–colored liquid with a distinct aromatic odor. The camphor aids in reducing the irritating effect of parachlorophenol.

Metacresyl acetate (Cresatin): an antiseptic-analgesic with a phenolic-acetic odor. This clear oily liquid is less irritating than all the others and not caustic.

Formocresol: a combination of formalin and cresol. It has been determined that this medicament is highly irritating and caustic.

■ **Describe the technique for sealing a master point into the canal.**

The sealer is mixed to a creamy consistency.

A small amount of sealer is placed into the canal with a reamer. Two applications are often inserted.

The master point is rolled into the sealer and placed into the canal. Care should be taken to avoid forcing sealer into the periapical space, which would cause discomfort.

Following seating of the master point, a spreader is placed alongside the point and forced toward the apex.

Auxiliary gutta-percha points are inserted into the space created by the spreader. The spreader is again used, and the procedure is repeated until firm resistance is met.

The canal is considered filled when the spreader does not penetrate beyond the cervical line.

A final x-ray film is taken to confirm the complete obturation of the canal.

With a heated instrument the excess gutta-percha is removed.

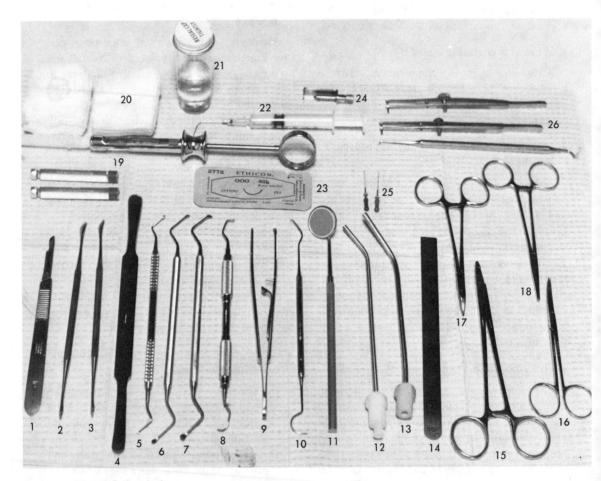

Fig. 10-8. Surgical tray setup.

 1. Scalpel
 2. Periosteal elevator
 3. No. 7 wax spatula
 4. Retractor
 5-8. Curets (three surgical and one periodontal)
 9. Locking pliers
 10. Explorer
 11. Mirror
 12, 13. Aspirator tips (two sizes)
 14. Millimeter ruler
 15. Hemostat-scissors

 16. Scissors
 17, 18. Hemostats (curved and straight)
 19. Anesthetic syringe and extra carpules
 20. Gauze and cotton pellets
 21. Biopsy bottle
 22. Irrigating syringe
 23. Suture material
 24. Bur changer
 25. Files (to aid in locating apex)
 26. Amalgam carriers and condenser

(From Bence, R.: Handbook of clinical endodontics, St. Louis, 1976, The C. V. Mosby Co.)

■ **Define apexification.**

Apexification is a method of inducing apical closure or the continued apical development of the roots of an incompletely formed tooth in which the pulp is nonvital, generally because of the formation of osteodentin or a similar hard tissue. Calcium hydroxide pastes are commonly used to bring about apexification.

■ **Define hemisection.**

Hemisection is a surgical procedure in which one root (or possibly two in maxillary molars) and the overlying crown may be removed. The tooth is cut buccolingually through the bifurcation into two separate parts. The diseased portion of the tooth is removed, and the remaining portion is restored.

■ **Describe an apicoectomy.**

An apicoectomy is a surgical procedure in which the root apex is removed and a periapical curettage is completed on the adjacent tissue.

■ **Identify the instruments included on an endodontic surgical tray setup.**

Fig. 10-8 lists and illustrates the instruments commonly used in an endodontic surgical procedure.

MULTIPLE-CHOICE QUESTIONS

1. A 7-year-old patient reports to a dental office following an accident in which the crown of a maxillary central incisor was fractured, grossly exposing the vital pulp. Treatment would be:
   a. Pulpotomy
   b. Extraction
   c. Pulp capping
   d. Apexification
2. Contraindications for endodontic treatment may be:
   a. Split roots
   b. Extreme mobility
   c. Nonrestorable teeth
   d. All of the above
3. A pulpectomy is treatment of a tooth involving:
   a. Removal of the pulp horns
   b. Partial removal of the pulp
   c. Total removal of the pulp
   d. None of the above
4. An apicoectomy is a surgical procedure that involves:
   a. The surgical removal of the apex or root tip
   b. Sterilizing the root canal
   c. Completing the treatment in one sitting
   d. None of the above
5. A pulpotomy is a procedure that involves:
   a. Removal of the pulpal tissue in the coronal portion of the tooth
   b. Treatment of the gingiva
   c. Amputation of the root
   d. None of the above
6. Which of the following instruments is not included on an endodontic tray?
   a. Round bur
   b. File
   c. Excavator
   d. Rongeur forceps
7. A bulbous growth of the pulp is called:
   a. An abscess
   b. A pulp stone
   c. A polyp
   d. None of the above
8. A fistula is an opening on the mucosa that provides drainage for:
   a. A site of infection
   b. A cyst
   c. An apical abscess
   d. None of the above
9. One of the best aids for obtaining a culture of a root canal is:
   a. Aspirating syringe
   b. Sterile absorbent paper point
   c. Sterile gutta-percha point
   d. None of the above
10. A nonvital tooth is said to be:

a. Necrotic
b. Hyperemic
c. Hemorrhaging
d. None of the above

11. The first procedure in the treatment of a tooth with a chronic alveolar abscess is to:
a. Open the apical foramen
b. Remove the necrotic pulp tissue
c. Establish drainage through the root canal
d. All of the above

12. The best instrument for enlarging the root canal is the:
a. Broach
b. Lentulo spiral
c. File
d. Bur

13. The instrument used to adapt gutta-percha points into the canal and the chamber of the tooth is the:
a. Spreader
b. Plastic instrument
c. Excavator
d. Plugger

14. Triangular wires twisted into gradual spirals used in pushing, twisting, and pulling in the canal are:
a. Files
b. Reamers
c. Broaches
d. Points

15. A temporary stopping material used in endodontic therapy is:
a. Beechwood creosote
b. Gutta-percha
c. Eugenol
d. Calcium hydroxide

16. Instruments designed to remove fragments of the pulp from the canal are:
a. Excavators
b. Reamers
c. Burs
d. Broaches

17. Inflammation of the pulp is referred to as:
a. Necrosis
b. Pulpitis
c. Cellulitis
d. Pulposis

18. A chemical agent used in bleaching a nonvital tooth is:

a. Hydrogen peroxide (Superoxol)
b. Carbolic acid
c. Beechwood creosote
d. Formocresol

19. What is placed snugly into the canal to close the space *not* occupied by the silver point?
a. Paper points
b. Cotton pellets
c. Gutta-percha points
d. Reamers

20. Identify the correct order for the procedures performed during a patient's first appointment with the endodontist.
a. Canals opened, canals irrigated, and walls of canal enlarged
b. Length of tooth measured, canals opened, debris removed, and canals irrigated
c. Length of tooth measured, canals opened, canals irrigated, and debris removed
d. Canals opened, debris removed, canals irrigated, and length of tooth measured

21. The major cause of failure following root canal treatment, as far as the placement of the root canal filling is concerned, is:
a. Underfilling of the root canal
b. Inadequate sterilization of the root canal
c. Inadequate sealing of the root canal
d. None of the above

22. During instrumentation the canal should be kept:
a. Dry
b. Moist
c. Both of the above

23. Which of the following instruments should be sterilized in dry heat?
a. Root canal broaches and files
b. Plastic instruments
c. Water syringe tip
d. All of the above

24. The best proof of sterility of a root canal is:
a. A radiograph
b. Clinical observation
c. Bacterial cultures
d. Symptoms

25. The mechanical removal of necrotic material from the root canal is:
a. Putrefaction

b. Pulp capping

c. Irrigation

d. Débridement

26. Discoloration of nonvital teeth is caused by:

a. Precipitated silver from an amalgam restoration

b. Use of medicaments in endodontic therapy

c. Hemorrhage of blood into the dentinal tubules

d. All of the above

27. The solutions used to irrigate and medicate the root canal include all *except* which one of the following?

a. Beechwood creosote

b. Sodium hypochlorite

c. Distilled water

d. Camphorated parachlorophenol (CPCP)

SUGGESTED READINGS

Bence, R.: Handbook of clinical endodontics, St. Louis, 1976, The C. V. Mosby Co.

Grossman, L. I.: Endodontic practice, Philadelphia, 1978, Lea & Febiger.

Ingle, J.: Endodontics, Philadelphia, 1970, Lea & Febiger.

Weine, F. S.: Endodontic therapy, St. Louis, 1976, The C. V. Mosby Co.

CHAPTER 11

Periodontics

JONI A. SELF and BETTY H. ZENDNER

■ **Define the specialty of periodontics.**

Periodontics is the specialty in dentistry concerned with prevention, diagnosis, and treatment of diseases affecting the hard and soft tissues surrounding the teeth.

■ **What is the purpose of periodontal therapy?**

Periodontal therapy is designed to instruct and motivate the patient toward optimum oral health care and to diagnose and treat diseases of the bone and gingiva surrounding the teeth for maximum retention of teeth throughout the adult lifetime.

■ **What are the tissues that make up the periodontium?**

The periodontium is composed of the gingiva, cementum, periodontal ligament, and alveolar bone.

■ **What is the purpose of the periodontium?**

The periodontium provides support to the teeth and holds the teeth within the alveolus (socket).

■ **Define the term gingiva and describe the location and appearance of normal gingiva.**

Gingiva is the mucous membrane surrounding the teeth and alveolar process. The color of gingiva varies with its thickness, blood supply, pigmentation, and disease processes. Healthy gingiva is often described as coral pink in color. The gingiva is divided in two parts: the free gingiva and the attached gingiva.

Free gingiva. This is the most coronal, unattached portion of the gingival tissues encircling the tooth. Its borders are formed apically by the free gingival groove, a shallow, linear depression running parallel to the gingival margin and occlusally by the free gingival margin. The space produced by the unattached, free gingiva against the tooth is termed the *gingival sulcus.*

Attached gingiva. That part of the gingiva extending apically from the free gingival groove to the mucogingival junction is called the attached gingiva. It is firmly attached to the underlying tooth and alveolar bone. Clinically, its surface is characterized by an orange peel–like appearance, called *stippling.*

Interdental papilla. This triangular shaped tissue fills the embrasure between the teeth and is continuous with both free and attached gingiva.

Mucogingival junction. This term refers to the demarcation between attached gingiva and alveolar mucosa.

Alveolar mucosa. This loosely connected, movable tissue covers the remainder of the alveolar bone.

■ **Identify the names and location of the principal fiber groups found within the periodontal ligament.** (For location refer to Fig. 11-2. The location of each group is identified by the letters that correspond to those below.)

A. Alveolar crest   D. Apical
B. Horizontal   E. Interradicular
C. Oblique   F. Transseptal

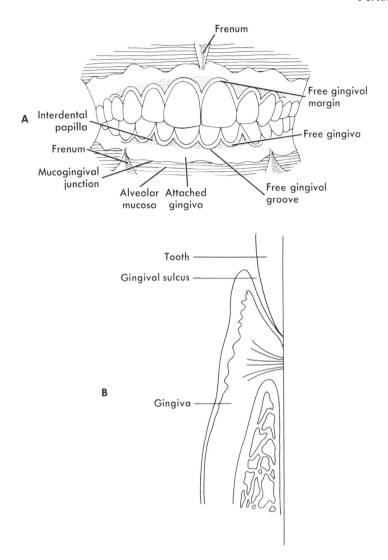

Fig. 11-1. A, The periodontium. **B,** Illustration of gingiva and gingival sulcus.

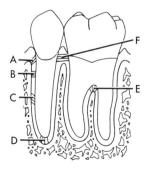

Fig. 11-2. Fiber groups found in the periodontal ligament. *A,* Alveolar crest; *B,* horizontal; *C,* oblique; *D,* apical; *E,* interradicular; *F,* transseptal.

■ **What is the function of each of the periodontal ligament fiber groups?**

Alveolar crest: counterbalances lateral occlusal forces (Fig. 11-2, *A*)

Horizontal: prevents lateral movement of tooth (Fig. 11-2, *B*)

Oblique: anchors and suspends tooth in socket; supports against masticatory forces (Fig. 11-2, *C*)

Apical: prevents tipping of tooth (Fig. 11-2, *D*)

Interradicular: attaches tooth to the bone within furcation areas (Fig. 11-2, *E*)

Transseptal: supports interproximal gingiva and holds adjoining teeth together (Fig. 11-2, *F*)

■ **Describe the location, characteristics, and functions of cementum.**

Cementum is a bonelike substance covering the outer root surface of teeth. There are two basic types of cementum: acellular cementum found in the cervical portion of the root and cellular cementum seen only in the apical part of the root. The main purpose of cementum is to provide attachment of periodontal ligament fibers to the tooth surface.

■ **Where is the alveolar bone (process) located, and what is its purpose?**

The alveolar process extends from the body of the mandible and maxilla and supports the teeth in the jaws.

■ **Describe the component structures of the alveolar bone (process).**

The outer surfaces of alveolar bone are composed of plates of compact cortical bone. Between the plates of cortical bone is a spongy, cancellous bone that is filled with a network of blood vessels, bone marrow, and nerve fibers. The alveolus (socket) is a cavity within the alveolar process to which the root of the tooth is held by the periodontal ligament. The alveolus is lined with thin compact bone called the *lamina dura*.

■ **Describe the causes, clinical signs, and symptoms of each of the following diseases.**

Gingivitis. Gingivitis is an inflammation of the gingiva caused by bacterial plaque and is characterized by swelling, bleeding, loss of stippling, redness, and pain. In chronic gingivitis, the gingiva turns bluish.

Periodontitis. Periodontitis is an inflammatory disease involving the gingiva and bony support of the teeth. Bacterial plaque is the primary cause; however, poorly constructed dental restorations, occlusal trauma, endocrine disturbances, and allergies are considered by some dentists to be contributing factors. Its appearance may resemble that of severe gingivitis with periodontal pockets, loss of supporting bone, and mobility.

Juvenile periodontitis (periodontosis). Juvenile periodontitis is a degenerative, noninflammatory disease of unknown origin, primarily found in 15- to 25-year-old patients. It is characterized by rapid bone loss seen mainly in the first molar and incisor areas.

Pericoronitis. Pericoronitis is an acute inflammatory condition of the tissue surrounding an incompletely erupted tooth. It is most commonly seen in mandibular third molar areas and is characterized by redness, swelling, and intense pain that is exaggerated by touch and that may radiate to the ear, throat, or mouth.

Periodontal abscess. Periodontal abscess is an acute, localized, inflammatory response usually associated with the presence of a periodontal pocket. It is characterized clinically by distention of the tissue over the area and is red to bluish red in color. There is usually a discharge of pus from the pocket or through a fistula.

Occlusal trauma. Occlusal trauma is abnormal stress on teeth that may occur from malpositioned teeth, improper restorations, or habits such as bruxism. It is characterized by pain on occlusion and destruction to the tooth-supporting tissues.

■ **Describe the role of the dental assistant during the evaluative procedures for periodontal disease.**

The dental assistant is responsible for obtaining a complete medical/dental history, charting the findings during the periodontal examination, taking impressions for study casts, and obtaining a complete radiographic survey. The dental assistant may also be required to obtain photographs and nutritional information.

■ **Why is a complete medical/dental health history critical in the diagnosis and treatment of periodontal disease?**

The medical/dental history is important in ascertaining the patient's present health status and whether systemic diseases, medications, allergies, or medical/dental conditions are contributing factors to the present periodontal conditions or would contraindicate specific treatment procedures.

■ **Describe the types of periodontal charting for which the dental assistant may be responsible.**

While the dentist is conducting the periodontal examination, the dental assistant will be responsible for charting all findings such as pocket depth, tooth mobility, recession, occlusion, soft or hard tissue pathology, and patient symptoms. The dental assistant may also be given the responsibility to check that all information regarding treatment has been entered in the patient's chart. In addition to notes on the specific procedure performed and the location in which the procedure was performed, information such as type of anesthetic used, dosage and patient reaction to anesthetic, type and number of sutures, periodontal dressing applied, prescriptions given, and postoperative instructions given to patient should be included.

■ **What basic instruments and equipment are needed for a periodontal examination?**

Essential
  Mouth mirror
  Explorer
  Periodontal probe
  Red/blue pencil
  Patient chart and radiographs
  Bib and chain
  2 × 2 inch gauze
Optional
  Articulating paper
  Cotton pliers
  Study casts
  Curet

■ **What procedures are usually performed during the periodontal examination?**

In addition to the basic dental examination such as identification of caries, missing teeth, and existing restorations, the dentist will measure and assess pocket depths, tooth mobility, recession, malocclusion, oral habits, condition of the gingiva, oral health care problems, furcation involvements, and abscess drainage. The dentist may also want to secure information on the patient's nutritional status.

■ **What are some of the periodontal conditions that can be diagnosed by properly angulated and processed radiographs?**

Resorption of alveolar bone
Vertical and horizontal bone loss
Widening or thinning of the periodontal ligament
Loss of lamina dura
Presence of heavy calculus
Periapical abscess
Hypercementosis
Root resorption or fractures
Caries and state of existing restorations as they relate to periodontal conditions
Degree of attrition
Furcation involvement

■ **Explain why study cast impressions are taken on patients with periodontal diseases.**

Study casts are useful for diagnosing traumatic occlusion, malpositioned teeth, location and extent of gingival recession, and tissue and bone contour.

■ **What benefits can be gained by taking photographs during the periodontal examination, and what precautions must be exercised?**

Photographs are extremely useful to the periodontist in that the actual appearance of the tissues can be observed without the patient being present. They are also used to follow the progress of healing or the degeneration process of periodontal conditions. They are useful as motivation and teaching aids; however, any photograph that shows the patient's full face must have the eye section blocked out, and written permission must be obtained from the patient before using the photograph for teaching purposes. Should it be necessary, photographs may be used for legal evidence.

■ **How might the dietary habits of the patient relate to their periodontal condition, and what is the dental assistant's role in dietary analysis and counseling?**

Although the role of nutrition has not been positively established in relation to periodontal health or disease, this information can be helpful in determining if the patient's diet could be a contributing factor to the periodontal conditions present. For optimum health, the patient's daily diet must include an adequate balance of the four basic food groups. The physical characteristics of the diet and the frequency of eating are also factors in dental health. The dental assistant plays an important role in instructing the patient in how to complete a dietary record, analyzing the dietary record, explaining to the patient where dietary problem areas are and how they can be corrected, assisting the patient in determining which foods could be used to replace those with high sugar content, and motivating and educating the patient toward an optimum diet for general health as well as dental health.

■ **What are some of the indications for periondontal treatment?**

The patient is motivated and capable of maintaining good oral hygiene.

A strict program of prevention, nutrition, and oral hygiene has not eliminated the periodontal problem.

The patient is receptive to periodontal treatment.

Generalized pocket depths of 5 mm or more cannot be eliminated by scaling, root planing, and adequate oral hygiene.

All signs and symptoms of periodontal disease are indications for treatment, such as mobility, exudate, bone loss, and presence of inflammation.

■ **What are some of the contraindications for periodontal treatment?**

Hopeless prognosis because of extensive bone loss and/or class III mobility

Patient disinterest and apathy

Systemic problems such as a recent myocardial infarction or uncontrolled diabetes

■ **What does the dental assistant have to know and be able to do to provide effective oral hygiene instructions for periodontal patients?**

The dental assistant must understand:

Human behavior and motivation techniques and be able to apply these to meet the needs of each individual patient

Plaque etiology and appearance

The purpose of plaque disclosing solution and how it is applied

Various toothbrushing methods and which method would be best for each patient

How to develop and operate a plaque control program

Different types and sizes of toothbrushes, different types of dental floss, and other oral health aids that are available to determine the most suitable oral hygiene aids for each patient and help the patient learn to use these aids effectively

■ **What is the purpose of scaling and root planing procedures?**

Scaling and root planing procedures are performed to remove soft and hard deposits from teeth and to attain smooth root surfaces, thus aiding in resolution of inflammation, readaptation of gingiva to the tooth, and maintenance of oral hygiene.

■ **What is the role of the dental assistant during scaling and root planing procedures?**

The dental assistant's most important functions are to maintain:

Clear field of vision

Patient comfort

Instrument exchange

■ **What instruments and equipment are required for scaling and root planing procedures?** (See Fig. 11-3 for description of periodontal instruments.)

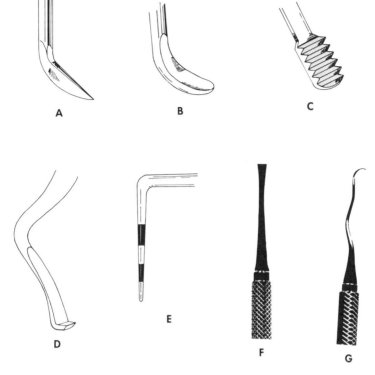

Fig. 11-3. A, Sickle (scaler); **B,** curet; **C,** file; **D,** hoe; **E,** periodontal probe; **F,** periodontal chisel; **G,** Gracey 11/12 curet.

The basic items needed are:
Mouth mirror
Explorer
Cotton pliers
Periodontal probe
Scalers
Curets
Saliva ejector
Evacuation tip
2 × 2 inch gauze
In addition to these items the dentist or dental hygienist may use:
Periodontal files
Periodontal hoes
Periodontal chisels
Local anesthetic setup

■ **What are some of the objectives of periodontal surgical procedures?**

Reduce or eliminate pocket depths
Reduce chronic inflammation
Improve gingival color, contour, and tone
Provide access for adequate plaque control
Finalize root planing
Facilitate regeneration of the attachment apparatus

■ **What is accomplished during a soft tissue curettage surgical procedure?**

The diseased epithelial lining of a periodontal pocket is removed, thus enhancing connective tissue attachment.

■ **What instruments and equipment may be included in a soft tissue curettage setup?**

Local anesthetic setup
Curets
Mouth mirror
Sterile 2 × 2 inch gauze
Evacuation tip
Sutures and/or periodontal dressings if indicated

■ **What are the steps in a periodontal flap procedure?**

Gingival tissue incised and reflected back
Curettage of remaining diseased soft tissue
Definitive scaling and root planing
Osseous contouring if indicated
Flap returned to desired position and sutured for stabilization
Periodontal dressing applied

■ **What instruments and equipment may be included in a periodontal flap procedure setup?**

Local anesthetic setup
Mouth mirror
Scalpel and blade
Curets
Periosteal elevators
Bone contouring burs
Evacuation tip
Sterile 2 × 2 inch gauze
Suture and needle sutures
Hemostat or suture needle holder
Suture scissors
Surgical scissors
Cotton pliers
Periodontal dressings
Periodontal probe

■ **What is the difference between a gingivoplasty and a gingivectomy surgical procedure?**

Gingivoplasty is the reshaping of the gingival tissue, but it is not necessarily performed to eliminate periodontal pockets. Gingivectomy is the resectioning or excision of tissue to eliminate periodontal pockets and to recontour the remaining gingiva. Both procedures are performed to provide optimum accessibility for patient oral health maintenance.

■ **What instruments and equipment may be included in a gingivectomy procedure setup?**

Local anesthetic setup
Mouth mirror
Periodontal probe
Cotton pliers
Pocket marker
Curets

Periodontal surgical knives and instruments
Scalpel and blade
Surgical hoe
Surgical scissors
Diamond stone
Evacuation tip
Sterile 2 × 2 inch gauze
Periodontal dressings

■ **What instruments and equipment may be included in a setup for a gingivoplasty procedure?**

Local anesthetic setup
Mouth mirror
Periodontal probe
Curets
Diamond stone
Evacuation tip
Sterile 2 × 2 inch gauze
Periodontal dressing

■ **What is the difference between a frenectomy and a frenotomy surgical procedure?**

A frenectomy is complete removal of a frenum, whereas a frenotomy is partial removal or severing and relocation of a frenum.

■ **What instruments and equipment may be included in a setup for frenum surgery?**

Local anesthetic setup
Mouth mirror
Surgical scissors
Suture holder, suture needle, and sutures for frenum relocation
Scalpel and blade
Hemostat
Evacuation tip
Periodontal dressings

■ **What types of surgical procedures are used to correct osseous (bony) defects?**

Osteoplasty: the reshaping of the bone with burs or diamond stone
Ostectomy: the removal and reshaping of supporting bone
Osteotomy: the removal of unsupporting bone
Bone implant: the use of an implant to fill bony defects

Root amputation: removal of one or more tooth roots

Hemisection: the sectioning in half of the tooth crown and root

■ **What is the purpose of periodontal splinting, and what types of splints are used?**

Splinting is used for temporary or permanent stabilization of mobile teeth. Temporary splints may be constructed of wire, acrylic, or etch-on composites; permanent splints are usually gold castings.

■ **What is the best procedure for providing postoperative instructions?**

The best procedure is to:

Provide the patient with complete printed instructions.

Go over each printed instruction with the patient and provide a rationale for why each must be done.

Demonstrate any procedure the patient may be required to do.

Ask questions to determine patient understanding of instructions.

Provide emergency telephone numbers that the patient can use after office hours.

■ **What is involved in periodontal maintenance procedures?**

Recall system. An effective recall system is crucial in providing continuing care at the appropriate intervals for each patient.

Reevaluation examination and charting. The dentist reexamines soft tissue for tone, color, and contour; pocket depths, recession, and mobility are remeasured; and bleeding points, exudate, and presence of plaque are noted. All these are written in the patient's chart for comparison with previous findings. Based on the findings in the reevaluation examination, a treatment plan is developed to meet the patient's needs.

Follow-up treatment. Follow-up treatment may include oral health care instructions, scaling, root planing, soft tissue curettage, or any surgical procedure necessary to provide for the optimum oral health of the patient.

ACKNOWLEDGMENT

We wish to thank Dr. Klaus D. Wolfram for his technical assistance in preparing this chapter.

MULTIPLE-CHOICE QUESTIONS

For questions 1 to 15, mark
a if the correct answer is **A** only
b if the correct answer is **B** only
c if the correct answer is both **A** and **B**
d if neither **A** nor **B** is the correct answer

    A. Periodontitis
    B. Juvenile periodontitis (periodontosis)

_____ **1.** Is an inflammatory disease
_____ **2.** Characterized by bone loss
_____ **3.** Caused by bacterial plaque
_____ **4.** Found mainly around incompletely erupted teeth
_____ **5.** Is of unknown origin

    A. Gingivoplasty
    B. Gingivectomy

_____ **6.** The reshaping of gingival tissue
_____ **7.** Done primarily to eliminate periodontal pockets
_____ **8.** The recontouring of bone
_____ **9.** A procedure in which a pocket marker is used
_____ **10.** A periodontal flap involved

A. Radiographs
B. Study casts

_____11. Used to determine bone loss
_____12. Used to determine tooth mobility
_____13. Shows level of recession
_____14. Shows widening and/or loss of periodontal ligament
_____15. Shows the lamina dura

For questions 16 to 32, mark
   a if **1, 2,** and **3** are the correct answers
   b if **1** and **3** are the correct answers
   c if **2** and **4** are the correct answers
   d if **4** only is the correct answer
   e if all the answers are correct

_____ 16. Which of the following are functions of periodontal ligament fibers?
1. Anchor and suspend teeth in sockets
2. Stabilize alveolar bone
3. Attach teeth to the bones within furcation areas
4. Control inflammatory process

_____ 17. Which of the following are part of the free gingiva?
1. Mucogingival junction
2. Gingival groove
3. Alveolar mucosa
4. Gingival margin

_____ 18. Which of the following comprise the periodontium?
1. Gingiva
2. Alveolar bone
3. Cementum
4. Enamel

_____ 19. The clinical signs of gingivitis include:
1. Swelling
2. Redness
3. Pain
4. Bone loss

_____ 20. Which of the following are types of surgical procedures used to correct osseous (bony) defects?
1. Osteoplasty
2. Ostectomy
3. Root amputation
4. Hemisection

_____ 21. Periodontal maintenance procedures include:
1. A recall system

2. Scaling and root planing
3. Reevaluation examination
4. Charting

_____ 22. Which of the following are component structures of the alveolar process?
1. Cortical bone
2. Cancellous bone
3. Alveolus
4. Periodontal ligament

To answer questions 23 to 28 refer to the following treatment plan sequence.

Appointment number	Treatment planned	Tooth number	Units required
1	Periodontal examination, radiographs, study casts		6
2	Consultation		2
3	Oral hygiene instruction No 1		2
4	Oral hygiene instruction No 2, scale, and root plane	1 to 8 25 to 32	6
5	Oral hygiene instruction No 3, scale, and root plane	9 to 16 17 to 24	6
6	Soft tissue curettage	22 to 27	2
7	Periodontal flap	13 to 15	3
8	Remove sutures		1
9	Reevaluation examination		3

_____ 23. What are the dental assistant's duties during the first appointment?
1. Pocket depth measurement
2. Tissue retraction
3. Postoperative instructions
4. Charting

_____ 24. What instruments and equipment are necessary for appointment 4?
1. Curets
2. Scalpel and blade
3. Evacuation tip
4. Periosteal elevator

_____ 25. What will be accomplished during appointment 6?
1. Recontour gingiva
2. Treatment charting
3. Remove periodontal pockets
4. Remove diseased epithelium

_____ 26. The setup for appointment 7 will include:
1. Periosteal elevator
2. Scalpel and blade
3. Sutures
4. Curets

_____ 27. What is the dental assistant's role during appointment 7?
1. Postoperative instructions
2. Tissue retraction
3. Oral evacuation
4. Suture removal

_____ 28. What is the dental assistant's role during appointment 9?
1. Chart mobility
2. Measure pocket depth
3. Maintain clear field of vision
4. Determine bleeding points

To answer questions 29 to 31 refer to the patient treatment record in column 1.

_____ 29. What information is missing from the 10-15-77 entry?
1. Toothbrushing method
2. Type of toothbrush
3. Type of floss
4. Type of fluoride solution

_____ 30. What information is missing from the 10-29-77 entry?
1. Number of sutures
2. Type of anesthetic
3. Length of procedure
4. Area involved

_____ 31. For legal purposes, what additional information should be included on the 11-24-77 entry?
1. Number and type of sutures
2. Postoperative instructions
3. Type of anesthetic
4. Type of medication prescribed and the instructions given to patient for taking medication

_____ 32. Which *one* group of the following groups of instruments would be used during a soft tissue curettage procedure?
1. Mouth mirror, periosteal elevator, curet
2. Explorer, scalpel, evacuation tip
3. Scalpel, anesthetic syringe, diamond stone
4. Anesthetic syringe, evacuation tip, curet

SUGGESTED READINGS

Peterson, S., editor: The dentist and the assistant, ed. 4, St. Louis, 1977, The C. V. Mosby Co.

Richardson, R. E., and Barton, R. E.: The dental assistant, ed. 5, New York, 1978, McGraw-Hill Book Co.

Stone, S., and Kalis, P. J.: Dental auxiliary practice, module 6, Periodontics, Baltimore, 1975, The Williams & Wilkins Co.

Torres, H. O., and Ehrlich, A.: Modern dental assisting, Philadelphia, 1976, W. B. Saunders Co.

Wilkins, E. M.: Clinical practice of the dental hygienist, ed. 4, Philadelphia, 1976, Lea & Febiger.

Date	Tooth number	Treatment completed	Fee
10-4-77		Complete periodontal examination, periapical and bite-wing radiographs, impressions for study casts	
10-11-77		Consultation	
10-15-77		Oral health instruction No 1: toothbrushing and flossing demonstrated	
10-22-77	1 to 8 and 25 to 32	Flossing and brushing lower anterior area redemonstrated Scaled and root planed	
10-29-77		Evaluated oral hygiene, demonstrated Perioaid, scaled and root planed, anesthetic administered	
11-10-77	22 to 27	Soft tissue curettage	
11-24-77	13 to 15	Periodontal flap, sutures, anesthetic administered, medication prescribed for pain	

CHAPTER 12

Prosthodontics

JANICE A. SCHWEITZER

■ **What is prosthodontics?**

Prosthodontics is that branch of dentistry that deals with the replacement of missing teeth and surrounding oral tissues.

■ **What are the two types of prosthodontics?**

The two types of prosthodontics are *fixed prosthodontics* that include crown and bridge procedures and *removable prosthodontics* that are complete and partial denture procedures.

■ **What is a bridge?**

A bridge is the name for the replacement of missing teeth, and it is attached permanently by cementation to the teeth on either side of the space being filled.

■ **What are the two major components of a bridge?**

The retainers or crowns and the pontics, which are the replacement teeth, are the two major parts of a bridge.

■ **How are the retainers and pontics joined together?**

The retainers and pontics are connected by a solder joint.

■ **What are the teeth called to which the retainer is cemented?**

These teeth are known as the abutment teeth.

■ **What are the advantages of placing a fixed bridge rather than leaving the space in the oral cavity?**

Replacement of missing teeth prevents drifting of the remaining teeth, prevents elongation of the opposing teeth, replaces the patient's ability to masticate his food properly, reduces the possibility of periodontal disease in the area, and is esthetically pleasing.

■ **What are the materials most commonly used in the construction of a fixed bridge?**

The material most commonly used is gold alloy. A nonprecious metal can also be used for the retainers. The material for a pontic may be plastic or porcelain with a metal backing, or the pontic may be cast in gold with the retainer.

■ **Why is an opposing model made at the time of the impression for a bridge?**

A model of the opposing teeth is necessary to fabricate the occlusal portion of the prosthesis. This model will provide articulation by determining how the opposing teeth contact in closed position and in lateral and protrusive movements.

■ **What is an articulator?**

An articulator is a mechanical device that represents the temporomandibular joint and arches to which maxillary and mandibular casts may be attached (Fig. 12-1).

■ **What is the most critical step in placing a fixed bridge?**

Cementation is the most critical aspect of placing a fixed bridge because that is when the final seating of the bridge is made. Contamination by saliva or any other alien material can be responsible for cutting the life span of the bridge.

■ **What is a complete denture?**

A complete denture is a dental prosthesis that

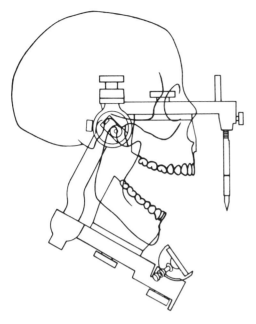

Fig. 12-1. An articulator simulating jaw movement. (Courtesy TeleDyne Hanau, Buffalo.)

is a substitute for the lost dentition and associated structures of the maxilla or mandible.

■ **What is an immediate denture?**

An immediate denture is a prosthesis that is placed when the last six anterior teeth are extracted. The advantage of an immediate denture is that the patient does not have to go without teeth. Another consideration is that the bandagelike effect of the denture prevents excessive bleeding, presents tongue restriction following the extractions, helps to retain the firmness of the lips and cheeks, and eliminates, to a great degree, the muscle fatigue that follows full arch extractions. One other advantage is that the immediate denture improves the mental attitude of the patient.

■ **What is an overdenture?**

An overdenture is a denture that has been constructed over several remaining roots that have been kept to serve as stops for the denture. Periodontal status, endodontic potential, caries status, and tooth position are the four criteria to be considered when abutment teeth are selected for this procedure.

■ **What are the advantages of an overdenture in comparison to a regular denture?**

The advantages of an overdenture are that (1) stress normally absorbed by the mucous membrane and alveolar ridge is reduced by the presence of the roots that act as stops, (2) the roots also serve as a retentive factor for the denture, and (3) the patient, although wearing a denture, is not completely edentulous.

■ **What are the indications for an overdenture?**

The factors that contribute to constructing an overdenture are (1) the condition of the alveolar ridge and mucosa (flat and flabby); (2) the opposing dentition, especially if this includes natural teeth; (3) the patient wishes to retain the natural teeth, but any other type of reconstruction process would prove ineffective; and (4) the patient has grinding or bruxing habits that will cause trauma to the ridge and tissues.

■ **What impression material is used for primary denture impressions?**

Alginate with a perforated tray or compound in an edentulous tray, if the ridges are extremely flat, are the two most frequently used materials for primary denture impressions.

■ **What are the advantages of taking a primary and secondary impression when constructing complete dentures?**

The secondary impression is taken using a custom-made acrylic tray that is border-molded or muscle-trimmed at the chair with impression compound. It is much more accurate than an alginate or compound primary impression taken in a stock tray. When the impression material is inserted in the acrylic tray, more control is kept over the amount of pressure exerted and subsequent displacement of the tissue.

■ **What is vertical dimension?**

Vertical dimension is the distance between the upper and lower jaws when the lower jaw is at rest.

■ **How is vertical dimension marked by the operator?**

Vertical dimension is marked by placing a small dot on the nose and chin. A ruler is used to connect the dots and measure the distance between them.

■ **What vertical dimension measurements are taken?**

The vertical dimensions taken are the rest and the occlusal measurements.

■ **What is the position of the mouth when the rest and occlusal vertical dimensions are taken?**

The rest vertical dimension is just that, when the jaws are at rest following a swallowing action. The occlusal vertical dimension is taken when the occlusal rims waxed on baseplates or teeth set in wax are seated. At this point the mouth is also in centric occlusion.

■ **What are the results of reduced vertical dimension?**

Creases and drooping of the corners of the mouth, puffy or flabby appearance because of loss of muscle tone, and change in proportion to the size of the head result from reduced vertical dimension.

■ **What are the functions of wax occlusal rims on baseplates in denture construction?**

The wax rims are used for numerous measurements in denture construction. The midline, the lip line, the corners of the mouth, the occlusal plane, and the vertical dimension are all measured using the wax rims with adjustment of and marking the same. The wax rim is also used to seat the face-bow for articulation of the casts.

■ **What is a face-bow?**

The face-bow is a caliper-like device that is used to record the relationship of the maxillae and mandible to the temporomandibular joint and to orient the casts in this same relationship to the opening axis of the articulator (Fig. 12-2).

■ **What are occlusion, centric relation, and protrusive relation?**

Occlusion is the relationship between the opposing surfaces of upper and lower teeth when they are in contact either in the mouth or on an articulator. *Centric relation* is the most posterior relation of the mandible to the maxilla at the established vertical dimension. *Protrusive relation* is the relation of the upper and lower teeth when the mandible is brought forward with the anterior teeth edge to edge.

■ **What three points form the plane of occlusion?**

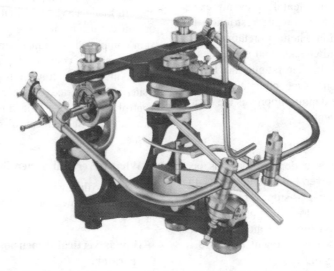

Fig. 12-2. Face-bow in relation to articulator. (Courtesy TeleDyne Hanau, Buffalo.)

The distobuccal cusps of the last molar bilaterally and the incisal edges of the anterior teeth form the plane of occlusion.

■ **Why are occlusal adjustments necessary?**

The following are the reasons for occlusal adjustments:

To protect the periodontal structures
To eliminate local trauma
To treat temporomandibular joint problems
To treat bruxism
To act as a prelude to reconstructive dentistry
To eliminate muscle spasm
To increase chewing efficiency
To promote bilateral chewing

■ **The dental assistant's contact with denture teeth most often involves ordering the teeth and cataloging them on arrival. How do the letters and numbers on the plastic cards identify the attached denture teeth?**

Each anterior mold number consists of a first number, a second number, and a letter. The first number on the card describes the classification or form of the tooth as follows: square, square tapering, square ovoid, tapering, tapering ovoid, ovoid, or square tapering ovoid. The second number on the card describes the proportion of the tooth—long, medium, or short—in relation to its width and/or whether the labial surface is straight or curved from gingival to incisal aspect. The letter on the card describes the width of the six anterior teeth on the

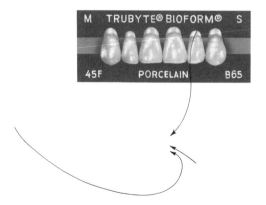

Fig. 12-3. Mold numbering system. (Courtesy Dentsply International, York, Pa.)

curve from canine to canine. Posterior teeth come in several molds, also anatomic, semi-anatomic, and mechanical or flat plane. Within each grouping is a degree used to determine the amount of chewing ability and cusp height (Fig. 12-3).

■ **Identify the differences between plastic and porcelain denture teeth.**

Porcelain anterior denture teeth are distinguished by their gold-covered pins projecting from the lingual surface. Pins provide a mechanical means of retention for porcelain teeth to the acrylic denture base. Porcelain posterior teeth have a "diatoric hole" that is molded into the ridge lap. "Vent holes" are also present that provide an escape for air as the denture base material flows into the diator hole. The only distinguishing mark on the plastic teeth is a small dot that appears on the lingual aspect of the posterior teeth (Fig. 12-4).

■ **What references are used in denture tooth selection?**

The most popular reference is old photographs, since patients wish to retain the image and individuality of their younger selves. Also age and sex of the patient and shape of the face determine the shape and shade of the teeth to be used.

■ **What are the advantages of acrylic resin teeth in denture construction?**

The plastic or acrylic resin teeth do not break as easily as porcelain teeth. They are easier to adjust to fit a particular denture case, and they bond well with the denture base material.

■ **What is meant by the term "milling-in" in reference to denture construction?**

Milling-in is the procedure of refining or perfecting the occlusion of teeth by the use of abrasives, while occluding surfaces are rubbed together either on the articulator or in the mouth.

■ **Why is milling-in necessary?**

Milling-in is necessary following the curing of the denture base material. This material has a tendency to warp in processing, and as a result the placement of the teeth may be altered.

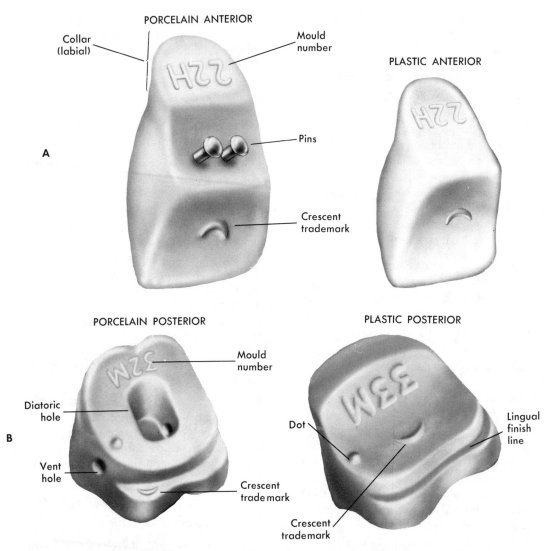

Fig. 12-4. Differences between plastic and porcelain tooth nomenclature. **A**, Anterior; **B**, posterior. (Courtesy Dentsply International, York, Pa.)

■ **In what position should the patient be seated for all impressions and face-bow registrations?**

The patient should *always* be seated in the upright position for impression taking. This is done to eliminate choking on the impression material. This same position is required for face-bow recording to reduce strain on the operator.

■ **What is the difference between relining a denture and rebasing a denture?**

Relining is actually the resurfacing of a denture base with new and additional material so that it will fit the alveolar bone more accurately. Rebasing goes beyond relining in that refitting of the denture base is done without changing the occlusal relationship of the teeth.

■ **List the instructions that should be given to patients regarding home care when they receive their first denture.**

Remove dentures at night to rest the tissues, and place them in water to prevent warping.

Rinse dentures after each meal.

When the denture is out of the mouth, handle it with care.

Avoid the use of powders to maintain denture stability.

Chew on both sides of the mouth at once.

Use the tongue as a stop to retain the lower denture.

Speak slowly and swallow often because of excess saliva caused by the new denture.

Read aloud to oneself to improve speech.

■ What is a partial denture?

A partial denture is a dental prosthesis that restores one or more, but less than all, of the natural teeth and/or associated parts and that is supported by the teeth and/or mucosa.

■ What are the components of a removable partial denture?

The parts of a partial denture are the rests, major connector, minor connector, retainers, base, and teeth.

■ What is meant by "surveying" in relation to dentistry?

Surveying is the procedure of locating and outlining the contour and position of abutment teeth and associated structures on the master cast before designing a removable partial denture. The purpose of surveying is to determine the most favorable path of insertion for the partial denture and to mark survey lines on the teeth to aid in the development of a suitable design for the metal framework.

■ What is the simple way of marking interferences when making a trial insertion of a partial framework?

The use of correction fluids or pastes painted on the underside of the frame and inserted on a dry field make high spots easy to detect.

■ What are the qualities of a good partial denture?

A good partial denture is stable, has good retention, and is esthetically pleasing.

■ How is direct retention of a removable partial denture obtained?

Direct retention of a partial denture is obtained with the attachments and clasps that are designed and built as part of the metal framework.

■ What are the disadvantages of a clasp partial denture?

The greatest disadvantage of a clasp partial denture is the possibility of caries developing on the tooth under the clasp. This is followed closely by the amount of strain which is put on the abutment teeth that may result in their mobility. Last, but not least, is the esthetics of the clasps showing on the facial surfaces of the teeth.

■ Why does the oral mucosa sometimes react to the metal of a removable partial denture?

The oral mucosa sometimes reacts unfavorably to a partial denture framework because of the great amount of pressure that is sometimes applied to the tissue as a result of the lack of support from the abutment teeth. The length of time that the partial is worn and the oral hygiene habits of the patient play a vital part in the continued oral health of the patient.

MULTIPLE-CHOICE QUESTIONS

1. The part of the bridge that is connected to the teeth is the:
   a. Abutment
   b. Retainer
   c. Both of the above
2. The greatest advantage of placing a fixed bridge rather than constructing a removable partial denture is:
   a. Kindness to the remaining teeth and oral mucosa
   b. Convenience to the patient
   c. Cost

3. The instrument that simulates jaw movement is:
   a. Face-bow
   b. Surveyor
   c. Articulator
4. A denture that is worn immediately after the extraction of the teeth is:
   a. Transitional
   b. Complete
   c. Immediate
5. When the mandible is brought forward, the teeth are in:
   a. Centric occlusion
   b. Protrusive relation
   c. Centric relation
6. The purpose of relining a denture is to:
   a. Adapt the denture to the alveolar bone more accurately
   b. Change the centric occlusion
   c. Alter the vertical dimensions
   d. Provide a bite registration
7. A face-bow is used to:
   a. Determine facial contour
   b. Articulate the bite rims
   c. Orient the patient to wearing dentures
   d. Record the relationship of the maxilla and mandible to the temporomandibular joint
8. The portion of a mandibular partial denture that rests on the ridge is referred to as the:
   a. Hamulus
   b. Saddle
   c. Connector
   d. Flange

9. Stippling refers to the:
   a. Tissue surface of a denture
   b. Milling-in of occlusion
   c. Simulated pits in the artificial gingiva
   d. Correcting of abnormal vertical dimension
10. Which of the following are markings found on porcelain anterior teeth:
   a. Vent hole
   b. Pins
   c. Diatoric hole

SUGGESTED READINGS

Castano, F. A.: Handbook of expanded dental auxiliary practice, Philadelphia, 1973, J. B. Lippincott Co.

Heartwell, C. M., Jr., and Rahn, A. O.: Syllabus of complete dentures, ed. 2, Philadelphia, 1975, Lea & Febiger.

Henderson, D., and Steffel, V. L.: McCracken's removable partial prosthodontics, ed. 4, St. Louis, 1973, The C. V. Mosby Co.

Instruments and equipment for better dentistry, Buffalo, 1978, Teledyne Hanau.

Johnston, J. F., Phillips, R. W., and Dykema, R. W.: Modern practice in crown and bridge prosthodontics, ed. 3, Philadelphia, 1971, W. B. Saunders Co.

Knop, F.: Occlusion, Milwaukee, 1972.

Simon, W. J.: Clinical dental assisting, New York, 1973, Harper & Row, Publishers, Inc.

Torres, H. O., and Ehrlich, A.: Modern dental assisting, Philadelphia, 1976, W. B. Saunders Co.

The trubyte primer, York, Pa., 1974, Dentsply International.

CHAPTER 13

Community dentistry

MARSHA N. MEYER and JUDITH A. McKAY

■ **Define dental public health.**

Dental public health is one part of total health planning. It is designed to promote, maintain, and improve the oral status of individuals or communities. These goals are accomplished through services that are organized, administered, or financed by governmental organizations or community groups.

■ **What is the concept of preventive dentistry?**

The concept of preventive dentistry is to avoid the occurrence of dental disease by educating the patient and by using recognized procedures and treatments. For example, caries control may be achieved by (1) the use of pit and fissure sealants, (2) fluoride treatments, and (3) nutritional counseling.

■ **What is the World Health Organization, and what is its significance in public health?**

The World Health Organization (WHO) is a special agency formed by the United Nations in 1948. It is designed to assist nations in solving health problems. WHO defines health as a state of complete physical, mental, and social well-being and not merely as the absence of disease and infirmity. Some services provided by WHO for member nations are helping countries find solutions to environmental problems, providing technical aid, providing teachers and teacher training, aiding research, and standardizing nomenclature.

■ **List three levels of public health in the United States.**

National. At the national level public health involves formulating and supervising health programs and funding state and local programs. The U.S. Department of Health, Education and Welfare is an example of an organization that functions on the national level.

State. The state acts in an advisory capacity to local departments and provides some direct services such as those of state hospitals. The state also assists in funding programs.

Local. At the local level direct services are offered to the public. The U.S. Office of Economic Opportunity authorizes the establishment of neighborhood health clinics (venereal disease, prenatal, visiting nurses, etc.), dental clinics, and public education.

■ **What are the responsibilities of the U.S. Department of Health, Education and Welfare?**

The U.S. Department of Health, Education and Welfare (HEW) contains many agencies such as the Bureau of Education, Social Security, Food and Drug Administration, Welfare Administration, Office of Economic Opportunity, etc. The department's concern is to formulate and enforce national policies in health, education, and welfare.

■ **What role has the U.S. Department of Health, Education and Welfare played in dental public health?**

Federal health legislation has provided that dentistry participate in intensified efforts to extend and improve the quality of the nation's overall public health. The Health Professions Education Act, which was enacted in 1963, has provided funds for the following:

Construction of new dental schools
Expansion of existing dental schools

Increase in enrollment and expansion of curricula

The addition of new teaching facilities for training the dentist, hygienist, assistant, and technician

Student loans

Expansion of research at dental colleges

■ **Have dental schools been the only facilities to receive federal aid for dental public health?**

Many universities, colleges, and junior colleges were granted federal assistance to improve the training of hygienists, assistants, and laboratory technicians. Apprenticeships in dental public health and residencies in preventive dentistry have also been provided with federal assistance.

■ **What are the U.S. Public Health Service and the National Institutes of Health?**

Although these two organizations are very similar, the National Institutes of Health (NIH) is mainly involved with research and the training of specialized personnel. The U.S. Public Health Service (USPHS), however, is concerned with the administration of national and international health problems and determines health policies for the United States. The USPHS also operates the Indian Health Service and provides research grants to institutions.

■ **What has the USPHS done to encourage the use of dental auxiliary personnel?**

As long as 30 years ago, the USPHS was promoting the efficient use of auxiliary personnel. This organization realized that existing dental schools probably would not produce enough graduates to meet an increased demand for dental services. The solution proposed was twofold:

Increase the number of dentists by expanding existing dental schools and building new ones

Increase the dentist's productivity through the effective and efficient use of dental auxiliaries

■ **What is meant by Dental Auxiliary Utilization and Training in Expanded Auxiliary Management?**

In 1960 the Division of Dental Health of the USPHS provided training grants to all dental schools for the purpose of creating programs in Dental Auxiliary Utilization (DAU). These programs were designed to increase the dentist's productivity by training the dental student to effectively utilize an educated dental assistant. The dental students would work with this dental assistant while performing the various procedures common to the daily general practice. All procedures were carefully planned and simplified to allow for maximum use of time and energy. DAU funding was phased out in 1972 and was replaced with the new Training in Expanded Auxiliary Management (TEAM) grant.

The TEAM grant's objective is to train dental students in the organization and management of a dental practice that uses a "team" for the delivery of dental health care.

Properly trained auxiliaries can perform many tasks previously left to the dentist. The patient receives the same quality of dental care, and the dentist has more time available for nonroutine procedures.

■ **What is the National Institute of Dental Research?**

The National Institute of Dental Research (NIDR), which is located at the NIH, was established in 1948 to initiate a program against oral disease. It is involved in:

Dental prevention through advancing disease control methods such as the fluoridation of community water supplies

Dental care through programs such as Head Start, Job Corps, and Volunteers in Service to America (VISTA)

Dental economics by helping in the design and operation of prepaid dental care programs

■ **What is a health maintenance organization?**

A health maintenance organization (HMO) is an alternative method of health care delivery that provides health care on a fixed prepaid basis. Eligibility is available for a specific enrolled membership.

■ **What is the function of a professional standards review organization?**

Professional standards review organizations (PSRO) function as peer groups to evaluate the quality and efficiency of care and treatment that is rendered in an HMO.

■ **What do the abbreviations "DMF" and "OHI" stand for?**

DMF expresses the accumulated dental caries in permanent teeth. D represents the number of decayed teeth; M the number of missing teeth; and F the number of filled teeth. OHI is a plaque index and is computed into a percentage as follows:

Oral hygiene index score (percent) =
$$\frac{\text{Number of teeth with plaque}}{\text{Total number of teeth}} \times 100$$

Both of these indices are used for comparison studies in public health programs.

■ **Define epidemiology.**

Epidemiology is the science dealing with factors that determine the frequency and distribution of disease in a community. When this is applied to dentistry, epidemiology could refer to a study of the incidence of caries in a given group of people in relationship to the components of their water supply.

■ **In what areas may the dental assistant be of service in the public health field?**

The dental assistant may be employed in school dental clinics.

The dental assistant may conduct educational seminars and programs and participate in Children's Dental Health Week.

The dental assistant may provide preventive treatment such as the topical application of fluoride and pit and fissure sealants if legally allowable.

■ **What is fluoride?**

Fluoride is an active chemical element known to make teeth less vulnerable to dental decay. In a compound, fluoride makes the tooth resistant to demineralization by bacterial acid when the fluoride is incorporated into the crystal structure of enamel.

■ **Give a brief history of the use of fluoride in dentistry.**

In the early 1900s a dentist in Colorado Springs observed that certain area residents had a remarkable freedom from tooth decay but that the enamel of their teeth had a brownish stained appearance. It was discovered that the water consumed by these residents contained more fluoride than did most water supplies. After experimentation with different concentrations of fluoride, it was established that a lower level of fluoride in the water would lower the incidence of tooth decay without staining or pitting the tooth enamel.

■ **Define ppm as it relates to the concentration of fluoride in a water supply.**

The amount of fluoride in relationship to the water supply is expressed as parts per million (ppm). The optimum amount of fluoride concentration is one part fluoride in one million parts of water or 1.0 ppm.

■ **List three forms in which fluoride can be used.**

Topical application. Fluoride is applied directly to the enamel surface. For optimum caries control this should be done once every 6 months. Commonly used types are

2% sodium fluoride. This type of fluoride is 40% effective, has a pleasant taste, does not discolor teeth, and is nonirritating to dental tissue. One disadvantage is that four appointments are needed to apply it.

8% stannous fluoride. Stannous fluoride is available in mouth rinse, gel, and/or liquid. It may be applied at a 6-month recall appointment. Disadvantages of this type are that it may mask caries on radiographs, it may cause discoloration of teeth, it has an unpleasant taste, and it may cause vomiting. Its effectiveness varies from 0% to 87%.

1.23% acidulated phosphofluoride. Acidulated phosphofluoride is available in a gel that can be painted on or used in trays, may be applied at the 6-month recall appointment, has an acceptable taste, is 35% to 45% effective, and does not cause discoloration. The only disadvantage is that it is stable only in plastic containers.

Dentifrice. This is only a supplement to routine topical fluoride applications.

Systemic. This consists of fluoridated water systems or fluoride tablets. Prior to prescription of fluoride tablets the water supply should be tested for natural fluoride content. Studies have shown that there is approximately a 60% reduction of caries if the optimum amount of fluoride is ingested during the age of tooth development.

■ **Define fluorosis and mottled enamel.**

Fluorosis is the discoloration of teeth during development caused by high concentrations of fluoride. Mottled enamel is a severe case of fluorosis recognizable by the dark stain and pitted surface of the enamel.

■ **List some side effects of fluoridation.**

Fluorosis
Mottled enamel
Prevention of osteoporosis (a weakening of the bone structure common in the elderly)
Possible prevention of calcification of the aorta (main artery of the body)

MULTIPLE-CHOICE QUESTIONS

1. At what level of public health in the United States are the most direct services offered to the public?
   a. National
   b. State
   c. Local
2. What is the name of the organization formed in 1948 that is designed to assist nations in solving health problems?
   a. National Institutes of Health
   b. World Health Organization
   c. U.S. Department of Health, Education and Welfare
3. Preventive dentistry is mainly concerned with treating existing disease.
   a. True
   b. False
4. Which of the following organizations is concerned with the administration aspects of national and international health problems.
   a. National Institutes of Health
   b. U.S. Public Health Service
5. What is the main objective of dental public health?
   a. To provide free services
   b. To promote oral health
   c. To maintain and improve the community awareness of dental disease
   d. a and b
   e. b and c

6. What is the most effective public health measure to reduce caries?
   a. Public Health Dentistry
   b. Pit and fissure sealants
   c. Fluoridated water supplies
7. The optimum level of fluoride in the water supply is:
   a. 0.7 ppm
   b. 1 ppm
   c. 2 ppm
   d. 10 ppm
8. What condition could be observed in the mouths of patients exposed to an excess of fluoride in their water supply?
   a. Extensive carious lesions
   b. Mottled enamel
   c. Osteoporosis
9. What is the approximate reduction of caries in children who have been exposed to fluoridated water since birth?
   a. 40%
   b. 60%
   c. 80%
10. The Health Professions Education Act provided funds for:
    a. Expansion and construction of dental schools
    b. The establishment of Dental Auxiliary Utilization and Training in Expanded Auxiliary Management programs
    c. Community fluoride programs

11. The agency most instrumental in initiating the fluoridation of water supplies is:
    a. The U.S. Public Health Service
    b. The National Institutes of Health
    c. The National Institute of Dental Research
12. What program teaches dental students to organize and manage a dental practice?
    a. Dental Auxiliary Utilization
    b. Training in Expanded Auxiliary Management

SUGGESTED READINGS

Caldwell, R. C., and Stallard, R. E.: A textbook of preventive dentistry, Philadelphia, 1977, W. B. Saunders Co.

Dental health education, Geneva, Switzerland, 1970, World Health Organization.

Fluoridation facts, 1974, The American Dental Association.

Guthrie, H. A.: Introductory nutrition, ed. 3, St. Louis, 1975, The C. V. Mosby Co.

Hanlon, J. J.: Public health: administration and practice, ed. 6, St. Louis, 1974, The C. V. Mosby Co.

Introduction to dental public health, Washington, D.C., 1964, U.S. Department of Health, Education, and Welfare.

Preventive dentistry and community health, Washington, D.C., 1966, U.S. Department of Health, Education, and Welfare.

Rothstein, T. J.: The dental health team, Philadelphia, 1970, J. B. Lippincott Co.

Stoll, F. A.: Dental health education, ed. 5, Philadelphia, 1977, Lea & Febiger.

Toward a comprehensive health policy for the 1970's, Washington, D.C., 1971, U.S. Department of Health, Education, and Welfare.

Training in expanded auxiliary management, Baltimore, 1976, University of Maryland.

CHAPTER 14

Four-handed dentistry

NANCY A. POLCYN

■ **What is the objective of four-handed dentistry?**

The objectives of four-handed dentistry are three-fold. Four-handed dentistry increases productivity of the dental practice while maintaining a high standard of quality in dental services with minimum fatigue and stress for the dental team.

These objectives can be achieved by use of equipment that allows the dental team to operate in a seated position and by standardizing all aspects of the dental practice.

■ **Explain the concept of operating zones.**

Relative to the patient's face, positions of the operating team and equipment can be stated in terms of positions on the clock. Visualizing the patient's face as a clock, 12 o'clock would be the middle of the forehead and 6 o'clock the chin.

The operating zones for a right-handed operator can be referred to as follows:

Operator's zone	7 to 12 o'clock
Static zone	12 to 2 o'clock
Assistant's zone	2 to 4 o'clock
Transfer zone	4 to 7 o'clock

For a left-handed operator the zones are transposed.

Operator's zone. This zone is used by the operator, and the operator's exact position depends on the quadrant and the surface of the tooth on which the procedure is being performed. The 11 o'clock position is considered universal except for the 8 to 9 o'clock position for the mandibular right quadrant and the 12 o'clock position for the anterior segments.

Static zone. This is reserved for equipment such as the mobile dental unit and the mobile cabinet. Accessory items such as preset tray, medicaments, an amalgamator, etc. would be on or within the cabinet.

Assistant's zone. This area is used by the assistant. The 2 o'clock position is used for procedures on the maxillary arch, and the 3 o'clock position is used for mandibular arch procedures.

Transfer zone. This zone is reserved for the transferring of instruments, medicaments, and restorative materials.

■ **What is the correct seated position for the operator?**

Correct posture of the operator should be considered to minimize fatigue and stress. Correct posture includes the following:

Shoulders and thighs parallel to the floor
Feet flat on the floor
Back straight and well supported
Minimal bending at the neck
Elbows close to the body
Operation at elbow height
Eye distance of 14 to 16 inches between operator and the site of operation

■ **What is the correct seated position for the assistant?**

The assistant's correct seated position should permit the assistant to see the field of operation and have easy access to the mobile cabinet, without causing fatigue or stress. Correct posture for the assistant includes the following:

Legs parallel to the patient's chair and toward the head of the chair
Shoulders and thighs parallel to the floor
Feet flat on foot ring
Back straight

Minimal bending at the neck

A firm stool with abdominal support

Eye level 4 to 6 inches above operator's eye level

Seating position higher for working in the mandibular arch and lower for working in the maxillary arch

■ **What is the correct positioning of the patient?**

Proper positioning of the patient is relative to the correct positioning of the operator. The patient should be comfortably seated in a supine position. The chair should be adjusted so that the patient's head is placed in the operator's lap. For work in the mandibular arch, the chair should be elevated 15 to 30 degrees, whereas for work in the maxillary arch the patient is completely supine with the chair elevated only 0 to 5 degrees.

■ **What are the basic types of instrument grasps?**

There are four basic types of instrument grasps: pen grasp, reverse pen grasp, palm grasp, and palm-thumb grasp.

Pen grasp. This type of instrument grasp is similar to holding a pen or pencil. It consists of the thumb and first finger on the handle with the second finger on the shank of the instrument for stability. The working tip of the instrument is held away from the operator. Examples of instruments for which the pen grasp is appropriate are explorer, excavator, scaler, amalgam condenser, etc.

Reverse pen grasp. This grasp is the same as the pen grasp except that the working tip of the instrument is held toward the operator which causes a slight rotation of the wrist. An example of an instrument for which the reverse pen grasp would be appropriate is the gingival margin trimmer.

Palm grasp. With this grasp the instrument is held in the palm of the hand. Examples of instruments handled with the palm grasp are rubber dam clamp holder, surgical forceps, cotton pliers, trimming knife, anesthetic syringe, etc.

Palm-thumb grasp. The handle or shaft of the instrument is grasped between the palm and four fingers. An example of an instrument handled with a palm-thumb grasp is a chisel.

■ **What are the principles for instrument exchange when working with a right-handed operator?**

Instrument exchange should occur in the area slightly anterior to the patient's chin. The instrument should be placed firmly into the operator's hand, and the instrument bevel or nib should be in the correct position for use. This will enable the operator to maintain correct posture, hand position, and visual activity. The only time it is necessary for the operator to relinquish the finger rest is when the grasp of the new instrument will be different.

When passing an instrument, the assistant positions the instrument between the thumb and forefinger of the left hand. At least three fourths of the instrument should extend beyond the fingertips. When the operator signals to exchange the instrument, the new instrument is held parallel with the instrument to be exchanged. The instrument is retrieved from the operator by the crook of the assistant's little finger or between the third and fourth fingers of the assistant's left hand. For ease of locating instruments during instrument exchange the preset tray should be placed to the extreme lower left side of the mobile cabinet. The instruments should be placed in order of use and returned to the same position.

Although it is the responsibility of the assistant to anticipate the operator's movements and to watch for the signal to begin the transfer, the assistant should be informed well in advance if there is to be a change in the standardized sequence.

When the operator is left-handed, the procedures for instrument exchange are transposed.

■ **What are the basic principles for high-velocity evacuation during high-speed cavity preparation?**

There are five basic principles for high-velocity evacuation:

The suction tip should be held in the assistant's right hand with a "thumb-to-nose" or "reverse palm-thumb" grasp. (The pen grasp is not recommended except for surgical procedures.)

The suction tip should be positioned distally and as close as possible to the tooth being prepared without injuring the soft tissue.

The bevel of the suction tip opening should be held parallel with the buccal or lingual surface of the tooth being prepared.

The edge of the suction tip should be placed even with the occlusal surface of the tooth being prepared.

■ How can retraction of the soft tissues be accomplished effectively?

During operative and surgical procedures retraction is necessary for better visibility, access, and protection of the cheeks, lips, and tongue.

Depending on the area of the mouth, retraction is accomplished by the operator, the assistant, or simultaneously by the operator and the assistant.

Maxillary right quadrant
Operator: retracts right cheek
Assistant: no retraction necessary
Maxillary left quadrant
Operator: no retraction necessary
Assistant: retracts left cheek
Mandibular right quadrant
Operator: retracts right cheek
Assistant: retracts right side of tongue
Mandibular left quadrant
Operator: retracts left side of tongue
Assistant: retracts right cheek

Suggested instruments for retraction are mouth mirrors, aspirating tips, tongue blades, and cheek retractors. Cotton rolls are sufficient for retracting the lips when operating on the anterior quadrants.

■ What is the purpose of preset trays?

The use of preset trays is essential in four-handed dentistry. After determining what instruments are necessary to complete a given procedure, enough preset trays should be duplicated to supply an average work day. Preset trays should be made up for the different procedures such as amalgam restorations, composite restorations, crown and bridge procedures, endodontics, etc. An easy way to identify each procedural tray is by color coding the trays and instruments.

The covered stainless steel or aluminum tray is the ideal tray because the tray and instruments can be autoclaved simultaneously. Stainless steel and plastic uncovered trays are also available. Trays with grooved slots are recommended. These enable the instruments to be placed and kept in the order of use. Grooved car mats may be used as an alternative if the trays do not have the fabricated grooves.

■ What major equipment is necessary for four-handed dentistry?

To carry out the objectives of four-handed dentistry, criteria for equipment selection should be reviewed.

The patient chair should have a thin, narrow back. This allows the dentist to sit closer to the patient. The patient's chair should also be contoured and provide complete body and arm support when the patient is in the supine position. Other considerations for the patient's chair are that it should have a low base and have independently powered back and seat segments. These adjustments should be accessible to both the operator and the assistant.

The operator's and assistant's stool should be completely mobile, with five casters and a broad stable base. The seats should be adequately padded with an adjustable back or front and left side abdominal support. The operator's chair should also have a minimum height of 14 inches. The assistant's chair should ideally have an adjustable foot ring.

The dental cabinet should be mobile and approximately 2 inches below the assistant's elbow. However, fixed cabinetry can be used in a limited capacity, and it also should be 2 inches lower than the assistant's elbow.

A *mobile* dental unit is superior to a *fixed* dental unit in that it can be moved around the chair when the operator is using different clock positions.

MULTIPLE-CHOICE QUESTIONS

1. Which of the following is/are objective(s) of four-handed dentistry?
   a. To increase productivity of the dental practice
   b. To minimize stress and fatigue
   c. To achieve high quality in dental service
   d. All of the above
2. The operating zone for a right-handed operator would be:
   a. 4 to 12 o'clock
   b. 7 to 12 o'clock
   c. 2 to 4 o'clock
   d. 7 to 2 o'clock
3. The static zone is reserved for:
   a. The assistant
   b. Transfer of instruments
   c. The patient
   d. None of the above
4. The operator's eye distance to the site of operation should be:
   a. 14 to 16 inches
   b. 6 to 8 inches
   c. 12 inches
   d. None of the above
5. In relation to the operator's eye level, the assistant should sit:
   a. 4 to 6 inches below eye level
   b. Even with eye level
   c. 4 to 6 inches above eye level
   d. None of the above
6. To reduce fatigue and stress the operating team should sit with:
   a. Back straight
   b. Minimal bending at the neck
   c. Shoulders and thighs parallel to the floor
   d. All of the above
7. Instrument exchange should occur in the area:
   a. Over the patient's left shoulder
   b. Slightly anterior to the patient's chin
   c. Over the patient's right shoulder
   d. Over the patient's stomach
8. When working with a right-handed operator, the assistant exchanges instruments with:

   a. The left hand
   b. The right hand
   c. Both hands
9. An example of a palm grasp instrument is a (an):
   a. Explorer
   b. Anesthetic syringe
   c. Chisel
   d. Gingival margin trimmer
10. When the index finger, thumb, and third finger are used to grasp and support an instrument, the grasp is referred to as:
    a. Reverse pen grasp
    b. Palm-thumb grasp
    c. Pen grasp
    d. Palm grasp
11. When the working tip of the instrument is held toward the operator, the grasp is referred to as:
    a. Reverse pen grasp
    b. Palm-thumb grasp
    c. Pen grasp
    d. Palm grasp
12. An example of a pen grasp instrument is a:
    a. Surgical forceps
    b. Spoon excavator
    c. Rubber dam clamp holder
    d. Scissors
13. For an operative procedure the assistant would hold the high velocity evacuator in the:
    a. Left hand with a pen grasp
    b. Right hand with a pen grasp
    c. Left hand with a reverse palm-thumb grasp
    d. Right hand with a reverse palm-thumb grasp
14. The suction tip should be positioned:
    a. Distal to the tooth being prepared
    b. Mesial to the tooth being prepared
    c. Parallel to the buccal or lingual surface being prepared
    d. Both a and c
15. Retraction of the soft tissues in the mandibular left quadrant is accomplished:
    a. By the assistant retracting the cheek only

b. By the assistant retracting the cheek and tongue
c. By the operator retracting the tongue and the assistant retracting the cheek
d. Without retraction

16. If the procedure is being performed on a maxillary right first molar, the suction tip should be positioned on:
   a. The lingual aspect of the maxillary right quadrant
   b. The buccal aspect of the maxillary right quadrant
   c. Distal to the maxillary right second premolar
   d. a and c
   e. b and c

17. Which instrument can be used for retraction of soft tissue?
   a. Mouth mirror
   b. Suction tip
   c. Tongue blades
   d. All of the above

18. A preset tray should:
   a. Use a color-coded system
   b. Include only a mouth mirror, explorer, and cotton pliers
   c. Be identical in all procedures
   d. None of the above

19. Mobile or fixed dental cabinetry should be _____ the assistant's elbow level.
   a. 5 inches above
   b. The same as
   c. 2 inches below
   d. 5 inches below

20. The preset tray should be located on the mobile cabinet in the:
   a. Upper left corner
   b. Lower left corner
   c. Upper right corner
   d. Lower right corner

SUGGESTED READINGS

Chasteen, J. E.: Four-handed dentistry in clinical practice, St. Louis, 1978, The C. V. Mosby Co.

Robinson, G., McDevitt, E., et al.: Four-handed dentistry manual, Birmingham, Ala., 1971, University of Alabama.

Torres, H., and Ehrlich, A.: Modern dental assisting, Philadelphia, 1976, W. B. Saunders Co.

CHAPTER 15

Expanded functions

JACK ELLIS SHOWLEY

The concept of expanded functions for dental auxiliaries is not new. Auxiliaries have been doing expanded functions since Dr. A. C. Fones delegated oral prophylaxis to his assistant in 1906. State dental practice acts and attitudes within the profession vary. Which functions are considered expanded, which auxiliary should perform expanded functions, how much education (training) should the auxiliary have in order to perform expanded functions, and how many intraoral tasks should be delegated are frequent topics of discussion. The following simple definition will clarify a number of issues. *Any task delegated to an auxiliary that involves an intraoral procedure may be considered an expanded function.* A rational categorization of tasks can be developed with this definition, and the profession may then specify tasks to delegate to each auxiliary according to that auxiliary's educational (training) level. Traditional hygiene tasks, that is, scaling, coronal polishing, and anticariogenic agent application are truly the earliest expanded functions, as is the exposure of radiographs by either the dental assistant or hygienist. These functions are so routinely delegated to auxiliaries that they are now considered traditional in many state practice acts, in educational programs, and in the dental profession.

It is important to realize that expanded function dental auxiliaries (EFDAs) are usually task oriented. It is the responsibility of the dentist to *treat* patients (that is, diagnosis, restorations, etc.) and in so doing use *procedures* (that is, new patient examination, restoration of a tooth) to complete a treatment. A certain *task* (that is, making impressions for study casts, making radiographs, placing a matrix, placing

and carving amalgam, etc.) is a portion of a treatment procedure. With the help of a qualified skilled EFDA the dentist is able to give more time to the critical functions of diagnosis and treatment planning and is able to concentrate on restorative preparation and surgery. The more functions an auxiliary, be it the assistant or hygienist, can legally perform in the dental office, the more valuable the auxiliary is to the profession and that office. The functions delegated must be completed to meet *high standards of performance.* The auxiliary must be required to meet educational criteria and standards of training equal to that of the dentist for each task performed. Just as the Dental Auxiliary Utilization programs had difficulties with definition of role understanding on the part of other members of the dental profession, and facility design in the late 1950s and early 1960s, so it is with the EFDA concept in the 1970s. As the dental profession members and auxiliaries better understand the definition of and rationale for expanded function dental auxiliaries, EFDAs may well become as traditional as present-day assistants and hygienists.

There are intraoral tasks in all categories of dental treatment that may be delegated, but it is impossible to cover all with detailed questions here. Skill tasks that are traditional are covered in other sections of this review, and procedure questions are discussed relative to EFDA skills. Questions relating to impressions for diagnostic study casts cover only that information which pertains to the intraoral impression task and not to pouring and trimming, since these acts are purely assisting or laboratory tasks.

The tasks of diagnosis (preparation of diagnostic aids) and preventive hygiene (scaling, polishing coronal surfaces, and applying topical anticariogenic agents) are some of the earliest expanded functions because of the number of these procedures completed every day in a dental practice. Other categories including restorative treatment, endodontics, prosthodontics, orthodontics, and surgery provide numerous opportunities for task delegation to a competent skilled EFDA. In the future, as needs are established and educational programs are developed, more of these tasks will be presented in EFDA task reveiws.

■ **Describe evaluation categories that can be used in evaluating the results of clinical restorative tasks.**

Specific categories of evaluation provide the evaluator, whether it be the EFDA or the responsible doctor, a method of determining whether criteria have been met in a specific assigned task.

Procedural results are important, since there is no way to evaluate certain tasks other than knowing that a specific order of steps has been completed. For such tasks the statement that the procedure has been completed is sufficient for the evaluator, that is, the application of two thin coats of copal varnish.

For a *measurable result* the evaluator can relate the result to criteria by using a measuring instrument, that is, the margin is submarginal by <0.2 mm.

A *sensory result* can be evaluated by a visual examination, that is, surface is smooth and shiny after polishing, surface has a dull lustre, restorative material has a homogenous color, etc., or by touch, that is, explorer catches on the restoration, to determine compliance with criteria.

■ **What are the three main restorative criteria for all completed restorations?**

All restorations—amalgam, zinc oxide–eugenol, tooth colored, gold, etc.—may be evaluated relative to the following:

With marginal adaptation the restorative material must be flush at the margins, not submarginal, overextended, or open.

Contour is critical because the restoration must approximate the original contour of the healthy tooth. This would include visual discrimination of overcontoured (undercarved) or undercontoured (overcarved) results. Contour evaluation should be modified to meet specific criteria of the tooth anatomic features, such as carving pits and fissures, reestablishing proper approximating contact in the correct area, and development of restored marginal ridge position and shape.

Appearance, texture, and/or color of the restorative material will give the evaluator (EFDA or dentist) an understanding of handling and use of the restorative material.

■ **Define the term "submarginal," and indicate how the operator (EFDA or dentist) may detect the deficiency in the restorative result.**

A restoration that is submarginal has too little restorative material to be flush at the margins. The restorative material is below the cavosurface margin of the prepared cavity. This may be detected by an explorer tip moving from restoration to tooth and catching on the cavosurface margin. A diagram is shown in Fig. 15-1. (A restoration may be improvable if it is submarginal [<0.2 mm].)

■ **Define the term "overextension," and indicate how the operator (EFDA or dentist) may detect this deficiency.**

Overextension is an excess of restorative ma-

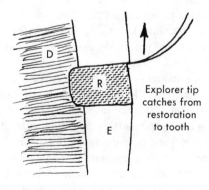

Fig. 15-1. Submarginal restoration. *D*, Dentin; *R*, restoration; and *E*, enamel.

terial above and/or beyond the cavosurface margin of the cavity preparation. The term *flash* is sometimes used to describe overextension on smooth or pit and fissure areas of the tooth. Overhangs are overextensions of restorative material at the cervical cavosurface margins of a class II restoration. It is important to visualize and remember the outline of all cavity preparations prior to placement of restorative material to help avert overextension. A diagram is provided in Fig. 15-2. A restoration with minimal overextension may be improvable to meet final criteria, depending on the cavity preparation location. Overextension may be detected by moving the tip of the explorer from tooth to restoration. If there is overextension, the tip of the explorer will catch on the restoration.

■ **Define the term "open margin," and indi-cate how the operator (EFDA or dentist) may detect the deficiency in the restorative result.**

Voids may be discovered in the body of restorative material, but a void at the cavosurface margin of the restoration is specifically defined as an *open margin*. It may be detected by moving an explorer tip from restorative material to tooth or tooth to restorative material; the explorer will catch both ways if there is an open margin. Fig. 15-3 depicts an open margin.

■ **Define the term "ditched margin," and in-dicate how the operator (EFDA or dentist) may detect the deficiency in the restora-tion.**

The term *ditched margin* should not be confused with open margin. A ditched margin is a product of time and therefore is a loss of either restorative material or tooth structure because

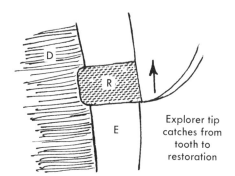

Fig. 15-2. Overextension of restoration. *D*, Dentin; *R*, restoration; and *E*, enamel.

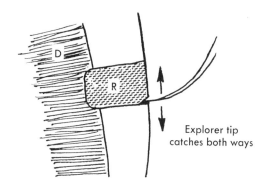

Fig. 15-3. Open margin. *D*, Dentin; and *R*, restoration.

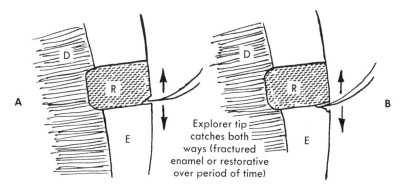

Fig. 15-4. A, Ditched restorative; **B,** Ditched enamel. *D*, Dentin; *R*, restoration; and *E*, enamel.

of wear or breakdown at the margins. It does leave a void at the margin and can be detected in the same manner as an open margin, but a ditched margin deficiency does not involve EFDA procedures (Fig. 15-4, *A* and *B*). An open margin should always be considered unacceptable and the restoration replaced. Replacement of a ditched margin is a diagnostic responsibility of the dentist.

■ **Define the term "overcontoured" (undercarved), and indicate how the operator (EFDA or dentist) may detect this deficiency in the restoration.**

A restoration should approximate the original contour of the healthy tooth. A tooth that is left overcontoured has not been carved or shaped sufficiently to meet this criteria. A visual comparison and evaluation of the final restoration are the principal manners of detection (Fig. 15-5). An overcontoured area of a restoration may be improved to meet final criteria.

■ **Define the term "undercontoured" (overcarved), and indicate how the operator (EFDA or dentist) may detect this deficiency in the restoration.**

An undercontoured restoration has been overcarved or shaped. There is too little remaining restorative material to achieve or meet final contour criteria. An undercontoured restorative should be considered unacceptable and should be redone. Detection of an undercontoured restoration is principally visual comparison

with the natural tooth contour of the restorative area (Fig. 15-6).

■ **Describe the prerequisite knowledge needed to perform a preliminary oral examination.**

Prior to attempting oral inspection a thorough knowledge is required of clinical anatomic features of the head, neck, oral cavity, as well as of the periodontium, tooth morphology, and occlusion classification.

In addition it is important to understand deviation from the normal clinical appearance of the aforementioned features. Classification of restoration and the clinical appearance of restorative materials should also be known.

■ **Describe instrumentation that may be required to complete the oral examination/inspection task.**

Minimal instrumentation is needed to provide a very thorough and complete preliminary oral examination/inspection. Cotton gauze squares, mirror, tongue blade, and explorer are all that is really required for this task. An additional instrument that may be of help is the periodontal probe.

■ **List a basic sequence for the oral examination/inspection.**

The sequence of examination for preliminary examination/inspection is a combination of extraoral and intraoral procedures; however, all involve EFDA type patient activity.

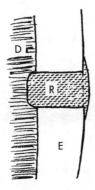

Fig. 15-5. Overcontoured (undercarved) restoration. *D,* Dentin; *R,* restoration, and *E,* enamel.

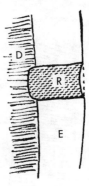

Fig. 15-6. Undercontoured (overcarved) restoration. *D,* Dentin; *R,* restoration; and *E,* enamel.

Observe and record the patient's general appearance—face, skin, eyes, lymphatic node areas, and temporomandibular joint.

Observe and record the information about lips, breath odor, mucosa, tongue and floor of the mouth, saliva, hard and soft palate, and tonsillar areas.

Observe and record the conditions existing in the periodontally associated soft tissues, missing teeth, surfaces of teeth restored, specific restorative material used in existing restorations, and any defects.

■ **Identify the general factors to be observed in the observation portion of the oral examination.**

An overall general observation of the patient will give information on the patient's general health status from the details of posture; hair; breathing; state of fatigue; general facial profile; jaw movement; color, texture, and defects of the skin; evidence of traumatic injuries; presence of neoplasms; and appearance of the eyes.

■ **Describe the results that may be obtained from the palpation portion of the oral inspection.**

Lymph nodes are to be observed for induration. General observation of the temporomandibular joint should take note of tenderness plus deviation from the norm and limitations of movement. The following sequence of inspection includes palpation as an aid in evaluation. The lips, labial and buccal mucosa, tongue and floor of the mouth, and hard and soft palate all should be observed for induration, swelling, and deviation from the normal.

■ **Identify the information that may be gained from "general observation" of the soft tissue, including lips, labial and buccal mucosa, tongue and floor of the mouth, hard palate, soft palate, and tonsillar areas.**

In general all tissues should be evaluated for color and texture plus size and/or contour. Also a general observation of changes in the normal appearance of mucosal surfaces from either abrasions or trauma, excess of tissue, and/or irritations should be listed. Any deviations from

one side of the mouth to the other of like tissue should be noted. Evidence of the effects of smoking, ulcers, and/or potential cancerous lesions should be recorded and brought to the attention of the treating doctor.

■ **What information is to be gained from the observation of saliva?**

The quantity of saliva, evidence of a dry mouth, and/or the quality of the saliva, whether it be watery, ropy, or mucoid in type are characteristics to observe.

■ **Describe what information is to be gained by the observation of teeth and restorations.**

Missing teeth, defects in tooth contour or anatomy, restored surfaces of the tooth, and what material was used for the restoration should be observed and recorded.

■ **List several impression tray criteria.**

The impression tray should clear all tissue by at least 4 mm.

The posterior border of an upper impression tray should not come in contact with the maxillary tuberosities or the hamular notch, but should be of sufficient length to cover the area.

The posterior border of the lower impression should cover all of the retromolar pad and not depress the anterior border of the ramus.

Tray sides should fall at least 4 mm short of the peripheral turn of the oral vestibule.

Tray sides should not severely depress the frenum.

The patient should not feel pain or excess pressure.

■ **Describe the loading and preparation of the impression tray.**

Impression trays vary, but it is important to provide retention of the impression materials in the tray. Various methods of retention are available: holes in the trays, wax or metal rims, and/or sticky chemical holding agents. The mix should be of a smooth, creamy consistency with no bubbles. Inadequate mixing gives a sponge-like appearance to the impression material.

When the tray is loaded, care must be taken to ensure that the material flows in from the side without entrapment of air. Material normally fills the tray to the level of the rim.

■ **Describe the seating of the mandibular impression tray.**

Make sure that the patient keeps the tongue relaxed. Keep the tray level with the arch, seat the tray straight down, and make sure that sufficient material flows around the vestibular tray periphery. Pull out the lip to allow flow of alginate and escape of air.

■ **Describe the seating of the maxillary impression tray.**

In seating an upper impression tray, seat the posterior portion of the tray first. Next, while holding the patient's lip out, seat the anterior portion. After making sure sufficient material has been expressed anteriorly, let the lip lie comfortably over the tray.

■ **Describe some methods that may be helpful in preventing the patient gagging.**

To prevent gagging the patient may be told to concentrate on something else, breath through the nose, hold a foot up, lean forward if upright, or in some instances lie in a prone position. The prone position lessens gagging because the soft palate and tongue fall away from the field of operation, and this position also improves visibility.

■ **After the initial gelation of a regular setting irreversible hydrocolloid impression material, how should the impression be removed from the mouth?**

The impression should be removed with a snap movement.

■ **Describe several criteria for completed maxillary and mandibular impressions.**

Removal of the tray should not produce distortion or fracture of impression material.
The impression should be accurate in detail in and around the dentition.
The distal extension of the impression should include the hamular notch on the maxilla and the retromolar pad on the mandible.
The buccal extension should have a smooth, continuous bubble-free roll.
The lingual extension should have a smooth, continuous bubble-free replica of the maxillary rugae and palate, and a mandibular lingual roll with no tongue interferences.
There should be no lip interference to prevent an accurate anterior roll.
The surface of impression material should be smooth, not spongy.
The tray should not be exposed in any area.

■ **List four factors or conditions that would make a tooth unsuitable for pulp testing.**

A primary tooth, a full metallic crown, metallic restorations covering or replacing more than three fourths of the tooth, and/or a tooth that has previously been treated endodontically are not suitable for pulp testing.

■ **Do anterior or posterior teeth require a higher intensity of current to elicit a pulpal response?**

Posterior teeth require a higher intensity of current as they have more insulative enamel.

■ **Explain why the gingival tissue surrounding the tooth, as well as the tooth itself, must be dried before pulp testing.**

The level of excitability of gingiva is higher than that of the tooth, and if moisture is present the current would pass to the gingiva and a false reading would be obtained.

■ **Describe the instrumentation and materials necessary for a pulp testing procedure.**

Pulp testers vary according to manufacturer, but the principle is basically the same for all: A battery powered or electrically powered current of low intensity is used to measure pulpal nerve excitability. The pulp tester is calibrated from a low to a high reading. The higher the number, the higher the current being delivered at the tip. A small amount of conductive material (tooth paste works well) is used to enhance proper contact with the dried tooth surface.

■ **Describe the procedure for a pulp test.**

The surface of the tooth to be tested is dried with a cotton gauze square. A small amount of conductive material is picked up on the tip of the pulp tester and placed in contact with the dried tooth, approximately 2 to 3 mm from the gingival border. Make sure that contact is made only with enamel. The dial or slide of the instrument is moved upward from the lowest reading until the first awareness of sensation is noted by the patient. This number is recorded for each trial of several similar teeth as well as the tooth to be tested. Care should be taken to move the calibration in small increments so as not to startle the patient.

■ **Describe the method of application of topical anesthetic to an injection site.**

The principles of application of a topical anesthetic are the same for all locations. In the placement of a topical anesthetic the EFDA is most often unassisted, and therefore placement may be completed from the assistant's work zone. The injection site is dried thoroughly with a gauze square, and care must be taken to place only moderate amounts of the topical material with a cotton-tipped swab to prevent the patient swallowing the anesthetic. Approximately 1 to 3 minutes should elapse for the topical anesthetic to take effect, and then the doctor should be notified that it is time to administer the local anesthetic injection.

■ **What characteristics of the tooth influence the selection of a rubber dam clamp?**

The mesiodistal width, curvature, gingivo-occlusal height, position of tooth, degree of eruption, and size all influence the selection of a clamp for rubber dam application.

■ **For what reason is a ligature attached to a rubber dam clamp when the clamp is placed on the tooth?**

The ligature is used to prevent the patient from accidentally swallowing or aspirating the clamp should it become dislodged.

■ **Why must the operator remove accumulations of plaque and calculus before a rubber dam is placed?**

If not removed, plaque and calculus may create inflammation and infection, bruise tissue, and possibly tear the rubber dam.

■ **What general criteria apply when isolating the field of operation with a rubber dam?**

Most texts recommend isolating the field of operation from the most posterior tooth on the treated side around to the premolar or at least the cuspid on the opposite side of the arch. The largest hole on the rubber dam punch is usually used for the clamp hole. This isolation yields maximum access; however, it may not always be indicated for less involved procedure such as one-surface occlusal restorations or anterior restorations. In the latter instance a premolar to premolar isolation might be more practical. A good rule of thumb is to isolate two teeth posterior and two teeth anterior to the treated teeth, unless otherwise specified. This gives adequate isolation whether dealing with a one-tooth treatment or a quadrant area.

■ **In what order should the operator seat the rubber dam clamp for maximum control and for the best view of the clamp jaws?**

The lingual jaw and then the facial jaw are seated to provide the best observation of clamp positioning.

■ **Why must the edges of the rubber dam be inverted into the sulcus around each tooth?**

Inverting the rubber dam into the sulcus will protect the gingiva, keep moisture out, and keep the rubber dam out of the work area. For these same reasons a wedge may be used when preparing the tooth in a proximal area.

■ **Describe the criteria to be met in placement of a rubber dam.**

The area isolated by the rubber dam provides access to the clinical site.

The holes are punched for correct number, size, position, and spacing.

A protective floss tie is properly attached to the clamp.

The clamp selected fits the clamped tooth and is stable.

The general placement of the rubber dam is smooth, and the proper tension has been used to prevent buckling or tissue discomfort.

The frame is placed properly to prevent discomfort to the patient and obstruction of the operator's view.

All contacts are clear of rubber dam, and the rubber dam retracts the interproximal papilla.

Ligation is completed when (where) necessary.

All tissue is protected by the invagination of the rubber dam.

The wedge is properly used to further isolate proximal teeth for cavity preparation if necessary.

■ **Explain how the hole position on the rubber dam should be altered to allow for use of the gingival retraction clamp.**

The hole should be displaced 3 to 6 mm facially for the tooth being treated on the facial surface. The opposite is true if treating a tooth on the lingual surface.

■ **For what two reasons should extreme care be taken when removing the gingival retraction clamp on completion of a restoration?**

The cementum can be gouged, and/or the completed restoration can be scratched or dented by careless removal of the retraction clamp.

■ **Identify eight criteria for placement of the gingival retraction clamp.**

Gingiva is retracted 0.5 mm to 1 mm below the proposed gingival margin of the preparation.

Retraction clamp does not trap the rubber dam or the gingiva.

Facial jaw of the clamp has full contact with tooth surface.

Bows of the clamp are parallel with the occlusal plane.

Compound surrounds the mesial and distal bows and is between the teeth.

Notches of the clamp are free of compound.

Access to the facial surface of the tooth is not impaired.

Clamp is stable.

■ **Give four reasons for the use of copal varnish in amalgam restorative treatment.**

Copal varnish reduces postoperative galvanic hypersensitivity, reduces potential irritation from the restorative material, decreases marginal leakage, and prevents discoloration from silver alloy restorative material.

■ **For what reason is copal varnish not used with tooth-colored restorative materials?**

There is the possibility of an unfavorable interaction between varnishes and resin restorative materials. Copal varnish will not allow resins to set and interferes with adaptation.

■ **Describe the placement of and criteria to be met with copal varnish.**

Copal varnish is placed over all surfaces in two thin coats. The second coat covers small porosities created during the drying of the initial coating. The criteria to be met are procedural and confirmed when two thin coats are placed.

■ **In what two areas of a cavity preparation should calcium hydroxide liners or bases "not" be placed?**

Unlike copal varnish that flows over all preparation surfaces, calcium hydroxide should not be placed on the enamel walls or in the retention grooves of the cavity preparation.

■ **Why is a calcium hydroxide liner applied only to the dentin walls and not to the enamel walls of the cavity preparation?**

The calcium hydroxide liner interferes with proper adaptation of the restorative material to the enamel walls, shows up as an unesthetic white line at the margins, and will eventually dissolve and leave a space resulting in marginal leakage.

■ **Copal varnish, calcium hydroxide liners, and bases serve varied functions. What is the purpose of a calcium hydroxide "liner" in restorations with tooth-colored materials?**

Calcium hydroxide liners are used as is copal varnish to cover cut dentinal tubules and therefore protect the pulp from temporary irritation from the restorative material. Since resins are nonconductive, galvanic action is not a factor when they are used, so calcium hydroxide liners do not reduce hypersensitivity to resins.

■ For what reasons are calcium hydroxide "bases" used?

A calcium hydroxide base will cover cut dentinal tubules to reduce potential irritation from restorative material, may be used with tooth-colored resin, promotes secondary dentin formation, acts as a thermal insulator, and provides strength to thin dentinopulpal floor when placed in a deeply excavated portion of the cavity preparation.

■ Describe the placement of and criteria to be met with use of calcium hydroxide.

Placement of calcium hydroxide can be done by one of two methods. A *liner* is a very *thin* coat of calcium hydroxide placed over cut dentinal tubules. Usually the calcium hydroxide placed in the cavity preparation is a suspension of calcium hydroxide particles in a liquid vehicle. A *base* of calcium hydroxide is a *thicker* coat or coats to actually build up a deeply excavated portion of a cavity. The base serves a dual purpose because it protects cut dentinal tubules and provides strength to the pulpal floor.

■ Matrices serve common functions whether they are used for amalgam or tooth-colored restorative materials. What four functions do they share?

Matrices reproduce missing contours of the tooth (a fourth wall), provide an ideal contact area with the adjacent tooth, prevent cervical overhang, and permit application of adequate placement or condensation pressures.

■ What are the purposes of the matrix band with "amalgam"?

The matrix band provides a surface to condense against, holds the rubber dam out of the preparation, and helps prevent overhang of the restorative material.

■ What are the purposes of the mechanical retainer in amalgam restorations?

The retainer aids in proper adaptation, holds the matrix in place at the gingival margin, holds the band securely, and allows the band to be tightened or loosened.

■ What purposes does the wedge serve in placement of a class II amalgam restoration?

The wedge aids in proper adaptation of the matrix band, holds matrix securely in place at the gingival margin, separates teeth, holds the rubber dam down, prevents overhang, and compensates for the thickness of the matrix.

■ What problems may result from improper placement of a wedge against a matrix band?

Poor placement of a wedge may lead to an open contact, indentation in the proximal surface of the restoration, restoration overhang, and/or displacement of the matrix band.

■ Give seven principal criteria for placement of the mechanical retainer and matrix band.

The retainer is adjacent to the facial surfaces of the teeth.

The matrix band is 0.5 mm to 1 mm gingival to the gingival margin of the cavity preparation and secure against the proximal surface.

The matrix band is 0.5 mm to 1 mm occlusal to the junction of the occlusoproximal cavosurface margins.

The matrix band approximates the contour of the mesial and distal surfaces.

The matrix band contacts the adjacent tooth.

The band and retainer are securely in place.

The band does not trap the rubber dam or gingiva.

■ Purposes of the wedge and matrix strip in a class III tooth-colored restoration are similar to an amalgam matrix in all aspects. What additional advantages does the matrix strip have with a tooth-colored (resin) restoration?

The matrix protects the restoration from air, holds the restoration in place during set of the restorative material, and provides pressure on the restoration to create a dense homogenous restoration.

■ **Before a restoration is placed, what can be done if a contact is so tight that you cannot pass a matrix strip between the teeth?**

Place a wedge to gain minimal access and separation for the matrix.

■ **Describe some variations of matrix techniques that may be helpful in restoration of a class IV cavity preparation. Indicate the criteria to be achieved for all techniques.**

There are three basic variations of matrix techniques for the class IV cavity preparation. A finger-held placement of a *routine class III matrix strip* leaves much to be desired as the operator must position the strips precisely to achieve restorative contour. All factors of placement with wedge and matrix are the same except that there is no incisal angle of the tooth to provide support when the band is positioned. The experienced operator may find this a workable technique; however, the EFDA will be better served using a *dead soft matrix* that allows placement of the restorative material. This technique of metal matrix also lends itself to ultraviolet light–polymerized resin. A small portion of copper matrix is trimmed, wedged, and compounded in place.

Another matrix suitable for class IV cavity preparations is *an incisal angle portion of clear plastic crown forms*. This allows the operator to position the matrix to the desired location and contour plus allowing the operator to generally observe the contours of the completed restoration. All three have merit, but the metal matrix and crown form lend themselves best to EFDA tasks.

■ **What are some reasons for placing a zinc oxide–eugenol temporary restoration?**

A zinc oxide–eugenol restoration is placed many times as a therapeutic filling material. Removal of gross caries allows the pulp a chance for regenerative healing. Also there may not be sufficient time to complete the restoration. Protection to the prepared tooth is provided by this temporary or therapeutic restoration.

■ **Describe the placement and criteria to be met by a zinc oxide–eugenol or similar intracoronal material used in a temporary restoration.**

The placement of an intracoronal temporary sedative restoration fills out the general contour of the prepared tooth. The material is only to be used for a very short term, unless it has been strengthened with additives. A stiff mix of zinc oxide paste is inserted in the cavity and adapted to all surfaces with a cotton pellet moistened with alcohol or water. Once initial set has commenced, it is carved to basic contour and occlusion is checked. No attempt is made to reestablish anatomy, but occlusal function must not be hindered by excess material.

■ **Describe how to determine occlusal contacts and the criteria of occlusion for a therapeutic intracoronal temporary restoration.**

The therapeutic sedative intracoronal temporary restoration should be contoured to approximate the natural tooth. Occlusal contacts are determined with occlusal marking paper for centric and excursive movements. The final temporary restoration should then be carved out of occlusion and therefore be devoid of any occlusal contacts.

■ **Describe three techniques for temporary protection of cavity or crown prepared teeth.**

Three principal techniques are used for temporary coverage or protection of prepared tooth structure while laboratory fabrication of inlays and/or crown restorations are being completed. The oldest method is the use of metal, usually *aluminum shells*. The shells are trimmed to fit gingival contour and shaped to functional occlusal contour with intraoral occlusal forces. Once contoured, the shells are temporarily cemented with a zinc oxide–eugenol cement. This technique of shell crowns has been replaced in more recent times by the use of *tooth-colored self-polymerizing resins*. These resins may be used to construct very esthetic and functional tooth contour; therefore, they provide a much more acceptable temporary protection. The technique uses an impression or plastic splint of the teeth prior to preparation. Once the teeth are prepared for inlays or crowns, tooth-colored self-curing resin is placed in the impression or splint. The void left by the removal of tooth structure is filled with resin and fills out to prepared contour. Excess resin is removed, and occlusion is adjusted. The temporary resin inlay or crown is then seated with a temporary cement luting agent. In similar fashion thin-walled *tooth-colored preformed crowns* may be purchased that only need to be trimmed and relined with self-curing resin.

■ **What difference would it make if the incisors were in occlusion prior to preparation but were in premature occlusion after a temporary crown was cemented in place?**

The temporary crown could be knocked loose because of occlusion and could cause extreme sensitivity of the prepared tooth. Also, supra-eruption of remaining teeth is possible.

■ **Why must the original occlusal pattern be replicated when the temporary crown is placed?**

Occlusion helps to maintain the original occlusal pattern and prevents teeth from shifting, as well as providing functional movement of tooth-to-tooth chewing movements.

■ **Why is undercontouring a temporary crown in the gingival one third preferred to overcontouring?**

An undercontoured temporary crown will reduce gingival pressure or irritation, and healing will be promoted.

■ **Describe the reasons that a polycarbonate crown is widely used for temporary crowns.**

Polycarbonate temporary crowns are strong yet flexible enough to contour, bond chemically to a self-curing acrylic resin when used to fill the shell, adapt to temporary cement without deteriorating, and provide satisfactory tooth-colored esthetics.

■ **Why must the temporary crown be removed from a preparation before the acrylic resin filler is completely polymerized during fabrication?**

Removing the crown during the soft state of polymerization prevents binding, allows the excess resin to be trimmed, and also reduces exothermic reaction that could sensitize the tooth and gingiva.

■ **What possible errors could distort the contours of a custom plastic temporary crown during polymerization?**

Movement of the crown or uneven pressure will create distortion during polymerization.

■ **When polishing a temporary crown, what three areas of the crown should "not" be polished?**

The centric stop areas, margins, and contacts should not be polished as they might be obliterated during this procedure.

■ **Give reasons for the placement of a temporary crown?**

A temporary crown helps reduce sensitivity, protects dentin from oral fluids, maintains occlusion (incisal length), prevents fracturing of finish line or breakdown of prepared teeth, prevents changes in gingival tissue or food impaction, provides for loss of function, gives suitable interim esthetics, allows the patient to begin to adjust to a permanent crown, and restores and/or improves the contour of the original tooth.

■ **A completed temporary crown should meet what three criteria?**

A temporary crown may be up to 0.5 mm short of the finish line.

Facial and lingual surfaces may be slightly overcontoured without disturbing healthy tissue.

Undercontouring in the gingival third on interproximal surfaces is preferable to overcontouring.

■ **Describe four conditions that must be met for any temporary crown to be satisfactory once it has been seated.**

The margins of a temporary crown must fit snugly to eliminate fluid seepage and contact adjacent teeth, and the occlusal pattern must be replicated for the crown to be satisfactorily seated.

■ **Why is a minimum of two increments of amalgam restorative material required to fill a cavity preparation?**

Two or more increments of amalgam reduce the chance of voids (better union of particles), give better adaptation to the walls of the preparation, and provide a sufficient overfill of amalgam.

■ **What are the purposes of condensing amalgam?**

Condensation decreases voids, provides better adaptation to walls, decreases residual mercury, creates a unified mass of alloy, and increases the strength of the final restoration.

■ **At what angle should the condenser be held when adapting alloy to the cavity walls of a preparation?**

As a general rule the condenser should be held at a 45-degree angle to the cavity walls during the adaptation of alloy.

■ **What are the reasons for overfilling the cavity preparation with amalgam?**

Overfill allows the final mercury-rich layer of alloy to be removed and provides adequate bulk to permit carving.

■ **What purposes does carving the alloy serve?**

Carving removes excess amalgam beyond the margins of the preparation, provides original contours (including anatomic), and removes the mercury-rich layer of alloy created during condensation of the overfill.

■ **What may result if an amalgam restoration is carved after the amalgam has begun to set?**

An uneven surface will be created that is difficult and time-consuming to finish; mercury will be pulled to the margins, and the chance of fracture will be increased which would result in poor anatomic features in the contour of the restoration.

■ **List the errors that would make it necessary to remove an amalgam restoration that has just been placed?**

The amalgam has set too long (cannot be carved or amalgam added).
Voids are present.
The amalgam is poorly condensed.
Submarginal areas created in carving are greater than 0.2 mm.
Open contact remains in a class II restoration.
Overextension of amalgam is unimprovable.

■ **Describe the technical steps in carving a class I amalgam restoration.**

The operator should first recall the original outline of the preparation. Next the operator should identify distal, mesial, lingual, and facial margins of the preparation in four strokes of the carver. The location of secondary grooves is marked, secondary grooves are refined and connected, and the central groove refined, the occlusal contour is refined, margins are checked, and remaining flash is removed. Finally the amalgam surface is cleansed and burnished to a dull luster.

■ **What are the class I carving criteria that should be achieved?**

The restoration should be flush at the margins, a contour that approximates original tooth contour should be reproduced, and the surface of the restorative material should have a dull luster and texture to achieve the carving criteria.

■ **What class I occlusion criteria should be evident when the restoration has been evaluated for occlusal markings?**

The markings of tooth and restoration should be of equal centric occlusion density, and the restoration should be free of excursive occlusal markings.

■ **Identify several ways one can judge the height of the marginal ridge to be restored when an adjacent proximal tooth is missing.**

Observation of the following anatomic factors will provide the operator clues to marginal ridge height:
Opposite side of mouth
Surrounding teeth

Incline of cusp arms of prepared teeth
Occlusal position of opposing teeth
Preoperative observation of the marginal
ridge prior to preparation

■ **Explain "why" and in "what direction" dental floss should be removed from the interproximal area after the contact area of a restoration is checked with the floss.**

If floss is forcefully brought occlusal to cervical or cervical to occlusal, it will destroy contact with the approximating tooth. Floss should be removed in a lingual or facial direction, never occlusally.

■ **What carving criteria should be achieved for a class II restoration?**

In addition to the criteria for a class I restoration, the following criteria must be achieved in a class II restoration:
The restoration should be flush at the margins.
Contact should be established in the correct area with the adjacent tooth.
Contour should be established approximating the original contour of the tooth.
The marginal ridge and contact should be undamaged by removal of the retainer and matrix.

■ **Why is it important to restore the original contour of the tooth on a class V restoration?**

An undercontoured restoration will cause plaque and debris to accumulate in the sulcus of the gingiva. An overcontoured restoration will create an irritation of the gingiva from reduced mechanical stimulation by food during mastication.

■ **What are the purposes of finishing and polishing an amalgam restoration?**

Finishing refines the contour and provides marginal adjustments to the restoration, that is, removes scratches, pits, and flash and corrects minute submarginal areas to increase the life of the restoration.

■ **Why should excessive heat be avoided in polishing amalgam?**

Excessive heat should be avoided in polishing amalgam restorations because mercury will be drawn to the surface and increase the danger of fracture and tarnish.

■ **How soon should an alloy be polished after it has been carved?**

An alloy should be polished no sooner than 24 hours after placement.

■ **Describe ways to minimize heat production during finishing and polishing procedures.**

The use of light pressure and intermittent strokes at low speed with the most abrasive agent feasible will reduce heat production.

■ **Describe a procedure for finishing and polishing a disto-occlusal amalgam on tooth 12 that has flash (overextension) on the buccal triangular ridge. Include in the description the burs or stones and polishing agents used.**

First, check the margins for finishing needs. Use a flame bur to remove the flash and a ½ round bur to sharpen the grooves if needed. Check the margins to see that the flash has been removed. Polish with a wet pumice on an occlusal bristle brush and floss on proximal surfaces. Wash, dry, and then polish with a fine polishing agent, that is, silica, tin oxide, or Amalgloss on a bristle brush. The polishing should be followed by flossing of the proximal surface. For the final step use a dry, fine polishing agent to bring out the final high luster and shine.

■ **What risk is there to the patient in finishing and polishing a class V restoration?**

The operator can gouge cementum, destroy the very thin enamel at the cementoenamel junction, and damage gingival tissues.

■ **Define the properties of unfilled resin restorations.**

Unfilled resins have a low degree of hardness, shrink more when set, percolate with temperature change, contain no fillers, can be polished easily to a high luster, and are capable of allowing more material to be added if the restoration is submarginal.

■ **Why must increments of unfilled resin be placed at approximately 15-second intervals?**

Fifteen-second intervals are necessary for unfilled resin placement to allow shrinkage away from the center of the mass and to form a good union between increments.

■ **What purposes does the protective film serve when applied to unfilled resin?**

Protective film prevents the monomer from evaporating and protects the restoration from air and moisture that inhibit the set and lead to a chalky surface.

■ **Why should a class IV mesioincisal restoration be out of occlusion?**

The class IV restoration should be out of occlusion to prevent fracture and prolong the life of the restoration.

■ **Describe conditions which might indicate that the auxiliary should not proceed with the removal of sutures?**

The following may be complications in removing sutures; (1) the wound is not sufficiently healed, and/or the tissue has grown over the wound site; (2) the dressing material has hardened over the sutures; and/or (3) there is inflammation or infection in the area.

■ **Why must the patient's chart be checked before sutures are removed?**

It is very important to know the number of sutures placed to determine that all sutures have been removed.

■ **What are the criteria for cutting and removing a simple suture?**

When sutures are removed from the mouth, care should be taken to assure that (1) all suture material is removed from the tissue, (2) all material is removed from the patient's mouth, and (3) the tissue is undamaged by the procedure.

■ **Why must the continuing (external) portion of a continuous suture be cut before the simple suture?**

It is important to cut the continuous portion first so that unnecessary stress is not placed on the tissue as the continuous portion is removed.

■ **Why must an exposed portion or a knot of a suture "never" be pulled through tissue?**

If the exposed portion of the suture and/or the knot is pulled through the tissue there is a possibility of injury to the tissue and an added possibility of infectious products being incorporated in the tissue.

■ **What various forms of medication are used to treat dry sockets?**

There are three basic forms of medication used in treating dry sockets: liquid medicaments, ointments, and self-hardening pastes (those incorporated into a gauze strip or gelatin sponge).

■ **Why is it important to irrigate the dry socket before applying medication?**

Removal of food debris and tissue particles is very important. Remaining particles would cause a continual irritation to the natural healing processes as well as the blockage of actual medication activity.

SUGGESTED READINGS

Extramural expanded functions training program, oral health instruction, Denver, Colo., 1975, Colorado Dental Association and University of Colorado School of Dentistry.

Miller, D. R., et al.: Expanded functions manual for on the job training, 1973, Florida State Board of Dentistry, Florida Department of Education, and The Florida Dental Association.

U.S. Department of Health, Education, and Welfare: Restoration of cavity preparations with amalgam and tooth colored materials, Project ACORDE, Washington, D.C., 1974, U.S. Government Printing Office.

U.S. Department of Health, Education, and Welfare: Taking an impression, Project ACORDE, Washington, D.C., 1975, U.S. Government Printing Office.

U.S. Department of Health, Education, and Welfare: Assisting with suture placement and removing sutures, Project ACORDE, Washington, D.C., 1976, U.S. Government Printing Office.

U.S. Department of Health, Education, and Welfare: Preformed plastic crown, and custom made acrylic crown, Project ACORDE, Washington, D.C., 1976, U.S. Government Printing Office.

Wilkins, E. M.: Clinical practice of the dental hygienist, ed. 4, Philadelphia, 1976, Lea & Febiger.

CHAPTER 16

Anatomy and physiology

RICHARD W. BRAND

■ **Identify the systems of the human body.**

There are seven systems of the human body: cardiovascular, respiratory, digestive, urinary, nervous, endocrine, and reproductive.

■ **What is the cardiovascular system?**

The cardiovascular system is composed of the heart and the blood vessels that carry the blood to and from the heart to all parts of the body. The blood vessels are arteries, veins, and capillaries.

■ **Trace the course of blood from the head to the heart and its return to the head.**

Blood returns from the head through the internal and external jugular veins into the brachiocephalic (innominate) veins. From there it enters the superior vena cava and then enters the right atrium of the heart. Blood flows from the right atrium to the right ventricle and then flows out of the heart through the pulmonary artery in which it is carried to the lungs to pick up oxygen again. It returns from the lungs through the pulmonary veins to the left atrium and then flows into the left ventricle. From the left ventricle it leaves the heart through the aorta. On the right side the brachiocephalic artery branches off the aorta, and the common carotid artery on the right side branches off the brachiocephalic artery. On the left side the common carotid artery branches off the arch of the aorta. The common carotid arteries divide into the internal and external carotid arteries that supply blood to the head.

■ **What regulates the heart rate?**

The heart rate is moderated by the autonomic nervous system.

■ **How does the autonomic nervous system affect the heart?**

There are two components to the autonomic nervous system, the sympathetic and the parasympathetic systems. The sympathetic nervous system increases the heart rate, whereas the parasympathetic nervous system slows the heart rate.

■ **What is the "fight or flight" mechanism?**

This is the resultant action when the sympathetic nervous system is stimulated. If you are suddenly frightened, your body begins to pump adrenaline from the adrenal gland into the bloodstream. This is because the sympathetic part of the nervous system is stimulated when you are frightened. Adrenaline makes the heart beat stronger, and the sympathetic nervous system causes the heart to beat faster. At the same time when you are frightened, you tend to become pale and feel a knot in the pit of your stomach. These two symptoms result from the capillaries near the skin shutting down and keeping the blood deeper in the body. The knot in the pit of the stomach is caused by the fact that the blood vessels of the stomach and gastrointestinal tract also shut down, and therefore the blood supply to that area is decreased. This tends to move most of the blood in the body toward the muscular system so that the individual can either fight or use this energy to run away.

■ **How does the parasympathetic nervous system affect the heart and body?**

The parasympathetic nervous system primarily aids the body in digestion. It slows down the heart, increases the blood supply to the stomach and gastrointestinal tract, causes the smooth muscle of the gastrointestinal tract to contract and thereby to move food through the system, and finally stimulates the salivary glands and other digestive glands to function in the digestion of food.

■ **What is shock, and what are some of the causes of shock?**

Shock is a depression of the central nervous system that may result in loss of consciousness. There are two main types of shock:

Neurogenic shock. When the nervous system is stimulated severely by something very traumatic, most of the capillaries in the body enlarge causing a large expansion in the capacity of the blood vessels. Because of this, most of the blood will tend to rush to the lower part of the body, and there will not be enough blood to supply the brain. Under these circumstances the individual will begin to lose consciousness. When this happens the patient should be placed in a horizontal position with the legs raised to cause the blood to rush to the head. The patient should be kept warm.

Hemorrhagic shock. When an individual is bleeding and loses so much blood that there is not enough blood to pump to the brain, the same symptoms are produced as with neurogenic shock. The treatment in this instance is basically the same. After an attempt is made to stop the bleeding, the patient is placed in a horizontal position with the feet raised to cause blood to flow to the brain.

■ **What are the components of the respiratory system?**

The components of the respiratory system include the nasal cavity; nasal, oral, and laryngeal pharynx; larynx; trachea; primary and secondary bronchi; terminal bronchioles; respiratory bronchioles; alveolar ducts and sacs; and finally alveoli.

■ **What do the terms "conducting" and "respiratory portions" refer to in the respiratory system?**

Conducting portions are those parts of the respiratory system that carry air into the lungs but do nothing about exchanging oxygen. In the list given in the previous discussion this would include everything from the nasal cavity to the terminal bronchioles. The respiratory portion is that part of the system engaged in the exchange of oxygen for carbon dioxide and includes the respiratory bronchioles, the alveolar ducts and sacs, and the alveoli.

■ **What allows gas exchange to take place in the lungs?**

The fact that the hemoglobin in the blood has a greater affinity for oxygen than carbon dioxide allows the exchange to take place. Also important to gas exchange is the fact that the separation between the lungs and the capillaries is only two thin membranes of cells, and the gases can pass readily between these membranes.

■ **Why are the lungs always expanded and filled with air?**

The lungs are expanded because the air in the lungs is at atmospheric pressure, whereas the space between the lungs and the ribs is an enclosed space that has a slight vacuum in relation to the atmospheric pressure. For this reason the lungs are always expanded just as a balloon full of air is always expanded.

■ **What is a pneumothorax?**

A pneumothorax is a collapsed lung. It results from the fact that a leak occurs in the space between the lung and the ribs. Air either enters from the lung into this space, or it enters from the outside into the space. The results are the same; if the pressure is the same on the outside as it is on the inside, the lung will not remain expanded but will collapse. To treat this collapse it is necessary to repair the leak and to withdraw air from this space between the lungs and ribs so once again there is a slight vacuum, then the lungs will once again expand.

■ **Why is it difficult to breathe during an asthma attack or during some allergic reactions?**

This breathing difficulty is due to the fact that the tissues of the respiratory tract become filled with plasma, and this causes the tissue to swell. In the area of the vocal cords there is very little space between the cords, and as the tissues swell the cords come in contact with one another, thus blocking the flow of air to and from the lungs.

■ **Why do the tissues of the respiratory tract become filled with plasma, and what can be done to treat this reaction?**

The reaction happens because certain cells in connective tissue called *mast cells* release a substance called *histamine* that causes small blood vessels to start to leak plasma. This leaking of plasma into the intercellular area causes swelling of the tissues, and this swelling obstructs the area. Treatment to stop the plasma leaking is use of a drug that combats the histamine reaction. These drugs are called antihistaminics and work rapidly to relieve the problem.

■ **What kind of regulatory control is there between the respiratory system and the cardiovascular system?**

At the beginning of the internal carotid artery there are two structures that regulate these systems. These structures are the carotid body and the carotid sinus. The carotid body measures the amount of oxygen in the blood and regulates both heart and lungs to maintain an adequate balance of oxygen at all times. The carotid sinus measures the blood pressure and regulates the heart to maintain a normal pressure.

■ **Name the components of the digestive system.**

In descending order the components of the digestive system include oral cavity, oral pharynx, laryngeal pharynx, esophagus, stomach, duodenum, jejunum, ileum, ascending colon, transverse colon, descending colon, sigmoid colon, rectum, and anal canal.

■ **What are the major glands associated with the digestive system?**

The liver, gallbladder, and pancreas are glands associated with the digestive system.

■ **What happens to food during each stage of the digestive process?**

Saliva in the oral cavity begins the breakdown of starches. As food reaches the stomach, gastric juices begin to break down proteins. As the food reaches the duodenum, secretions of the duodenum, pancreas, and gallbladder all mix with the food and most of the breakdown occurs at this point. The breakdown continues as the food moves on into the jejunum and ileum. By the time the food has reached the large intestine, most of the digestion and absorption of nutrients have taken place. The primary function of the large intestine is the reabsorption of water.

■ **What precautions must be taken regarding diet when a patient has had his gallbladder removed?**

The gallbladder's function is to concentrate bile that aids in the breakdown of fat. When the gallbladder has been removed, bile can still reach the duodenum, but it will be in smaller quantities at any one time and it will be less concentrated. This means that the individual will have decreased ability to break down fat, and so the patient will have to decrease the amount of fat taken into the body at one time. It is not necessary to give up fatty foods but simply to decrease the intake. These individuals may also be instructed to eat smaller but more frequent meals.

■ **What are some of the problems that may occur when food and drugs are absorbed through the intestinal wall?**

Several things may happen. The first problem may be diarrhea. With this condition the peristaltic contractions of the intestinal tract are sped up, and food and drugs move through the tract so fast that there is not enough time to absorb them. The food also moves through the tract so fast that there is not enough time for water reabsorption, and this accounts for the consistency of the feces. Also the cell lining of the intestinal tract may be unable to absorb the nutrients or drugs. These problems can lead to dehydration and starvation even though the person is eating and drinking a sufficient amount of nutrients.

■ **What are the components of the urinary system?**

The kidneys, ureters, urinary bladder, and urethra are the components of the urinary system.

■ **What is a nephron, and what are its two divisions?**

The kidney is made up of millions of nephrons that form the histologic unit responsible for the production of urine and the retention of fluid and electrolytes such as sodium and potassium. The two functional units of the nephron are the secretory portion that is extremely active and the excretory portion that does not change the fluid product to any great extent but simply carries it to the ureter.

■ **What is the importance of sodium in maintaining fluid and electrolyte balance in the kidney?**

Sodium moves out of the nephrons into the connective tissue around them and by the process of osmosis pulls water out of the nephron and concentrates the urine, thereby keeping water loss at a minimum. This process, which is also referred to as a "sodium pump," in addition aids in the retention of electrolytes.

■ **What is the significance of changes in urinary patterns?**

In general the two major changes in urinary patterns are an increase or a decrease in urination. An increase in urination leads to dehydration of the body unless there is a corresponding increase in water consumption. The classic signs of diabetes are polyphagia (increased hunger), polydipsia (increased thirst), and polyuria (increased urination). Decreased urination is seen in a number of conditions, however, the most common of which is kidney disease in which the nephrons do not pull water out of the blood as they normally do. In actuality the nephrons pull out more than water from the blood. If the kidneys do not produce urine, then one of the main components of urine, uric acid, begins to build up in the bloodstream, and the patient could be poisoned by this uric acid. This condition is referred to as uremic poisoning.

■ **What are endocrine glands?**

Endocrine glands are glands that release their products into the bloodstream because of the absence of a duct system. In general, products of the endocrine glands are known as hormones. Hormones are substances that affect the functioning of other organs in more distant parts of the body.

■ **What organs make up the endocrine system?**

The organs within the endocrine system are the pituitary gland, thyroid gland, parathyroid glands, adrenal glands (suprarenals), islets of Langerhans in the pancreas, thymus, and pineal body.

■ **What is the function of the thyroid gland?**

The thyroid gland controls the basal metabolic rate of the body. Its function is balanced by the hormone thyrotropin produced by the pituitary gland.

■ **Where are the parathyroid glands located, and what is their function?**

The tiny parathyroid glands are buried in the posterior surface of the thyroid gland and control the use of calcium in the body.

■ **Where are the adrenal glands located, and what is their function?**

These glands are located on the upper surface of the kidney. They have an outer area, the cortex, that controls protein and carbohydrate metabolism, sodium and potassium balance, and some of the sex hormones. There is also a central area, the medulla, that produces epinephrine (adrenaline), which speeds up and strengthens the heart beat and provides a source of instant "energy."

■ **What are the islets of Langerhans, and where are they located?**

The islets of Langerhans are part of the pancreas. The pancreas is both an exocrine gland that produces digestive enzymes and an endocrine gland that produces insulin in the islets of Langerhans. Insulin controls storage and use of glucose and glycogen in the body, primarily in the liver.

■ **What hormone is produced by the testes, and what is the function of this hormone?**

Testosterone is produced by the testes as well as by the adrenal gland. This hormone regulates the secondary sex characteristics in the male.

■ **What hormones are produced by the ovaries, and what is their function?**

The ovaries plus the placenta produce several estrogens that affect sexual drive, secondary female sex characteristics, and salt and water retention. The ovaries and placenta also produce progesterone that aids in the control of ovarian follicle development as well as in the control of the changes in the uterine endometrium that occur during the menstrual cycle.

■ **What is the function of the thymus gland, and what happens to this gland as the body develops?**

The thymus provides antibody protection for the newborn and young individual. As part of this it is also an early blood-forming organ, providing lymphocytes for the body. As other areas of the body take over its function, it begins to shrink until it almost disappears and is nonfunctional.

■ **What are the meanings of the terms "neurocranium" and "viscerocranium," and**

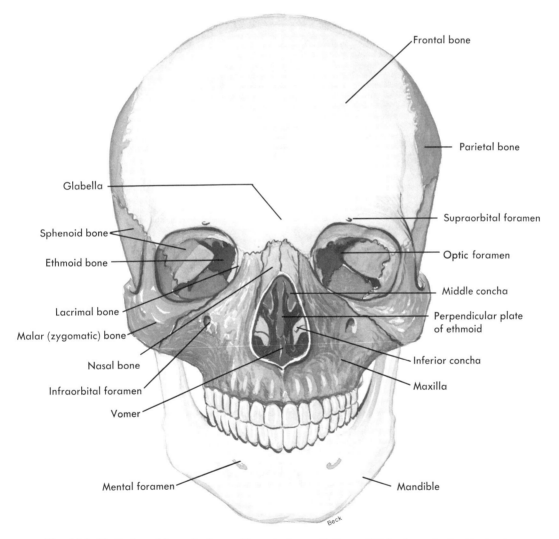

Fig. 16-1. Skull viewed from the front. (From Anthony, C. P., and Thibodeau, G. A.: Textbook of anatomy and physiology, ed. 10, St. Louis, 1979, The C. V. Mosby Co.)

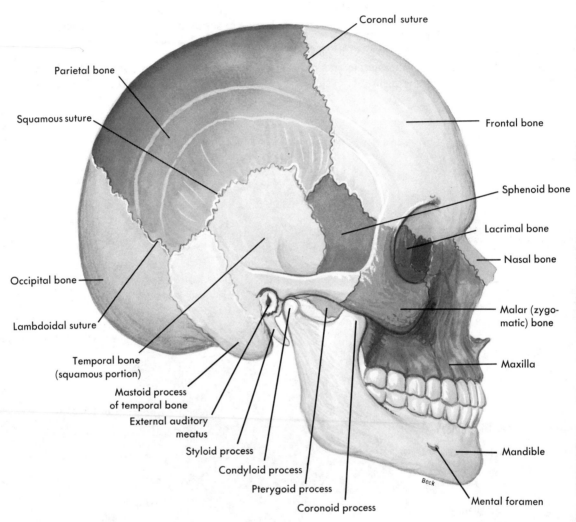

Fig. 16-2. Skull viewed from the right side. (From Anthony, C. P., and Thibodeau, G. A.: Textbook of anatomy and physiology, ed. 10, St. Louis, 1979, The C. V. Mosby Co.)

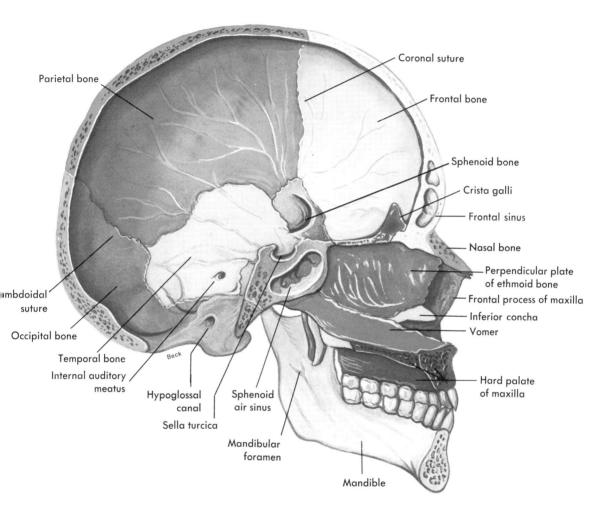

Parietal bone

Coronal suture

Frontal bone

Sphenoid bone

Crista galli

Frontal sinus

Nasal bone

Perpendicular plate
of ethmoid bone

Frontal process of maxilla

Inferior concha

Vomer

Lambdoidal
suture

Occipital bone

Temporal bone

Internal auditory
meatus

Hypoglossal
canal

Sella turcica

Sphenoid
air sinus

Mandibular
foramen

Mandible

Hard palate
of maxilla

Beck

Fig. 16-3. Left half of skull viewed from within. (From Anthony, C. P., and Thibodeau, G. A.:
Textbook of anatomy and physiology, ed. 10, St. Louis, 1979, The C. V. Mosby Co.)

what bones contribute to each? (Figs. 16-1 to 16-3)

The term *neurocranium* refers to the eight bones that surround and protect the brain. These are the parietal bones, temporal bones, and frontal, occipital, sphenoid, and ethmoid bones. The bones of the *viscerocranium* are the maxillae, palatine bones, zygomatic bones, nasal bones, inferior nasal conchae, lacrimal bones, vomer, and mandible.

■ **What are the various parts of the maxilla, and what is their role or function?**

The body of the maxilla is the major bulk of bone that contributes to general facial form and contains the maxillary sinus within it. The frontal process of the maxilla is a slender ridge of bone that contacts the frontal bone and forms the lateral contours of the base of the nose. The zygomatic process of the maxilla contacts the zygomatic bone and helps form the floor of the orbit and part of the lower rim of the orbit. The alveolar process of the maxilla forms the sockets for the upper, or maxillary, teeth. This process is frequently lost following the loss of teeth or as a consequence of periodontal disease. The palatal process of the maxilla along with the horizontal process of the palatine bone form the hard palate.

■ **What are the three major components of the mandible?**

The ramus is the posterior vertical component of the mandible. The body is the lower half of the horizontal component of the mandible. The alveolar process is the upper half of the horizontal component of the mandible and forms the sockets for the mandibular teeth.

■ **What are the major landmarks, or points of study, on the mandible?**

The ramus contains the condyle and its neck, the coronoid process, and notch. From a medial view, the ramus can also be seen to contain the mandibular foramen and lingula. The ramus meets the body at the angle of the mandible. The external and internal oblique lines run from the ramus down onto the alveolar process and body. On the body can be found the mental foramen on the lateral side and the mylohyoid line, genial tubercles (mental spines), and the digastric fossae on the medial side (Figs. 16-1 to 16-3).

■ **What are the pterygoid processes, and what is their function?**

The pterygoid processes are a downward projection of the spenoid bone lying immediately posterior to the maxillary tuberosity. Each of these processes has a pair of thin bony plates running posteriorly known as the medial and lateral pterygoid plates. Between these plates is a depression known as the pterygoid fossa. These pterygoid processes serve as a point of origin for portions of the medial and lateral pterygoid muscles, which are important muscles of mastication (Fig. 16-4).

■ **Name the muscles of mastication, their origin, insertion, action, and nerve and blood supply.**

The muscles of mastication are the *paired* temporal, masseter, and medial and lateral pterygoid muscles (Figs. 16-5 and 16-6). (See Table 16-1 for the origin, action, and nerve and blood supply of the muscles of mastication.)

■ **How is a lateral excursive movement of the mandible accomplished?**

Basically lateral excursive movement of the mandible is accomplished by contraction of the lateral pterygoid muscle on the opposite side, that is, to move the mandible to the left, contract the right lateral pterygoid muscle while the muscles of mastication on the left side stabilize the left condyle and hold it in place.

■ **What are the hyoid muscles?**

The hyoid muscles include two groups of muscles—the *suprahyoid* muscles running between the hyoid bone and the mandible and skull above it and the *infrahyoid* muscles running from the hyoid bone downward to the larynx, sternum, and shoulder blade (scapula).

■ **What is the function of the hyoid muscles?**

These muscles help depress and retrude the mandible as well as elevate the larynx during swallowing.

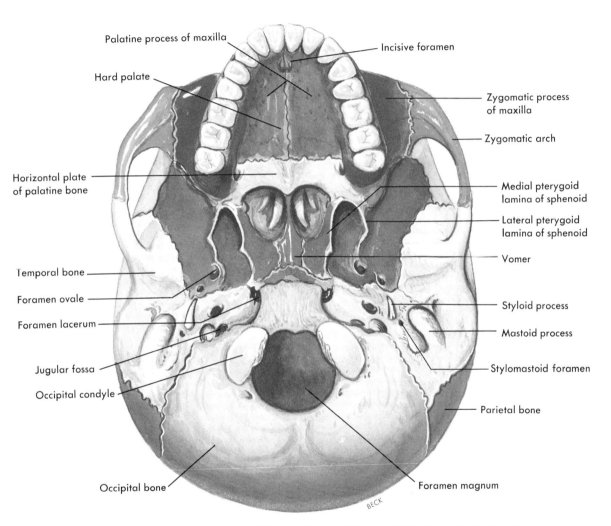

Palatine process of maxilla

Incisive foramen

Hard palate

Zygomatic process of maxilla

Zygomatic arch

Horizontal plate of palatine bone

Medial pterygoid lamina of sphenoid

Lateral pterygoid lamina of sphenoid

Vomer

Temporal bone

Foramen ovale

Foramen lacerum

Styloid process

Mastoid process

Jugular fossa

Occipital condyle

Stylomastoid foramen

Parietal bone

Occipital bone

Foramen magnum

BECK

Fig. 16-4. Skull viewed from below. (From Anthony, C. P., and Thibodeau, G. A.: Textbook of anatomy and physiology, ed. 10, St. Louis, 1979, The C. V. Mosby Co.)

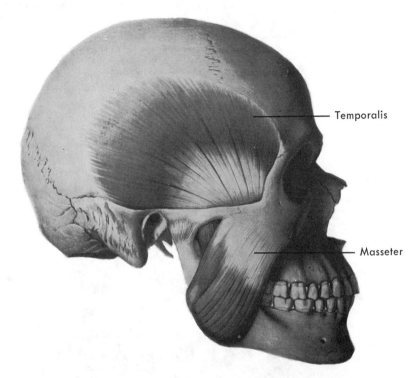

Fig. 16-5. Masseter and temporal muscles. (Sicher and Tandler: Anatomie für Zahnärzte.) (From Sicher, H., and DuBrul, E. L.: Oral anatomy, ed. 6, St. Louis, 1975, The C. V. Mosby Co.)

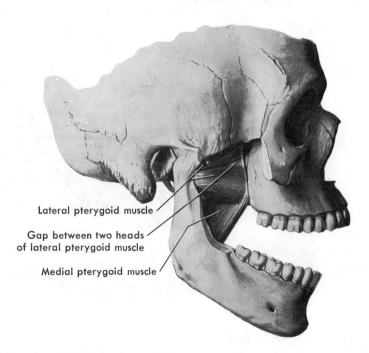

Fig. 16-6. Lateral and medial (external and internal) pterygoid muscles, lateral aspect, after removal of zygomatic arch and coronoid process. (Sicher and Tandler: Anatomie für Zahnärzte.) (From Sicher, H., and DuBrul, E. L.: Oral anatomy, ed. 6, St. Louis, 1975, The C. V. Mosby Co.)

Table 16-1. Muscles of mastication

Muscle	Origin	Insertion	Action	Nerve supply	Blood supply
Temporal	Entire temporal fossa on side of skull	Anterior fibers proceed vertically downward Posterior fibers run horizontally forward over the ear All fibers insert into the coronoid process of mandible	Overall contraction elevates mandible and closes the mouth If only the horizontal fibers are contracted, the mandible will retrude	Third division of trigeminal nerve (V_3)	Second part of maxillary artery
Masseter	Superficial portion from inferior border of anterior two thirds of the zygomatic arch Deep portion from inferior border of posterior one third of zygomatic arch and most of the medial surface of zygomatic arch	Into angle of mandible on lateral surface	Elevates mandible	Third division of trigeminal nerve	Second part of maxillary artery
Medial pterygoid	Major portion from medial wall of lateral pterygoid plate and adjacent fossa Also a small group of fibers from maxillary tuberosity	Into angle of mandible on medial surface	Elevates mandible	Third division of trigeminal nerve	Second part of maxillary artery
Lateral pterygoid	Minor (superior) origin from infratemporal crest of greater wing of sphenoid Major (inferior) origin from lateral wall of lateral pterygoid plate	Minor head into disc of temporomandibular joint and neck of condyle Major head into neck of condyle	Pulls disc and condyle forward in protrusive movement	Third division of trigeminal nerve	Second part of maxillary artery

■ **Which nerve innervates the muscles of facial expression?**

The muscles of facial expression are innervated by cranial nerve VII.

■ **Which muscle of facial expression plays an important role in the mastication of food?**

The buccinator muscle aids in moving food from the buccal vestibule back up onto the occlusal tables.

■ **To which parts of the oral cavity does the lingual artery supply blood?**

The lingual artery supplies blood to the tongue and the mucosa of the floor of the mouth including the mandibular lingual gingiva.

■ **Which branches of the maxillary artery supply blood to the oral cavity and the structures therein? List the area supplied by each branch.** (Fig. 16-7)

Inferior alveolar artery. This artery supplies all mandibular teeth and the marrow area of the mandible as well as the periodontium for those teeth.

Mental artery. This is a branch of the inferior alveolar artery coming out through the mental foramen. It supplies the facial gingiva of anterior teeth and the labial mucosa of the lower lip.

Buccal artery. The buccal artery supplies the mucosa of the cheek and the buccal gingiva for the maxillary and mandibular posterior teeth.

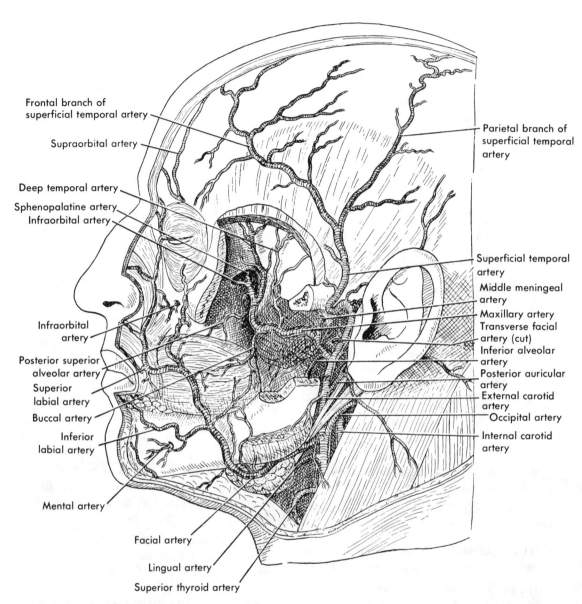

Frontal branch of
superficial temporal artery

Supraorbital artery

Deep temporal artery

Sphenopalatine artery
Infraorbital artery

Infraorbital
artery

Posterior superior
alveolar artery

Superior
labial artery

Buccal artery

Inferior
labial artery

Mental artery

Facial artery

Lingual artery

Superior thyroid artery

Parietal branch of
superficial temporal
artery

Superficial temporal
artery

Middle meningeal
artery

Maxillary artery

Transverse facial
artery (cut)

Inferior alveolar
artery

Posterior auricular
artery

External carotid
artery

Occipital artery

Internal carotid
artery

Fig. 16-7. Superficial and deep arteries of the face. (Modified and redrawn after Tandler: Lehrbuch der Anatomie.) (From Sicher, H., and DuBrul, E. L.: Oral anatomy, ed. 6, St. Louis, 1975, The C. V. Mosby Co.)

Table 16-2. Cranial nerves and their general function

Number	Name	Function
I	Olfactory	Sense of smell
II	Optic	Sense of sight
III	Oculomotor	Some movement of the eye
IV	Trochlear	More eye movement
V	Trigeminal	Sensation to skin of the face and oral mucosa; nerve supply to aid movement of jaw
VI	Abducent	More eye movement
VII	Facial	Muscles of facial expression, some salivary glands, and taste to anterior two thirds of tongue
VIII	Statoacoustic	Hearing and equilibrium
IX	Glossopharyngeal	Some salivary glands, taste, and sensation on posterior one third of tongue
X	Vagus	Speech, heart, and digestive tract
XI	Accessory (spinal accessory)	Muscles of posterior neck
XII	Hypoglossal	Muscles of tongue

Posterior superior alveolar artery. This artery supplies the maxillary molars and possibly the premolars as well as the marrow in that area and the periodontium of those teeth.

Descending palatine artery. This artery divides into a lesser palatine artery that supplies the soft palate and a greater palatine artery that supplies the hard palate and maxillary lingual gingiva.

Infraorbital artery. The infraorbital artery has a branch, the anterior superior alveolar artery, that supplies the anterior teeth and possibly the premolars as well as the marrow and periodontium of these teeth.

■ **What are the two main veins that drain the head and neck?**

The internal and external jugular veins supply drainage from the head and the neck.

■ **What is the pterygoid plexus of veins, and why is it important?**

The pterygoid plexus is an interconnecting network of veins posterior to the maxillary tuberosity that may be injured during a posterior superior alveolar injection with a hematoma developing as the result of this injury.

■ **What are the parts of the central nervous system (CNS) and the peripheral nervous system (PNS)?**

The central nervous system (CMS) is composed of the brain and spinal cord; the peripheral nervous system (PNS) is composed of the cranial nerves and the peripheral nerves or branches that come segmentally off of the spinal cord at vertebral levels.

■ **What are the names of the 12 pairs of cranial nerves, and what is the general function of each pair?**

The 12 pairs of cranial nerves (identified by Roman numerals) are given in Table 16-2.

■ **What are the branches of the second division of the trigeminal nerve that supply the oral cavity?** (See Fig. 16-8.)

The branches of the second division of the trigeminal nerve are

Posterior superior alveolar: the nerve supply to the second and third maxillary molars and all but the mesiobuccal root of the maxillary first molar

Middle superior alveolar: the nerve supply to the maxillary premolars and the mesiobuccal root of the maxillary first molar

Anterior superior alveolar: the nerve supply to the maxillary anterior teeth

Descending palatine nerve:

    Lesser palatine nerve—the nerve supply to the mucosa of the soft palate

    Greater palatine nerve—the nerve supply to the mucosa of the hard palate except for the area immediately lingual to the maxillary incisors

Nasopalatine nerve: the nerve supply to the

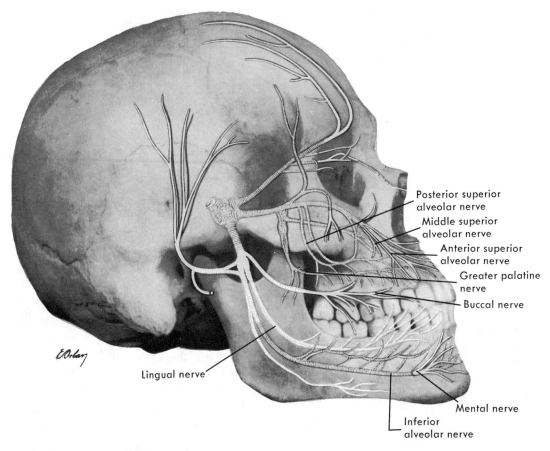

Posterior superior
alveolar nerve

Middle superior
alveolar nerve

Anterior superior
alveolar nerve

Greater palatine
nerve

Buccal nerve

Lingual nerve

Mental nerve

Inferior
alveolar nerve

Fig. 16-8. Diagrams of main sensory branches of trigeminal nerve. (From Sicher, H., and DuBrul, E. L.: Oral anatomy, ed. 6, St. Louis, 1975, The C. V. Mosby Co.)

mucosa immediately lingual to the maxillary incisors

Infraorbital nerve: the nerve supply to the labial mucosa and lip of maxillary anterior region

■ **What are the branches of the third division of the trigeminal nerve that supply the oral cavity and associated structures?**

The inferior alveolar nerve supplies all of the lower or mandibular teeth. It has two branches:

The mylohyoid nerve leaves the inferior alveolar nerve before it enters the mandibular foramen to supply the mylohyoid muscle and the anterior belly of the digastric muscle.

The mental nerve comes out through the mental foramen and supplies the facial gin-

giva and mucosa from the mandibular first premolar forward to the midline. It also supplies the mucosa of the lower lip.

The lingual nerve supplies general sensation to the anterior two thirds of the tongue and the mucosa of the floor of the mouth as well as the mandibular lingual mucosa. It also carries some fibers from nerve VII.

The buccal nerve supplies the buccal mucosa of the cheek as well as the buccal gingiva of mandibular and maxillary teeth.

The auriculotemporal nerve supplies the skin over the ear.

There are also branches for the muscles of mastication: the temporal and masseter muscles and the medial and lateral pterygoid muscles.

■ **What branches of cranial nerves VII, IX, and X supply the oral cavity?**

Facial nerve (cranial nerve VII). The *chorda tympani nerve* has two functions. First it carries taste from the anterior two thirds of the tongue, and it also carries parasympathetic (secretomotor) fibers to the submandibular gland and the sublingual gland. The *greater petrosal nerve* carries secretomotor fibers to the minor salivary glands of the roof of the mouth (palate) and the tonsil area.

Glossopharyngeal nerve (cranial nerve IX). The *lingual branch* of the glossopharyngeal nerve provides general sensation and taste to the posterior one third of the tongue. The *lesser petrosal nerve* joins with the auriculotemporal nerve of the third division of the trigeminal nerve and carries parasympathetic fibers to the parotid gland for secretomotor function.

Vagus nerve (cranial nerve X). The internal branch of the *superior laryngeal nerve* provides general sensation and taste to the base of the tongue.

■ **What are parasympathetic nerves, and what is their function in the head and neck region?**

The parasympathetic nerves are part of the autonomic, or automatic, nervous system that originates from cranial nerves III, VII, IX, and X as well as from sacral nerves in the lower back region. These nerves are primarily concerned with glandular secretion in the head and neck as well as with the supply of some smooth muscle located in the eye.

■ **In what two ways may infection spread in the head and neck?**

Infection may spread through a series of interconnected tubes and bean-shaped structures known as lymph nodes. Infection may also spread in the fascial spaces that are in between the muscles in the head and neck.

■ **What are the four major groups of lymph nodes associated with drainage of the structures of the oral cavity?** (See Fig. 16-9.)

The four major groups of lymph nodes are the submental, submandibular, upper deep cervical, and lower deep cervical.

■ **What happens to an infection in the area of the oral cavity that spreads by way of the fascial spaces?**

In general infection spreads in the spaces between muscles and from the oral cavity region down to the sides of the neck. From there the infection may travel behind the esophagus and downward into the posterior mediastinum or chest region. If the infection reaches this area, it will generally cause death. Most infections are treated with antibiotics before reaching the chest region.

■ **What are primary, secondary, and tertiary nodes?**

Primary, secondary, and tertiary refer to the lymph nodes involved in the spread of infection and the order in which they become involved. A primary node is the first node or group of nodes involved. If an infection is not stopped or overcome by the primary node, it will spread to secondary nodes. If it is not stopped by this group of nodes, it will spread to a third, or tertiary, group of nodes. An example of this would be infection of a mandibular central incisor. The submental nodes would be the primary nodes involved. From there an infection would spread to the submandibular nodes (secondary nodes). The infection would spread from there to the upper deep cervical nodes (tertiary nodes). By comparison, if a mandibular premolar was initially infected, the primary nodes of involvement would be the submandibular nodes, the secondary nodes of involvement would be the upper deep cervical nodes, and the tertiary nodes of involvement would be the lower deep cervical nodes. Therefore, nodes may be primary, secondary, or tertiary depending on the original source or focus of infection.

■ **Where are the major salivary glands located, and where do their ducts open?** (See Fig. 16-10.)

Parotid glands. This pair of glands is located on the side of the face in front of the ear and on the surface of the masseter muscle. Their ducts run forward and medially and open into the oral cavity on a small elevation of tissue opposite the maxillary second molar.

Submandibular glands. These glands are lo-

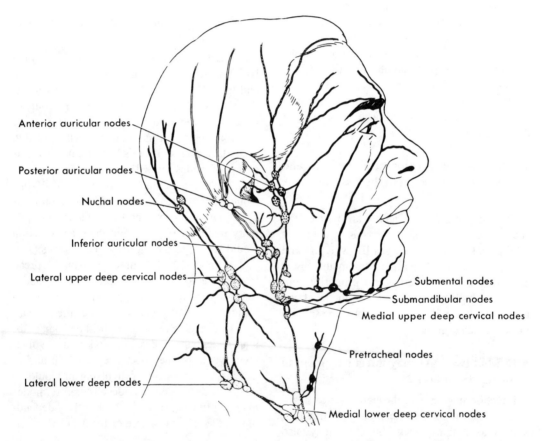

Anterior auricular nodes

Posterior auricular nodes

Nuchal nodes

Inferior auricular nodes

Lateral upper deep cervical nodes

Lateral lower deep nodes

Submental nodes

Submandibular nodes

Medial upper deep cervical nodes

Pretracheal nodes

Medial lower deep cervical nodes

Fig. 16-9. Regional lymph nodes and lymph vessels of superficial structures of head and neck. (Modified after Tandler: Lehrbuch der Anatomie.) (From Sicher, H., and DuBrul, E. L.: Oral anatomy, ed. 6, St. Louis, 1975, The C. V. Mosby Co.)

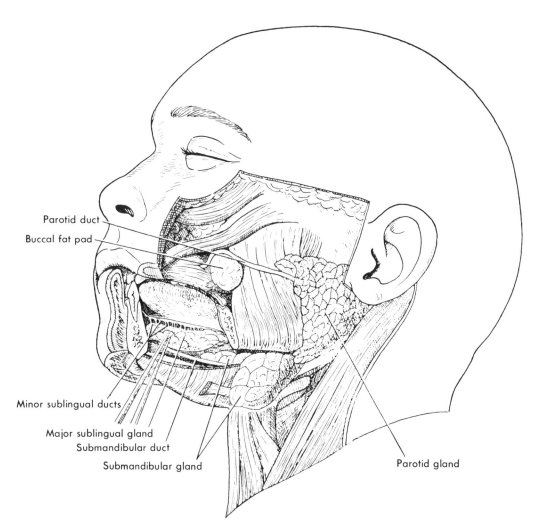

Fig. 16-10. Major glands of oral cavity after removal of part of left mandibular body. (Modified and redrawn after Sicher and Tandler: Anatomie für Zahnärzte.) (From Sicher, H., and DuBrul, E. L.: Oral anatomy, ed. 6, St. Louis, 1975, The C. V. Mosby Co.)

cated in the posterolateral part of the floor of the mouth beneath the angle of the mandible. The ducts run forward in the floor of the mouth and open onto the small elevations at the base of the lingual frenum. These elevations are known as the *sublingual caruncles*.

Sublingual glands. The sublingual glands are located in the floor of the mouth just lingual to the mandibular canines. They have multiple ducts that open into the floor of the mouth along a small fold of tissue beneath the tongue known as the *sublingual fold*. Each of these two glands may also have one duct that is larger than the rest which opens along with the submandibular duct onto the sublingual caruncle.

■ **Where are the minor salivary glands located, and what is their duct arrangement?**

Labial glands: located in the upper and lower lip

Buccal glands: located in the cheeks

Sublingual glands: located in the floor of the mouth

Glossopalatine glands: located in the tonsillar pillars

Palatine glands: located in the posterior hard palate and in the entire soft palate

Lingual glands: located in the tongue

These minor glands all have multiple ducts instead of one or two large ducts.

■ **What are the papillae of the tongue, where are they located, and what is their function?**

The papillae are raised, or elevated, areas of the tongue. There are four groups and their location and function are as follows:

Filiform papillae. These are small pointed projections all over the upper, or dorsal, surface of the tongue. They function for general sensation. In the cat's tongue they are very elongated and give it the rough texture that you feel when a cat licks your hand.

Fungiform papillae. These small rounded elevations cover the anterior two thirds of the tongue on the dorsal surface. Many times these will appear reddened. A few taste buds are located in the fungiform papillae, and therefore these papillae provide some sensations of taste.

Vallate, or circumvallate, papillae. These are a V-shaped row of about 13 large, rounded, raised papillae that divide the anterior two thirds of the tongue from the posterior one third of the tongue. Many taste buds are located in these papillae.

Foliate papillae. Several vertical rows of foliate papillae are located on the lateral surface of the tongue about two thirds of the way back. In lower forms of animals a number of taste buds are located in these papillae, but in man the foliate papillae are poorly developed, or rudimentary, and have no taste buds.

■ **What are the intrinsic and extrinsic muscles of the tongue?**

The *intrinsic* muscles of the tongue are the muscles that begin and end within the tongue. They are named according to their grouping: superior longitudinal, inferior longitudinal, vertical, and transverse. The *extrinsic* muscles of the tongue are those muscles that originate outside the tongue and end within it. They are the genioglossus, hyoglossus, styloglossus, and palatoglossus muscles.

■ **What are the three types of mucosa found in the oral cavity?**

The mucosa of the oral cavity include

Specialized mucosa: refers to the dorsum of the tongue and the papillae discussed previously

Masticatory mucosa: the mucosa of the hard palate and the gingiva surrounding the teeth

Lining mucosa: includes all other mucosa of the oral cavity

■ **What are the subdivisions of the gingiva?**

The subdivisions of the gingiva include

Free gingiva. This gingiva forms the gingival sulcus. It is about 2 mm in length.

Attached gingiva. This gingiva runs from the free gingiva toward the vestibule and changes into alveolar mucosa.

Interdental papillae. These projections of gingiva between the teeth protect the interproximal spaces.

■ **What are frenula, and where are they located?**

Frenula are folds of tissue that extend from

the lips, tongue, and cheeks and attach to the gingiva. They are located labially at the midline of the mandible and maxilla, as well as lingually in the mandible and in the canine region in both maxilla and mandible. They are less well developed in these latter areas.

■ **What is the vestibule?**

The vestibule is the space between the lips or cheeks and the teeth. Its upper and lower boundaries are known as the *mucobuccal folds* or *mucolabial folds*.

■ **What are the posterior boundaries of the oral cavity?**

The posterior boundaries of the oral cavity are the *fauces,* or *anterior* and *posterior palatine pillars*. These are the folds of tissue in front of and behind the palatine tonsil that are formed by the palatoglossus and palatopharyngeal muscles, respectively.

■ **What forms the floor of the mouth?**

Although the floor of the mouth is formed by the mucous membrane, in reality it is the mylohyoid muscle beneath it that actually forms and supports the floor of the mouth.

MULTIPLE-CHOICE QUESTIONS

1. Venous blood flows from the internal jugular vein into the _____ vein.
   a. External jugular
   b. Maxillary
   c. Brachiocephalic (innominate)
   d. None of the above

2. Which of the following does *not* happen when the sympathetic nervous system is stimulated?
   a. The skin blanches.
   b. One experiences the sensation of a knot in the stomach.
   c. The heart rate slows.
   d. The muscles receive more blood.

3. Which of the following should *not* be done for hemorrhagic shock?
   a. Attempt to stop the bleeding.
   b. Keep the patient's head raised slightly higher than rest of body.
   c. Keep the patient warm.
   d. Keep the patient still.

4. In the respiratory system, air passing into the lungs passes from the secondary bronchi directly into the:
   a. Primary bronchi
   b. Terminal bronchiole
   c. Alveolar ducts
   d. Respiratory bronchiole
   e. None of the above

5. What separates the blood from the air in the lungs?
   a. A single cell wall
   b. Two cell walls
   c. Three cell walls
   d. Four cell walls
   e. None of the above

6. Why are the lungs always somewhat expanded?
   a. The lungs are under negative pressure.
   b. The pleural spaces are under pressure.
   c. The pleural spaces are the same pressure as the lungs.
   d. None of the above.

7. A pneumothorax is:
   a. A bacterial disease of the lung
   b. A collapsed lung
   c. An oversized rib cage
   d. None of the above

8. An allergic reaction can be treated by administering:
   a. Antihistaminic
   b. Histamine
   c. Procaine hydrochloride (Novocain)
   d. Lidocaine (Xylocaine)
   e. None of the above

9. Which of the following structures help to control blood pressure?
   a. Carotid body
   b. Phrenic nerve
   c. Hypoglossal nerve
   d. None of the above

10. Which of the following glands is *not* associated with the digestive system?
    a. Pancreas

b. Pituitary
c. Gallbladder
d. Liver
e. None of the above

11. The gallbladder functions to break down:
    a. Sugar
    b. Carbohydrates
    c. Proteins
    d. Fats
    e. None of the above

12. The main functioning unit of the kidney is the:
    a. Ureter
    b. Calyx
    c. Nephron
    d. None of the above

13. Increase in urination, hunger, and thirst are classic signs of:
    a. Nephritis
    b. Cancer
    c. Diabetes
    d. Epilepsy

14. Which of the following is *not* part of the endocrine system?
    a. Parotid gland
    b. Thyroid gland
    c. Adrenal (suprarenal) gland
    d. Pancreatic islets of Langerhans

15. The basal metabolic rate of the body is primarily controlled by the:
    a. Adrenal gland
    b. Thyroid gland
    c. Parathyroid gland
    d. Pineal body

16. The islets of Langerhans in the pancreas produce:
    a. Insulin
    b. Adrenaline
    c. Bile
    d. Ptyalin

17. Which of the following bones is *not* a part of the neurocranium that surrounds the brain?
    a. Parietal
    b. Zygomatic
    c. Occipital
    d. Frontal

18. Which of the following is a muscle of mastication:
    a. Buccinator

b. Digastric
c. Medial pterygoid
d. Mylohyoid

19. Lateral excursions of the mandible are primarily accomplished by contraction of the _____ muscle.
    a. Temporal
    b. Digastric
    c. Lateral pterygoid
    d. Masseter

20. The muscles of facial expression are innervated by cranial nerve:
    a. V
    b. VII
    c. IX
    d. X

21. The major blood supply to the oral cavity and its structures is through the:
    a. Maxillary artery
    b. Lingual artery
    c. Facial artery
    d. Pterygoid artery

22. Which of the following teeth is frequently supplied by two different nerves?
    a. Mandibular second molar
    b. Maxillary second molar
    c. Maxillary first molar
    d. Maxillary first premolar
    e. None of the above

23. The muscles of mastication are supplied by branches of the:
    a. First division of the trigeminal nerve (V_1)
    b. Second division of the trigeminal nerve (V_2)
    c. Third division of the trigeminal nerve (V_3)
    d. None of the above

24. Which of the following nerves does *not* supply part of the oral cavity?
    a. Cranial nerve VII
    b. Cranial nerve VIII
    c. Cranial nerve IX
    d. Cranial nerve X

25. The sublingual caruncle is the primary opening of which gland?
    a. Parotid
    b. Submandibular
    c. Sublingual
    d. None of the above

26. Which of the following papillae of the tongue contain the most taste buds per papilla?
    a. Filiform
    b. Foliate
    c. Fungiform
    d. Circumvallate
27. The mucosa of the hard palate is an example of _____ mucosa.
    a. Lining
    b. Specialized
    c. Masticatory
    d. None of the above
    e. All of the above
28. The muscle that forms the floor of the mouth is the _____ muscle.
    a. Diagastric
    b. Mylohyoid
    c. Geniohyoid
    d. Omohyoid

SUGGESTED READINGS

Anthony, C. P., and Kolthoff, N. J.: Textbook of anatomy and physiology, ed. 9, St. Louis, 1975, The C. V. Mosby Co.

Brand, R. W., and Isselhard, D. E.: Anatomy of orofacial structures, St. Louis, 1977, The C. V. Mosby Co.

Dunn, M. J., and Shapiro, C.: Dental auxiliary practice, Module 1, Dental anatomy, head and neck anatomy, Baltimore, 1975, The Williams & Wilkins Co.

Fried, L.: Anatomy of the head, neck, face, and jaws, Philadelphia, 1976, Lea & Febiger.

Greisheimer, E., and Wiedeman, M.: Physiology and anatomy, ed. 9, New York, 1975, Macmillan, Inc.

Langley, L., Cheraskin, E., and Sleeper, R.: Dynamic anatomy and physiology, ed. 2, New York, 1973, McGraw-Hill Book Co.

Pansky, B.: Review of gross anatomy, ed. 2, New York, 1975, Macmillan, Inc.

Reed, G., and Sheppard, V.: Basic structure of head and neck, Philadelphia, 1976, W. B. Saunders Co.

Taylor, N., and McPhedran, M.: Basic physiology and anatomy, New York, 1965, G. P. Putnam's Sons.

CHAPTER 17

Dental anatomy

SHIRLEY A. WILSON

■ **Which structures are to be considered when studying dental anatomy?**

Dental anatomy is the study of the teeth and their supporting structures.

■ **A tooth is composed of both hard and soft tissues. Name these tissues.**

The hard tissues are enamel, dentin, and cementum. The pulp is the soft tissue (See Fig. 17-1.)

■ **What is enamel?**

Enamel is the hardest, most calcified, and most brittle of the body tissues. Its chemical composition is 96% inorganic matter and 4% organic matter and water. Enamel covers the coronal portion of the tooth. Its color depends on the translucence of the enamel or the color of the underlying dentin, and the color can vary from yellow to white to greyish white.

■ **What is dentin?**

Dentin is a yellow hard calcified tissue that is harder than bone but softer than enamel. Its chemical composition is 70% inorganic matter and 30% organic matter and water. Dentin makes up the bulk of the tooth structure. It surrounds the pulp cavity and is covered by enamel in the anatomic crown and by cementum in the root.

■ **What is cementum?**

Cementum is another hard tissue whose chemical composition is 50% inorganic matter and 50% organic matter. It covers the dentin of the root of a tooth and along with the peri-

odontal ligament functions as a means of attaching the tooth to the alveolar bone.

■ **What is the dental pulp?**

The pulp is the soft connective tissue organ found in the central portion of a tooth surrounded by dentin. It contains an abundant nerve, vascular, and lymph supply. Although the pulp is one continuous tissue it may be divided into two areas:

Pulp chamber. This is the enlarged portion of the pulp cavity that is found in the coronal portion of the tooth and that has pulpal horns which correspond to and extend toward the cusp tips and incisal edges.

Pulp canal. That portion of the pulp cavity located in the root area is the pulp canal. The constricted opening(s) at or near the root apex through which the nutrient and nerve supply enter and exit is called the *apical foramen.*

■ **What are the supporting structures of a tooth?**

The supporting structures, also referred to as the *periodontium,* are divided into two sections referred to as the gingival unit and the attachment apparatus.

Gingival unit	Attachment apparatus
Gingivae (free and attached)	Cementum
	Periodontal ligament
Alveolar mucosa	Bone

■ **Explain the functions of teeth.**

Tooth design is related to the following functions:

Efficient mastication of food

Esthetics

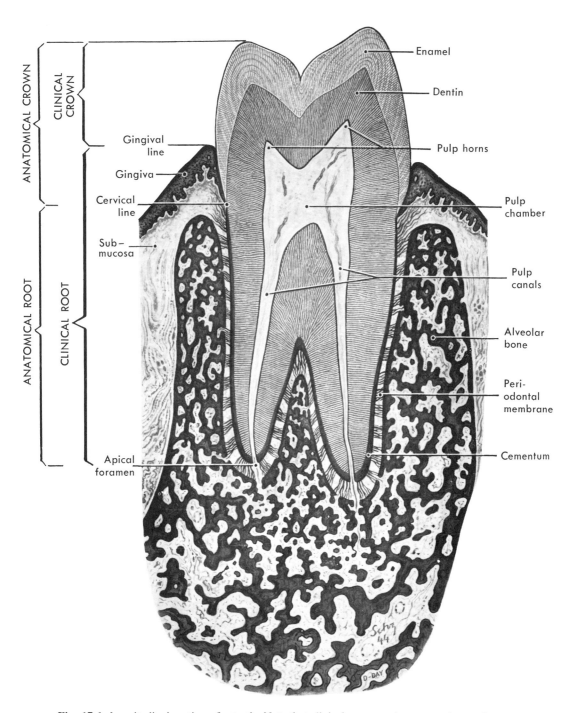

Fig. 17-1. Longitudinal section of a tooth. Note that clinical crown and root can change, but anatomic crown:root ratio must always remain the same. (Zeisz and Nuckolls.) (From Brand, R. W., and Isselhard, D. E.: Anatomy of orofacial structures, St. Louis, 1977, The C. V. Mosby Co.)

Table 17-1. Primary dentition eruption schedule

Tooth	Age of eruption (months)	
	Mandible	**Maxilla**
Central incisor	6	7½
Lateral incisor	7	9
Canines	16	19
First molar	12	14
Second molar	20	24

Table 17-2. Permanent dentition eruption schedule

Tooth	Age of eruption (years)	
	Mandible	**Maxilla**
Central incisor	6 to 7	7 to 8
Lateral incisor	7 to 8	8 to 9
Canines	11 to 12	11 to 12
First premolar	10 to 12	10 to 11
Second premolar	11 to 12	10 to 12
First molar	5 to 6	5½ to 7
Second molar	11 to 13	12 to 13
Third molar	17 to 21	17 to 21

Speech production
Protection of the supporting structures
Maintain stability of adjacent teeth

■ **What is the eruption pattern of the primary dentition?**

As a general rule, the mandibular primary dentition precedes its maxillary counterpart in eruption (Table 17-1).

■ **What are the fundamental differences between primary and permanent dentition?**

The crowns of the primary anterior teeth are wider mesiodistally in comparison to their cervicoincisal length than are the crowns of the permanent anterior teeth.

The roots of the primary anterior teeth are longer and narrower compared to the roots of the permanent anterior teeth.

The labial and lingual surfaces of the anterior primary teeth have more prominent cervical ridges, when viewed from the mesial or distal surfaces, than do the labial and lingual surfaces of the permanent anterior teeth.

The crowns of the primary molars, when viewed from the buccal surface, are narrower at the cervical third area than are the crowns of the permanent molars.

The cervical ridge on the buccal surface of the primary molars is quite pronounced.

The buccal and lingual surfaces of the primary molars are flatter above the cervical ridge. This taper causes a narrowing of the occlusal surface of the primary molars.

The roots of the primary molars are narrower and longer in comparison to those of the permanent molars, with a flare that extends beyond the crown outline. This flare facilitates room between the roots for development of the permanent tooth.

The pulp chambers are larger and the pulpal horns are higher in the primary dentition than in the permanent dentition.

The enamel of the primary teeth is thinner than that of the permanent teeth.

The color of the primary dentition is generally lighter than that of the permanent dentition.

■ **What is root resorption?**

The phenomenon is thought to occur when the permanent tooth root is developing and increasing in length causing pressure on the root of the primary tooth. It is felt that this pressure causes *osteoclasts* to form and begin destroying the primary root dentin and cementum. This is a progressive but intermittent process. It is important to point out that it is possible for a primary tooth to undergo root resorption without the presence of an underlying developing permanent tooth being present as well as when a primary tooth is retained in the presence of a permanent tooth.

■ **What is the eruption schedule for the permanent dentition?**

Again, it is important to note that the mandibular teeth normally erupt before their maxillary counterparts (Table 17-2).

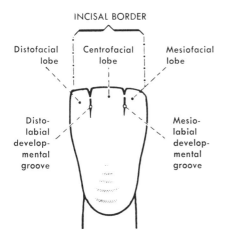

INCISAL BORDER

Distofacial lobe | Centrofacial lobe | Mesiofacial lobe

Disto-labial developmental groove

Mesio-labial developmental groove

Fig. 17-2. Incisal edge of three labial lobes are formed from mamelons. (Zeisz and Nuckolls.) (From Brand, R. W., and Isselhard, D. E.: Anatomy of orofacial structures, St. Louis, 1977, The C. V. Mosby Co.)

■ How many lobes form an anterior tooth?

All anterior teeth develop from four lobes, three labially and one lingually. The three scalloped lobes (mamelons) (Fig. 17-2) on the newly erupted incisal edges are worn away soon after eruption. Developmental lines separate these labial lobes. The lingual lobe is called a *cingulum.*

■ How many lobes form a posterior tooth?

The number of lobes necessary in the development of a tooth depend on the number of cusps the tooth will have. For example, the maxillary premolars and the mandibular first premolar form from three buccal lobes and one lingual lobe. The mandibular second premolar may have two cusps or three cusps. If it has two cusps, it will have the same arrangement as the mandibular first premolar; however, if it has three cusps, it will have three buccal lobes and two lingual lobes. All molars have two buccal and two lingual lobes with the exception of the first molars which have a fifth lobe.

■ What are succedaneous teeth?

Succedaneous teeth are permanent teeth that replace or succeed the primary teeth. The permanent molars are nonsuccedaneous teeth because they do not replace primary teeth.

■ Define "line angles."

A *line angle* is the angle formed by the junction of two surfaces and derives its name from the two surfaces it joins. In the anterior teeth the line angles are

Mesiolabial	Distolabial
Mesiolingual	Distolingual
Linguoincisal	Labioincisal

In posterior teeth the line angles are

Mesiobuccal	Distobuccal
Mesiolingual	Distolingual
Mesio-occlusal	Disto-occlusal
Bucco-occlusal	Linguo-occlusal

■ Define "point angles."

A *point angle* is formed by the junction of three surfaces and also derives its name from the surfaces that join to form it. In the anterior teeth the point angles are

Mesiolabioincisal
Distolabioincisal
Mesiolinguoincisal
Distolinguoincisal

In posterior teeth the point angles are

Mesiobucco-occlusal
Distobucco-occlusal
Mesiolinguo-occlusal
Distolinguo-occlusal

■ Identify and define the anatomic landmarks of a tooth.

Anatomic crown: the whole crown of a tooth covered by enamel (Fig. 17-1).

Clinical crown: the part of the crown that is visible above the gingiva. Any nonerupted area is not part of the clinical crown (Fig. 17-1).

Cementoenamel junction (CEJ): the line around the external surface of a tooth where the cementum and enamel meet. It is also referred to as the cervical line, neck, or cervix of a tooth (Fig. 17-1).

Contact area: the area in which the mesial and distal surfaces of adjacent teeth make contact. All teeth have two contact areas except the most distal tooth which has no distal contact area (Fig. 17-3).

Embrasure: the triangular-shaped space that widens out from the contact area labially, buccally, or lingually. It serves as a spillway for the escape of food and makes the teeth self-

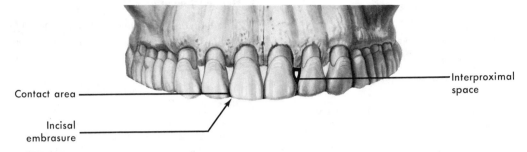

Contact area

Incisal embrasure

Interproximal space

Fig. 17-3. Arrow points to incisal embrasure. Area cervical to contact area is gingival embrasure, also called interproximal space. Interproximal space is outlined as triangle. (Zeisz and Nuckolls.) (From Brand, R. W., and Isselhard, D. E.: Anatomy of orofacial structures, St. Louis, 1977, The C. V. Mosby Co.)

cleansing because the rounded coronal surface is exposed to the cleansing action of oral fluids and the friction of the cheeks, lips, and tongue (Fig. 17-3).

Cusp: the elevated projection on the crown of a tooth that makes up a divisional portion of the occlusal surface.

Tubercle: a small elevation on a crown produced by an extra formation of enamel.

Cingulum: a large rounded eminence of enamel located on the cervical third of the lingual surface of the primary and permanent anterior teeth (Fig. 17-4).

Ridge: any linear elevation on the surface of a crown. It is named by location. Examples of ridges are the following:

Marginal ridges. These rounded elevations are found on the mesial and distal margins of the occlusal surfaces of premolars and molars and on the mesial and distal margins on the lingual surfaces of the incisors and canines (Fig. 17-4).

Triangular ridge. These ridges descend from the tips of the cusps on posterior teeth toward the central portion of the occlusal surface. They are labeled triangular because the slopes on either side of the ridge appear as two sides of a triangle (Fig. 17-5).

Transverse ridge. The union of two triangular ridges, one from a lingual cusp and the other from a buccal cusp crossing the occlusal surface of a posterior tooth is called a transverse ridge.

Oblique ridge. A ridge formed by the union

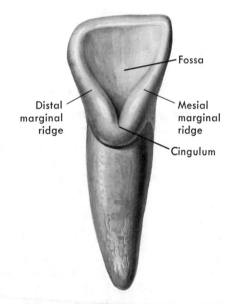

Fossa

Distal marginal ridge

Mesial marginal ridge

Cingulum

Fig. 17-4. Lingual view of central incisor. (Zeisz and Nuckolls.) (From Brand, R. W., and Isselhard, D. E.: Anatomy of orofacial structures, St. Louis, 1977, The C. V. Mosby Co.)

of two triangular ridges but crossing the occlusal surface of the maxillary molars obliquely from the mesiolingual to distobuccal cusps.

Inclined plane. The sloping area between cusp ridges is called an inclined plane and is generally labeled by the combined names of the two cusp ridges between which it lies.

Fossa. The fossa is an irregular depression or concavity on the tooth surface (Fig. 17-4).

Sulcus. The sulcus is a long depression in the surface of a tooth between ridges and cusps. In

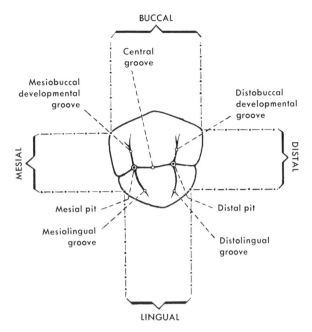

Fig. 17-5. Occlusal surface, H type (two-cusp variety). (Zeisz and Nuckolls.) (From Brand, R. W., and Isselhard, D. E.: Anatomy of orofacial structures, St. Louis, 1977, The C. V. Mosby Co.)

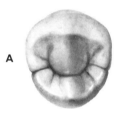

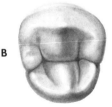

Fig. 17-6. A, Occlusal view, U type; **B,** occlusal view, H type; **C,** occlusal view, Y type. (Zeisz and Nuckolls.) (From Brand, R. W., and Isselhard, D. E.: Anatomy of orofacial structures, St. Louis, 1977, The C. V. Mosby Co.)

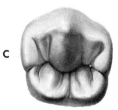

cross section the sulcus is V shaped, with a developmental groove found at the bottom.

Developmental groove. This groove or line designates the junction of the lobes on the crown of the tooth (Figs. 17-2, 17-5, and 17-6).

Supplemental groove. This shallow depression is irregular in direction or extent, is less distinct than a developmental groove, and does *not* denote the junction of the lobes.

Pit. This is a small pinpoint depression located where developmental grooves intersect or at the termination of a single developmental groove (Fig. 17-5).

Fissure. This crevice or fault in a tooth surface results from the failure of the enamel of the primary parts to fuse.

■ **Review the major characteristics of the permanent dentition.**

The important characteristics of each permanent tooth are given in Tables 17-3 to 17-7.

Text continued on p. 156.

Table 17-3. Incisor characteristics

Maxillary central	Maxillary lateral*	Mandibular central	Mandibular lateral
Labial aspect			
Wide mesiodistally	Narrow mesiodistally	Narrow mesiodistally	Slightly wider mesiodistally
Mesial outline nearly straight	Mesial outline slightly	Mesial outline straight	than mandibular central
Mesioincisal angle sharp	rounded	Mesial contact near the in-	Distoincisal margins slope
Distal outline convex	Mesioincisal angle slightly	cisal edge	slightly toward gingiva,
Distoincisal angle slightly	rounded	Mesioincisal and distoincisal	which causes a more
rounded	Distal outline more round-	angles quite sharp	rounded angle and creates
Labial surface flat with the	ed than on central incisor	Three mamelons present on	short distal outline com-
height of contour on the	Distoincisal angle noticeably	newly erupted teeth, but	pared to mesial outline
cervical third	more rounded than that of	incisal edges wear quickly	
	central incisor	and evenly	
	Labial surface rounded with	Flat labial surface	
	height of contour in the		
	cervical third		
Lingual aspect			
Lingual fossa moderately	Mesial and distal marginal	Mesial and distal marginal	Landmarks on this surface
deep and bordered by	ridges and cingulum more	ridges not prominent	also are not prominent as
heavy marginal ridges, the	prominent and lingual	Cingulum low and broad	on the mandibular central
cingulum and the incisal	fossa deeper than central	Fossa shallow	incisor
edge	incisor		
Height of contour is at the	A linguogingival groove with		
greatest convexity of the	a pit near the center is		
cingulum	common		
	Height of contour is with		
	greatest curvature of the		
	cingulum		
Mesial aspect			
Cervical line curves evenly	Cervical line shallower than		
and has greatest depth of	on maxillary central incisor		
curvature of all teeth	Contact area larger and wider		
Contact area in incisal third	and located at junction of		
near incisal edge	the incisal and middle		
Only mesial contact area in	thirds		
maxilla that contacts an-			
other mesial contact sur-			
face			

*Anomalies are common to this tooth.

Table 17-3. Incisor characteristics—cont'd

Maxillary central	Maxillary lateral	Mandibular central	Mandibular lateral
Distal aspect			
Less cervical line curvature Contact area at junction of incisal and middle thirds	Smaller and more convex in all dimensions than mesial aspect Contact area at middle third		Contact area at junction of incisal and middle thirds and is only mandibular incisor contact area not located in incisal third
Incisal aspect			
General outline triangular Portions of lingual fossa and cingulum visible Lingual surface narrower mesiodistally than labial surface Labial surface slightly convex	General outline ovoid Labial and lingual surfaces quite convex from this view	Straight incisal edge Mesial and distal symmetrical from this view	Crown appears twisted distolingually
Root			
Single, cone shaped, and relatively straight with rounded apex	Single, narrow, and flattened mesiodistally; thick labiolingually Apex sharper than on maxillary central incisor and inclined distally	Single and straight with sharp apex	Single; longer, slightly thicker, and wider than mandibular central incisors

Table 17-4. Canine characteristics

Maxillary canine	Mandibular canine
Labial aspect	
Labial outline convex in all directions, but more pronounced mesiodistally	Labial surface appears longer cervicoincisally than on maxillary canine because of narrow mesiodistal measurement and height of contact areas
Mesial outline convex from contact area to cervical line with short, rounded mesioincisal angle	Labial ridge not as prominent as on maxillary canine
Distal outline concave from cervical line to contact point	Mesial outline is straight from contact to cervical line
Labial ridge on well-developed middle labial lobe extending from cervical line to incisal edge with slight developmental depression on either side of ridge	Mesial contact area in incisal third near mesioincisal angle
	Distal outline convex cervicoincisally
	Distal contact at junction of middle and incisal thirds
Lingual aspect	
Cingulum bulky and similar to a small cusp	Entire surface flatter than that of maxillary canine
Well-developed marginal ridges	Landmarks less prominent
Lingual ridge extending from below cingulum to incisal edge dividing fossa into two fossae	
Mesial aspect	
Wider labiolingually than any other incisor	Appears triangular in shape, but narrower labiolingually than maxillary canine
Appears triangular in shape	Flattened area above cervical line
Contact area at the junction of the middle and incisal thirds	
Distal aspect	
Contact area located in middle of the middle third	Similar to mesial surface except smaller in all dimensions
	No flattened area above cervical line as on mesial aspect
Incisal edge	
Crown not symmetrical; mesial portion thicker and more convex; the distal, thinner and somewhat concave	Similar to that of maxillary canine
Root	
Single; tapered, slightly blunt apex; and tipped distally	Normally single and straight
Longest root in mouth with mesial and distal developmental grooves that provide anchorage	Narrow mesiodistally and thick labiolingually
	Labial and lingual surfaces convex; mesial and distal surfaces concave which causes concavities that extend entire root length
	Occasionally bifurcation with labial and lingual roots

Table 17-5. Premolar characteristics

Maxillary first	Maxillary second	Mandibular first	Mandibular second
Buccal aspect			
Resembles both maxillary canine and second premolar	Buccal cusp not as long or as sharp as that of first premolar	Resembles both mandibular canine and second premolar	Resembles first premolar from this aspect only except that crown is larger
Prominent buccal ridge extending from cervical line to buccal cusp tip resulting from the considerable development of middle buccal lobe	Mesio-occlusal slope shorter than disto-occlusal slope	Buccal cusp tip pointed and off center to the mesial aspect	buccal cusp is shorter
Mesiobuccal and distobuccal developmental depressions on either side of ridge		Mesial slope straight	Mesio-occlusal and disto-occlusal slopes are symmetrical
		Slight concavity of distal slope	

Table 17-5. Premolar characteristics—cont'd

Maxillary first	Maxillary second	Mandibular first	Mandibular second
Lingual aspect			
Crown convex in all directions Lingual cusp shorter than the buccal cusp; as a result both cusp tips visible from this view	Similar to first premolar except that lingual cusp is longer, which causes less visibility of occlusal surface from this view	Crown convex in all directions Lingual cusp much smaller than buccal cusp Occlusal surface visible from this view Mesiolingual developmental groove	Lingual cusp or cusps well developed If there are two lingual cusps, a lingual groove will separate them
Mesial aspect			
Concavity in cervical third, referred to as a mesial developmental depression Well-defined mesial developmental groove that extends from occlusal surface over mesial marginal ridge Contact area located at junction of occlusal and middle third	Both cusps appear to be the same height No mesial marginal developmental groove No mesial concavity in cervical third; it is convex Contact area in junction of occlusal and middle third	Occlusal surface inclined lingually Contact area close to occlusal surface Mesiolingual developmental groove	Contact area close to occlusal surface Marginal ridge horizontal Mesial marginal groove
Distal aspect			
Contact area located in middle third	Both cusps appear to be the same height Contact area in middle third	Distal marginal groove Contact area closer to middle third	Contact area near occlusal surface
Occlusal aspect			
Occlusal outline is hexagonal Two cusps Buccal cusp more prominent than lingual cusp Mesiobuccal and distobuccal ridges have sharp slopes Transverse ridge Central developmental groove extends mesiodistally from mesial pit to distal pit over mesial marginal ridge Central, mesial marginal, and buccal grooves create trait design Supplemental grooves are rarely present	Occlusal outline more rounded and less angular Two cusps Central groove short with several supplemental grooves that often give a folded or wrinkled effect Well-developed marginal ridges	Diamond-shaped occlusal outline Large buccal cusp centered over long axis of the root Lingual cusp appears to be more of a tubercle than a real cusp Transverse ridge Mesial marginal ridge slopes from buccal to lingual Distal marginal ridge is longer and more prominent	Square-shaped occlusal outline Three-cusped type (Y type): buccal cusp, mesiolingual cusp, and distolingual cusp Two-cusped type (U type; H type is rare): buccal cusp and lingual cusp "Y", "H", and "U" relate to general groove pattern (Fig. 17-6) Buccal and lingual cusps almost the same size
Root			
Normally two roots, one buccal and one lingual Bifurcation in apical third Occasionally a single root	Normally single, tapered to a blunt apex, and slightly tipped to distal aspect	Normally single and straight with sharp apex	Normally single with tapered blunt apex slightly tipped to distal aspect

Table 17-6. Maxillary molar characteristics

First molar	Second molar	Third molar
Buccal aspect		
Two cusps; the mesiobuccal cusp is broad mesiodistally and the distobuccal cusp is sharp Buccal developmental groove Crown is short cervico-occlusally	Crown smaller in all dimensions than that of first molar Mesiobuccal cusp is large because buccal groove is located distally more than that of first molar; this creates smaller distobuccal cusp	Most variable tooth in maxillary arch; difficult to describe a standard design Crown smaller in all dimensions than crowns of preceding molars Occlusal outline generally heart shaped Generally only three cusps: mesiobuccal, distobuccal, and mesiolingual Variable groove pattern with many supplemental grooves
Lingual aspect		
Two cusps; the mesiolingual cusp is larger than the distolingual cusp Distolingual developmental groove Fifth cusp or tubercle cusp of Carabelli is evident on lingual portion of mesiolingual cusp	Distolingual cusp smaller in all dimensions No cusp of Carabelli	
Mesial aspect		
Wider at the cervical area than at the occlusal area Convex in the cervical third, becoming slightly concave in the middle third, and then relatively straight to the occlusal surface Well-developed marginal ridge	Cervical concavity as seen on first molar often not apparent on this tooth Contact area larger because of contact with adjacent molar	
Distal aspect		
Marginal ridge less prominent than the mesial; it tips cervically so more of the occlusal surface can be seen from this view	Small distobuccal and distolingual cusps allow more occlusal surface to be visible	
Occlusal aspect		
Occlusal outline rhomboidal Four main cusps (listed according to size, largest to smallest): mesiolingual, mesiobuccal, distobuccal, and distolingual Oblique ridge extending from mesiolingual cusp to distobuccal cusp	Two types of occlusal outline, rhomboidal and heart shaped: rhomboidal is most common and resembles first molar; heart-shaped outline is similar to third molar with a small distolingual cusp that occasionally is missing Occlusal ridge Cusps, grooves, and pits similar to first molar	
Root		
Three well-developed roots: mesiobuccal, distobuccal, and lingual Lingual root longest and strongest Mesiobuccal second largest with blunt apex Distobuccal smallest	Shape and number of roots similar to first molar Buccal roots parallel each other and occasionally are fused All inclined distally	Generally three short roots fused together with a distinct distal inclination

Table 17-7. Mandibular molar characteristics

First molar	Second molar	Third molar
Buccal aspect		
Crown has widest mesiodistal width Three cusps (ranked according to size largest to smallest): mesiobuccal, distobuccal, and distal Cusps divided by mesiobuccal groove and distobuccal groove	Crown smaller in all dimensions than first molar and tips distally Two buccal cusps, mesiobuccal and distobuccal, divided by buccal developmental groove	As with all third molars, it is difficult to describe a standard pattern Normally crown is smallest of all molars, but occasionally can be oversized Occlusal outline generally oval; variations include four-cusped type similar to second molar An irregular groove pattern with more supplementary grooves than in second molar
Lingual aspect		
Two cusps, mesiolingual cusp slightly wider than distolingual cusp Cusps divided by lingual developmental groove	Two cusps, mesiolingual and distolingual, of approximately the same size divided by a lingual developmental groove	
Mesial aspect		
Well developed marginal ridge with mesial marginal groove Contact area at occlusal and middle third junction	Little curvature of the cervical line View similar to that of first molar	
Distal aspect		
Crown shorter cervico-occlusally than on mesial surface Distal marginal ridge has developmental groove crossing it		
Occlusal aspect		
Occlusal outline pentagonal Five cusps (listed according to size, largest to smallest): mesiolingual, mesiobuccal, distolingual, distobuccal, and distal Two buccal grooves and lingual groove form ''Y'' pattern in central area of surface Central groove extends from mesial pit to distal pit Many supplemental grooves	Occlusal outline rectangular All four cusps generally are of equal size Developmental grooves cross occlusal surface in a + pattern Transverse ridge from mesiobuccal to mesiolingual cusp tips and from distobuccal to distolingual cusp tips	
Root		
Two well-developed roots bifurcated mesially and distally Both inclined distally	Two roots, one mesial and one distal Roots parallel to each other and inclined distally	Two roots shorter than those of second molar, fused, and inclined distally

MULTIPLE-CHOICE QUESTIONS

1. Which incisor has the smallest crown mesiodistally?
   a. Maxillary central
   b. Maxillary lateral
   c. Mandibular central
   d. Mandibular lateral

2. What is the proximal boundary of the lingual fossa on the maxillary central incisor called?
   a. Cingulum
   b. Marginal ridge
   c. Lingual ridge
   d. Incisal edge

3. What is the V-shaped space between two adjacent teeth that are in contact called?
   a. Dorsum
   b. Cingulum
   c. Proximal
   d. Embrasure

4. When the mesial surfaces of the maxillary central incisors are separated, the condition is known as:
   a. Microdontia
   b. Anterior crossbite
   c. Diastema
   d. None of the above

5. The teeth that are anatomically designed for tearing are:
   a. Molars
   b. Cuspids
   c. Incisors

6. A rounded, wide, and relatively shallow depression on a tooth surface is a:
   a. Fossa
   b. Sulcus
   c. Fissure
   d. Embrasure

7. A ridge extending from the tip of a cusp to the central groove is a(an):
   a. Oblique ridge
   b. Secondary ridge
   c. Transverse ridge
   d. Triangular ridge

8. Rounded elevations of enamel found on the incisal edges of anterior teeth at the time of eruption are known as:
   a. Lobes
   b. Cusps

   c. Enamel pearls
   d. Mamelons

9. When a primary tooth erupts, it is covered by an enamel cuticle called:
   a. Andrecovich's membrane
   b. Nasmyth's membrane
   c. Edward's membrane
   d. Carabelli's membrane

10. Which tooth has the most prominent labial ridge?
    a. Maxillary central incisor
    b. Maxillary lateral incisor
    c. Maxillary canine
    d. Mandibular canine

11. Which is the first succedaneous tooth to take its place in the dental arch?
    a. Maxillary central incisor
    b. Mandibular central incisor
    c. Mandibular first molar
    d. Maxillary first premolar

12. In which of the following classifications would a cavity in the lingual pit of the maxillary lateral incisor be put?
    a. Class I
    b. Class II
    c. Class III
    d. Class IV

13. In which of the following classifications would a cavity along the cervical line on the buccal surface of the mandibular first molar be put?
    a. Class I
    b. Class II
    c. Class III
    d. Class IV
    e. Class V

14. Usually two roots are found on the:
    a. Maxillary first premolars and mandibular molars
    b. Maxillary second premolars and mandibular molars
    c. Maxillary and mandibular molars and maxillary canines
    d. Maxillary molars and mandibular second premolars

15. Which premolar may have three cusps?
    a. Maxillary first
    b. Maxillary second

c. Mandibular first

d. Mandibular second

16. Which molar normally has two buccal developmental grooves?

    a. Maxillary first

    b. Maxillary second

    c. Mandibular first

    d. Mandibular second

17. Aging affects the pulp by:

    a. Enlarging the apical foramen

    b. Enlarging the pulpal horns

    c. Reducing the dentinal wall

    d. Reducing the size of the pulp

18. Cells that cause internal resorption of the primary teeth are:

    a. Osteoclasts

    b. Odontoblasts

    c. Ameloclasts

    d. Alveoblasts

19. Bifurcated roots would normally be found on maxillary:

    a. Molars

    b. Premolars

    c. Canines

    d. Incisors

20. The roots of the maxillary second molar are:

    a. Mesiolingual, distolingual, and buccal

    b. Mesiobuccal, distobuccal, and lingual

    c. Mesial, distal, and lingual

    d. Mesiolingual, mesiobuccal, and distal

21. The cusp of Carabelli generally is found on the:

    a. Distobuccal cusp

    b. Distolingual cusp

    c. Mesiolingual cusp

    d. Mesiobuccal cusp

22. The smallest cusp on the mandibular first molar is the:

    a. Mesiobuccal cusp

    b. Mesiolingual cusp

    c. Distolingual cusp

    d. Distal cusp

23. The oblique ridge extends from the:

    a. Mesiobuccal cusp to the distobuccal cusp

    b. Mesiolingual cusp to the distobuccal cusp

    c. Mesiolingual cusp to the distolingual cusp

    d. Mesiobuccal cusp to the mesiolingual cusp

24. Which permanent tooth is frequently congenitally missing from the arch?

    a. Maxillary lateral incisor

    b. Mandibular lateral incisor

    c. Maxillary canine

    d. Mandibular canine

25. When root apices are inclined, they will generally incline toward the _____ aspect.

    a. Mesial

    b. Distal

    c. Buccal

    d. Lingual

26. How many permanent teeth of a 9½-year-old child are usually fully erupted?

    a. 10

    b. 12

    c. 8

    d. 14

SUGGESTED READINGS

Brand, R. W., and Isselhard, D. E.: Anatomy of orofacial structures, St. Louis, 1977, The C. V. Mosby Co.

Dunn, M. J., and Shapiro, C.: Dental auxiliary practice. Module 1. Dental anatomy, head and neck anatomy, Baltimore, 1975, The Williams & Wilkins Co.

Fuller, J. L., and Denehy, G. E.: Concise dental anatomy and morphology, Chicago, 1977, Year Book Medical Publishers, Inc.

Kraus, B. S., Jordan, R. E., and Abrams, L.: Dental anatomy and occlusion, Baltimore, 1969, The Williams & Wilkins Co.

Wheeler, R. C.: Dental anatomy, physiology, and occlusion, Philadelphia, 1974, W. B. Saunders Co.

CHAPTER 18

Histology and oral pathology

CAROL M. BROBST

■ **What is oral histology?**

Oral histology is the microscopic study of the structures and tissues of the oral cavity.

■ **Define the term "tissues."**

Cells that are similar in structure and that cooperate to perform one or more functions are termed *tissues*.

■ **List the basic types of tissue.**

All tissue of the human body can be classified as epithelial, connective, muscle, or nerve tissue.

■ **What are the structural components of tissue?**

All body tissue contains cells, intercellular substances, and tissue fluid.

■ **What are the primitive embryonic cellular layers?**

Three primitive embryonic cellular layers form body tissue. These are the ectoderm, outer layer; the mesoderm, middle layer; and the entoderm, inner layer.

■ **What are the three components of a tooth bud?**

Each tooth bud or tooth germ develops in three parts: the enamel organ from which the tooth's enamel develops, the dental papilla from which the dentin and pulp develop, and the dental sac from which the cementum and the periodontal ligament develop.

■ **Which embryonic cellular layers contribute to the development of the teeth and the oral cavity?**

Structures of the oral cavity derive principally from the ectoderm and the mesoderm.

■ **What is the dental lamina?**

When the embryo is about 6 weeks old, two bands of thickened oral epithelium develop from the ectodermal cells to begin the formation of the oral cavity and dental arches. This thickened epithelium is termed the *dental lamina*. Subsequent tooth development begins within the dental lamina.

■ **At what time does the cap stage of tooth development occur?**

The enamel organ assumes the shape of a cap at about the ninth embryonic week. At this time specialized cells of the enamel organ, called *ameloblasts*, begin the production of enamel.

■ **What is the significance of the bell stage of tooth development?**

During the bell stage of tooth development, the enamel organ begins to form the outline of the shape of the crown of each subsequent tooth.

■ **What is the composition of enamel?**

Enamel is 96% mineralized and 4% organic matter and water. It is the most highly mineralized tissue in the body.

■ **What is the neonatal line that appears in enamel?**

During the formation of enamel an accentuated incremental line of Retzius marks the boundary between enamel formed prenatally and that formed postnatally. This line is referred to as the *neonatal line*.

■ **Diagram the development of dental structures from their embryonic initiation.**

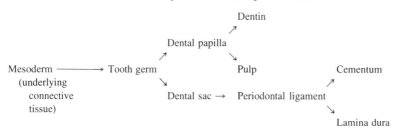

Ectoderm → Dental lamina → Tooth germ → Enamel organ → Enamel

■ **Why is enamel incapable of self-repair?**

Formative ameloblasts are lost in the process of tooth eruption, and tooth enamel contains no living cells.

■ **What is the histologic structure of enamel?**

Enamel is composed of enamel rods, rod sheaths, and interrod substances.

■ **What are the striae of Retzius?**

Enamel rods are formed in a pattern of incremental growth that results in lines in the enamel. These lines are termed the *striae of Retzius*.

■ **List the dental structures according to degree of mineralization.**

Enamel is the most highly mineralized structure followed by dentin and cementum. The dental pulp is not a mineralized structure.

■ **What is the composition of dentin?**

Dentin is approximately 70% mineralized and 30% organic substances and water.

■ **Why is dentin able to repair itself?**

Dentin is formed by odontoblasts. These specialized cells remain living in the pulp after the initial dentin has been formed. In response to irritation from attrition, erosion, or dental caries, the odontoblasts form reparative secondary dentin. As a result, the size of the pulp slowly decreases.

■ **What are Tomes' fibers?**

Odontoblastic processes found in the dentinal tubules are termed *Tomes' fibers*.

■ **What is interglobular dentin?**

In some areas of the tooth, poorly mineralized or unmineralized areas occur because of the joining and overlapping of odontoblastic processes. Such an area is termed *interglobular dentin*. It is primarily found near the dentino-enamel junction in the crown and just beneath the cementum in the root portion of the tooth.

■ **What is Tomes' granular layer?**

The interglobular dentin found in the root portion of the tooth just beneath the cementum is termed *Tomes' granular layer*.

■ **What is the difference between predentin and mature dentin?**

Predentin is only partially mineralized. It is found nearest the dental pulp. As the structure becomes more mineralized, it becomes mature dentin.

■ **What is sclerotic dentin?**

When dentinal fibers degenerate and the tubule fills with mineralized salts, the subsequent tissue is called *sclerotic dentin*. Sclerosis is the hardening of a body part, and sclerotic dentin is more highly mineralized than mature dentin.

■ **Compare the mineralization of cementum and bone.**

Cementum is approximately 50% mineralized, and bone is 60% mineralized in structure.

■ **What are cementoblasts?**

Specialized cells that form cementum are termed *cementoblasts*.

■ **Where are cementoblasts located?**

Cementoblasts are located in the periodontal ligament.

■ **Differentiate between cellular and acellular cementum.**

Acellular (primary) cementum lacks cells and is located toward the coronal portion of the tooth where the cementum meets the enamel. Cellular (secondary) cementum is located in the apical portion of the tooth root where cementoblasts are trapped in the developing cementum.

■ **What are Sharpey's fibers?**

Sharpey's fibers are fibers from the periodontal ligament that are embedded in the cementum and attach the tooth to the alveolar bone.

■ **What is the relationship of the pulp tissue to the formation of dentin?**

Pulpal tissue contains odontoblasts that respond to stimuli and form new predentin. Nerves in the pulp assist the tooth in responding to the need for this new dentin formation.

■ **What is the zone of Weil?**

The zone of Weil is a cell-free layer in the pulp located just below the odontoblasts.

■ **What are fibroblasts?**

Cells for protection of the nerve and blood network of the tooth, which are located in the dental pulp, are termed *fibroblasts*.

■ **Differentiate between cortical and cancellous bone.**

Cortical bone is dense bone located on the outer surface of bone. Between the areas of cortical bone is another type of less dense spongy bone known as *cancellous bone*.

■ **What are osteoblasts?**

Osteoblasts are specialized bone-forming cells.

■ **Describe the haversian system of bone formation.**

Fibers of bone formed after birth are organized into definite layers called lamellae. Intervening between the exterior and interior lamellae of bone are haversian canals around which are arranged haversian lamellae in concentric circles. This circular arrangement of bone around a central nutritional vessel is termed a *haversian system*. There are many other possible arrangements of bone.

■ **What is the lamina propria of the gingiva?**

The gingiva is composed of an outer epithelial tissue layer and an underlying connective tissue layer termed the *lamina propria*. The lamina propria contains fibroblasts and a detailed nerve and blood supply.

■ **What is the purpose of the periodontal ligament?**

The periodontal ligament supports the teeth by connecting the tooth to the alveolar bone. This process is called *gomphosis*. The periodontal ligament consists of fibers that allow the tooth to yield to the forces applied to it.

■ **List the principal fibers of the periodontal ligament.**

The fibers of the periodontal ligament are named by their location. They are principally classified as apical, oblique, horizontal, interradicular, transseptal, and alveolar crest.

■ **List the stages and periods in the development and continuing life of a tooth in the order in which they occur.**

The stages of tooth development are initiation, proliferation, histodifferentiation, morphodifferentiation, apposition, calcification, eruption, and attrition.

■ **Define oral pathology.**

Oral pathology is that area of pathology that concerns itself with disease and disease processes related to the oral cavity, teeth, and jaws.

■ **What is etiology?**

Etiology is the study of the causative factors or agents of disease.

■ **What are the cardinal signs or symptoms of inflammation?**

The cardinal signs of inflammation are pain, heat, redness, and swelling.

■ **Discuss the clinical symptoms of inflammation.**

Redness and heat are caused by increased blood flow to an injured area of the body. Swelling results from an increased escape of fluid into the tissue. In addition to these symptoms, the pressure of fluids on sensory nerves in the affected area causes pain.

■ **What are examples of injurious agents that may cause pathologic changes in tissues?**

Heat, cold, trauma, chemicals, radiation, and pressure may all cause adverse reactions and response from body tissues.

■ **What is tissue degeneration?**

Degeneration refers to deterioration of body tissues. As part of the normal aging process, degeneration is normal. Degeneration can also take place as a result of injury to developing cells and tissues. When this occurs, degeneration is abnormal, and the consequences are serious. Tissues may respond and recover from degeneration if the injurious agent is withdrawn soon enough.

■ **What is hyperplasia?**

Hyperplasia is an abnormal increase in number of cells. It may result as a response to irritation, and the involved tissue will show a thickening or enlargement.

■ **What is hypertrophy?**

Hypertrophy is an increase in the size of cells. It may occur as a reaction or response to injury or irritation. Either hyperplasia or hypertrophy may result in an increase in the overall size of a tissue or organ.

■ **What is hypoplasia?**

Hypoplasia is defective or incomplete development of any tissue or structure. A disturbance during the formative and developing stages of cells and tissues may cause a defect in the mature tissue.

■ **What is neoplasia?**

Neoplasia is new growth of cells and tissues that does not serve any useful purpose. It is caused when cells multiply in excess of the tissue's need for them.

■ **What is the difference between a benign and a malignant neoplasm?**

A *benign* neoplasm does not have the ability to metastasize or spread. Benign neoplasms generally do not cause death of the individual unless they occur in a specific area or location that causes further complications. *Malignant* neoplasms (tumors) always cause death of the individual if they are allowed to continue untreated. They metastasize and spread to other body parts and organs.

■ **What is metastasis?**

Metastasis is the transfer or spread of disease from one organ or region to another. Malignant tumor cells metastasize.

■ **What is a carcinoma?**

A carcinoma is a malignant epithelial neoplasm.

■ **What is a sarcoma?**

A sarcoma is a malignant neoplasm originating in connective tissue.

■ **Define anodontia.**

Anodontia is the congenital absence of teeth. It is also referred to as *hypodontia*. The condition tends to be hereditary and may occur as the absence of all teeth or the absence of some teeth. In either complete or partial anodontia, the teeth do not develop.

■ **What are supernumerary teeth?**

Supernumerary teeth are extra teeth that develop in addition to the normal number of teeth. This condition is also referred to as *hyperdontia*. Supernumerary teeth may occur in any tooth-bearing area of the oral cavity, but they are most frequently located in the maxillary anterior and molar areas.

■ **What is macrodontia?**

Macrodontia is the term used to describe the development of exceptionally large teeth.

■ **What is microdontia?**

Microdontia is the development of abnormally small teeth.

■ **What is enamel hypoplasia?**

Enamel hypoplasia is an incomplete formation of the organic matrix during the development of the teeth. In enamel hypoplasia, a disturbance in tooth formation causes the enamel to be defective. The cause of this condition may be birth trauma, vitamin deficiency, or certain drugs, such as forms of tetracycline, taken by the mother prenatally or by the child during the period of tooth development.

■ **What is the clinical appearance of enamel hypoplasia?**

Enamel hypoplasia will appear as small pits and grooves on the surface of teeth. In some severe cases it may alter the complete crown formation of the tooth as is the case in mulberry molars. Only those teeth developing at the time of the disturbance will show evidence of the condition.

■ **What is amelogenesis imperfecta?**

Amelogenesis imperfecta is a condition of severe hypoplasia caused by a reduction in the amount of enamel formed during development of that structure. It is generally inherited.

■ **What is dentinogenesis imperfecta?**

Dentinogenesis imperfecta is a disturbance of the dentin during formation characterized by early calcification of the pulp chambers and root canals and by an opalescent color of the teeth. These teeth will show evidence of marked attrition. The condition is hereditary and is also known as *hereditary opalescent dentin*.

■ **What are Hutchinson's teeth?**

Hutchinson's teeth refers to a developmental defect sometimes evidenced in the incisors of patients who have a history of congenital syphilis. The biting edge of the tooth is often notched and is described by some as screwdriver shaped.

■ **Define dental fluorosis (mottled enamel).**

Dental fluorosis is a form of enamel hypo-plasia caused by the ingestion of water containing excessive amounts of fluorine during the time of enamel formation. Teeth with mottled enamel usually have brownish stains.

■ **What is attrition?**

Attrition is the normal loss of tooth structure because of the forces of mastication and occlusion or because of the interaction of one tooth with another tooth.

■ **What is abrasion?**

Abrasion is the abnormal or pathologic wearing away of tooth substance. Abrasion may be a result of mastication, incorrect methods of brushing, bruxism, or other similar causes.

■ **What is erosion?**

Erosion is the progressive and localized decalcification of tooth substances of nonoccluding surfaces. Erosion is often evidenced on the labial and buccal surfaces of the teeth near the cementoenamel junction. It is probably caused by chemical action.

■ **Define dental caries.**

Dental caries is the process of progressive destruction of the hard structures of teeth. Caries initiation is caused by the presence and action of acids produced by bacteria on the surface of teeth. The process of dental caries is irreversible. The presence of plaque, which is composed of mucin derived from the saliva and bacteria present in the oral flora, contributes to the inception of dental caries and to gingivitis that results in periodontal disease.

■ **What is periodontal disease?**

Periodontal disease refers to any of several conditions involving the periodontium. Therefore periodontal disease includes gingivitis, periodontitis, periodontosis, and other such inflammatory and diseased conditions.

■ **What is gingivitis?**

Any inflammation of the gingiva is termed *gingivitis*. It may be further diagnosed and identified by the causative agent or by the region in which the condition is localized, that is, marginal gingivitis, herpetic gingivitis, fusospiro-chetal gingivitis, etc.

■ What is periodontitis?

Periodontitis is an inflammation of the periodontium that includes the periodontal ligament and the supporting alveolar bone.

■ What is periodontosis?

Periodontosis is a degenerative form of periodontal disease of unknown etiology in which inflammation apparently plays no causative role.

■ Define pulpitis.

Pulpitis is an inflammation of pulpal tissue. It is caused by bacteria from a carious lesion that enter into the pulp through the dentinal tubules and inflame the pulp. The pulp may also respond to inflammation caused by thermal shock from a deep restoration.

■ What is a pulp polyp?

A pulp polyp is a mass of pulpal tissue that may appear in a large carious lesion of a tooth. It usually occurs in a primary tooth with a large pulp chamber. The pulp becomes bulbous and extends into the cavity.

■ What is hyperemia?

Hyperemia is an increase in the blood flow to a localized area causing pressure on the sensory nerves in that area. It may occur in the pulp of a tooth.

■ Define fistula.

A fistula is a passageway through which pus drains from an abscess.

■ What is a parulis?

When pus drains into the oral cavity, the area of the gingiva may become swollen and inflamed causing an abscess of the gingiva. This abscess in the mouth is termed a *parulis*. These abscesses are more frequently seen in children than in adults and are commonly referred to as ''gum boils.''

■ Describe necrotizing ulcerative gingivitis (NUG).

Necrotizing ulcerative gingivitis, known also as Vincent's infection and trench mouth, is an infection of the oral mucous membrane and gingiva. It is caused by bacterial invasion of a mouth exhibiting poor oral hygiene when an individual is susceptible to stress and fatigue. The observable symptoms of the disease are profuse bleeding of the gingiva, gray and yellow ulcerated areas, and foul breath. If allowed to continue untreated, the interdental papilla will show evidence of being cut off and shortened. Soon after onset the condition becomes quite painful, and the individual may show overall symptoms of physical illness—fever, weakness, pallor, and insomnia. Although the condition may infrequently develop when oral hygiene habits are good, its treatment requires increased attention and effort in maintaining good oral hygiene, proper diet, and rest. The dentist may prescribe an antibiotic for the patient to inhibit the bacterial growth.

■ What is pericoronitis?

Pericoronitis is inflammation of the gingival tissue surrounding the coronal portion of the tooth. It is most frequently observed in the area of the mandibular second or third molars when a flap of tissue occurs over the partially erupted tooth.

■ What characterizes an impacted tooth?

When an unerupted tooth is wedged against another tooth or teeth or located where the tooth cannot erupt in a normal manner, it is termed *impacted*. Eruption of such a tooth is prevented because of some physical barrier in its path.

■ What is ankylosis?

Ankylosis is the fusion of cementum with the alveolar bone of the tooth socket. The condition occurs when the periodontal ligament of the tooth is absent.

■ What is ankyloglossia?

Ankyloglossia is a fusion between the tongue and the floor of the mouth.

■ Describe periapical abscess.

An abscess is a localized collection of pus in the tissue. When this condition develops at the apex of the tooth root, it is termed a *periapical abscess.* The area will be characterized by an accumulation of pus and swelling, and the tooth will be sensitive to pressure from occlusion, etc.

■ **What is a cyst?**

A cyst is a pathologic space in bone or soft tissue that contains fluid. In the oral cavity the cyst is almost always lined with epithelial tissue.

■ **Define granuloma.**

When an individual has enough resistance to counteract a developing abscess, the abscess may enter a chronic stage. New connective tissue will develop as a result of the chronic state of inflammation. This new outgrowth of granulation tissue is termed a *granuloma.*

■ **What are aphthous ulcers?**

Aphthous ulcers are circumscribed small ulcers possessing necrotic yellow centers with red inflammation around them. The exact cause of the condition is not determined. These areas are commonly referred to as *canker sores.*

■ **What is herpes simplex?**

Herpes simplex is a disease that causes a single or multiple lesions on the lips—*herpes labialis.* The cause of herpes simplex is believed to be a virus. These lesions are commonly called fever blisters or cold sores.

■ **What is moniliasis?**

Moniliasis is an oral infection caused by a fungus, *Candida albicans.* It affects the oral mucosa and appears as creamy white or bluish-white patches or dots.

■ **Define leukoplakia (hyperkeratosis).**

Leukoplakia is a condition characterized by white raised patches on the mucous membranes of the mouth. It may vary from smooth irregular patches to rough, raised, horny areas. It has often been associated with smoking and may be referred to by some as "smoker's patches." This condition, if left untreated, may become cancerous, and a biopsy should be performed.

■ **Describe lichen planus.**

Lichen planus is a skin disease that may also affect the oral cavity. Like leukoplakia, it is characterized by white, smooth, raised patches on the inner surfaces of the cheeks and lips and on the tongue. This condition is harmless; however, because of its characteristics and similarity to leukoplakia, a biopsy should be performed for a correct diagnosis.

■ **What is cheilosis?**

Cheilosis is a condition characterized by cracks, redness, and irritation of the skin at the corners of the mouth. It is caused by a nutritional deficiency.

■ **What are the oral manifestations of syphilis?**

Syphilis, an infectious disease, caused by *Treponema pallidum* is transmitted by direct contact with infected individuals. The disease is evidenced by certain oral manifestations. During the first phase of syphilis, an oral *chancre* may be found on the lips. The second stage of the disease is the most highly contagious and may be evidenced in the mouth by oral *mucous patches.* The third stage of the disease is characterized by the appearance of a lesion known as a *gumma,* which is generally located in the area of the nose and palate.

■ **What is cellulitis?**

When inflammation is not controlled within a localized area and the infection spreads through an organ or tissue, the resulting condition is known as cellulitis.

■ **Define osteomyelitis.**

Osteomyelitis is inflammation of the bone. It may occur as the result of advanced inflammation in the oral cavity. It may develop into deep inflammation of the jawbone.

■ **Describe a torus.**

A torus is a bulging projection of bone. These projections are also correctly termed *exostoses.*

■ **What is a papilloma?**

A papilloma is a soft tissue tumor with a warty appearance.

■ **What is a fibroma?**

A fibroma is a soft tissue tumor with a smooth pink appearance. Fibromas are the most frequently occurring tumors of the oral cavity.

■ **What is an epulis?**

Any benign tumor of the gingiva is termed an *epulis*.

■ **Describe geographic tongue.**

Geographic tongue is a harmless condition characterized by loss of the filiform papillae in irregularly shaped patches on the surface of the tongue. These areas become smooth and appear to change their pattern across the surface.

■ **What is black hairy tongue?**

Black hairy tongue is a condition in which there is hypertrophy of the filiform papillae of the tongue resulting in a thick discolored matter on the dorsal surface of the tongue. It usually appears brown or black in color.

■ **What is squamous cell carcinoma (epidermoid carcinoma)?**

Squamous cell carcinoma is the most frequently occurring malignancy of the oral cavity. It appears as a raised hard lesion with rolled borders and a necrotic center.

MULTIPLE-CHOICE QUESTIONS

1. From which embryonic cellular layers do the structures of the oral cavity develop?
   a. Dental papilla and dental sac
   b. Mesoderm and ectoderm
   c. Mesoderm and entoderm
   d. Dental lamina and dental sac
2. The first evidence of tooth formation is the appearance of thickened bands of epithelial cells termed the:
   a. Tooth germ
   b. Dental organ
   c. Dental lamina
   d. Dental sac
3. The components of the tooth bud are:
   a. Odontoblasts, cementoblasts, and ameloblasts
   b. Ectoderm, mesoderm, and entoderm
   c. Enamel organ, dental papilla, and dental sac
   d. Dental lamina, dental papilla, and dental sac
4. The ectoderm gives rise to which dental structure?
   a. Enamel
   b. Dentin
   c. Cementum
   d. Pulp
5. Each primary tooth forms from a/an:
   a. Tooth germ
   b. Anlage
   c. Dental papilla
   d. Osteoblast
6. Each anterior tooth forms from _____ developmental lobe(s).
   a. One
   b. Two
   c. Three
   d. Four
7. Succedaneous teeth form from:
   a. Tooth buds
   b. Anlages of primary tooth buds
   c. The dental lamina directly
   d. Fibroblasts
8. Which of the following statements is accurate concerning the development of a tooth?
   a. The cap stage of development precedes the bell stage.
   b. Eruption of a tooth begins after the root is fully formed.
   c. Apposition follows eruption.
   d. Tooth development begins 6 months after birth.
9. In the development of a tooth, the period when cells multiply is called:
   a. Initiation

b. Apposition
c. Differentiation
d. Proliferation

10. In the development of a tooth, the period when cells arrange themselves in the pattern of a tooth is called:
    a. Apposition
    b. Histodifferentiation
    c. Morphodifferentiation
    d. Proliferation

11. Which of the following terms does *not* refer to enamel?
    a. Striae of Retzius
    b. Lamellae
    c. Nonreparative
    d. Dead tract

12. The thickness of enamel is greatest:
    a. On the occlusal areas of cusps that are subject to greatest wear
    b. At the cementoenamel junction
    c. At the incisal edge of anterior teeth
    d. At the dentinoenamel junction

13. The primary cuticle formed as the last function of ameloblasts is termed:
    a. Tomes' granular layer
    b. Nasmyth's membrane
    c. Pellicle
    d. None of the above

14. Small faults or cracks that run through enamel are termed:
    a. Striae of Retzius
    b. Enamel tufts
    c. Enamel rods
    d. Enamel lamellae

15. Portions of odontoblasts that are caught during the mineralization of enamel are termed:
    a. Striae of Retzius
    b. Enamel spindles
    c. Enamel tufts
    d. Interglobular dentin areas

16. Odontoblasts form:
    a. Dentin
    b. Pulp
    c. Enamel
    d. Sclerotic dentin

17. Bone-forming cells are termed:
    a. Cementoblasts
    b. Osteoblasts

c. Osteocytes
d. Ameloblasts

18. Which of the following statements accurately states the structure of dentin?
    a. Dentin is composed of rods, rod sheaths, and interrod substances.
    b. Dentin is both cellular and acellular depending on its location within the tooth.
    c. Dentin is composed of mineralized tubules, Tomes' fibers, an intertubular cementing material, and collagen fibers.
    d. All of the above are accurate regarding the structure of dentin.

19. Which of the following statements describes interglobular dentin?
    a. Interglobular dentin is highly mineralized.
    b. Interglobular dentin is poorly mineralized.
    c. Interglobular dentin and sclerotic dentin are synonymous.
    d. None of the above statements is accurate.

20. The process of dental caries is often _____ by the presence of sclerotic dentin.
    a. Accelerated
    b. Retarded
    c. Stopped completely
    d. Unaffected

21. Cellular cementum most closely resembles bone and is located:
    a. In the coronal portion of cementum
    b. In cementocytes
    c. In the apical portion of the tooth root
    d. Near the cementoenamel junction

22. Which of the following possible relationships of enamel and cementum occurs most frequently?
    a. Cementum overlaps the enamel.
    b. Enamel overlaps the cementum.
    c. Cementum simply meets the enamel.
    d. Cementum does not contact the enamel.

23. Which of the following statements is accurate regarding pulp tissue?
    a. The sensory activities of the tooth are accomplished by nerves located in the pulp.
    b. Pulp tissue is unmineralized.

c. Pulp tissue contains fibroblasts that aid in defense of the tooth.

d. All of the above statements are accurate.

24. Pulp tissue is important to the formation of:
a. Enamel
b. Cementum
c. Dentin
d. Alveolar bone

25. The bone lining the tooth socket is termed the:
a. Lamina propria
b. Dental lamina
c. Lamina dura
d. Cancellous bone

26. A haversian system is an arrangement that refers to:
a. Flat layers of bone
b. Circular formation of bone
c. Density of bone
d. None of the above

27. The gingiva is composed of which types of tissue?
a. Connective and nerve
b. Epithelial and connective
c. Muscle and nerve
d. Epithelial only

28. Which of the following is *not* a sign of inflammation?
a. Swelling
b. Pain
c. Pallor
d. Heat

29. A causative factor in a disease or condition may be termed the:
a. Pathologic manifestation
b. Etiologic agent
c. Symptom
d. None of the above

30. The study of disease processes, the causes of disease, the manifestations and effects of disease on a living organism, and the alterations in structure resulting from the disease is the study of:
a. Histology
b. Etiology
c. Pathology
d. Microscopic anatomy

31. Which of the following conditions may be normal or abnormal depending on the time it occurs during an individual's lifetime?
a. Degeneration
b. Fluorosis
c. Hyperplasia
d. Hypoplasia

32. In the life cycle of a tooth when the chewing surface becomes worn through normal processes, the condition is identified as:
a. Attrition
b. Exfoliation
c. Apposition
d. Eruption

33. An abnormal increase in the number of cells is:
a. Hypertrophy
b. Hyperplasia
c. Atrophy
d. Hypoplasia

34. Which of the following is an example of a sarcoma?
a. Torus
b. Papilloma
c. Fibroma
d. None of the above

35. The most frequently occurring malignant oral condition is:
a. Ameloblastoma
b. Odontoma
c. Squamous cell carcinoma
d. Osteogenic sarcoma

36. Small ulcers with necrotic centers and areas of inflammation surrounding them may be found in the oral cavity. These areas are known by the lay person as:
a. Herpes simplex
b. Lichen planus
c. Gum boils
d. Canker sores

37. Mulberry molars are an example of:
a. Enamel hypoplasia
b. Hereditary opalescent dentin
c. Anodontia
d. Enamel hyperplasia

38. When inflammation is present in the pulp chamber of a tooth, the pathway through which pus drains into the mouth is called a:
a. Periapical abscess
b. Granuloma

c. Cyst

d. Fistula

39. Which of the following conditions is synonymous with dentino-genesis imperfecta?

a. Amelogenesis imperfecta

b. Congenital syphilis

c. Odontoblastic regeneration

d. Hereditary opalescent dentin

40. An inflammation of pulpal tissue is:

a. A periapical abscess

b. Osteomyelitis

c. Cellulitis

d. Pulpitis

41. A condition in which the tongue is characterized by a wandering pattern of smooth areas resulting from a loss of the epithelium is:

a. Black hairy tongue

b. Aphthous ulcers

c. Herpes simplex

d. Geographic tongue

42. The clinical symptoms of lichen planus resemble which of the following conditions?

a. Leukoplakia

b. Geographic tongue

c. Dental fluorosis

d. Squamous cell carcinoma

43. A space lined with epithelial tissue and filled with fluid is a/an:

a. Granuloma

b. Cyst

c. Odontoma

d. Ameloblastoma

44. An inflammation of the parotid glands is:

a. Measles

b. Salivary duct calculi

c. Mumps

d. Tetanus

45. Which of the following is characteristic of the initial stage of syphilis?

a. Oral mucous patches

b. Gumma

c. Chancre

d. Hutchinson's teeth

46. Phenytoin (Dilantin) is a drug that may cause which of the following conditions?

a. Dental caries

b. Squamous cell carcinoma

c. Mottled enamel

d. Gingival hyperplasia

47. Tetracycline taken by a small child may result in which of the following conditions?

a. Dental caries

b. Squamous cell carcinoma

c. Mottled enamel

d. Enamel hypoplasia

48. Koplik's spots are associated with which of the following systemic diseases?

a. Leukemia

b. Diabetes

c. Measles

d. Pernicious anemia

49. The practitioner observes areas of white raised and smooth patches on the patient's buccal mucosa. The likely procedure to be performed for a definite diagnosis is:

a. Exfoliative cytology

b. Biopsy

c. Questioning the patient to establish duration of the condition

d. Observing the area again in 2 weeks and recording the changes in the patient's condition

50. A patient complains of bleeding and painful gums and of a foul breath odor. There is evidence of poor oral hygiene throughout the mouth. The condition is most likely:

a. Periodontal disease

b. Acute necrotizing ulcerative gingivitis

c. Leukoplakia

d. Geographic tongue

51. A 6-year-old boy has a swollen red area on the gingiva near his second primary molar. When the swelling is touched gently, pus seeps from the bulbous tissue. His condition is called:

a. An aphthous ulcer

b. A papilloma

c. A parulis

d. Herpes simplex

52. A patient with a history of convulsive seizures has been treated with Phenytoin (Dilantin) for the past 3 years. The resultant condition that may be manifested in the oral cavity is:

a. Rampant dental caries

b. Enamel hypoplasia

c. Gingival hyperplasia

d. None of the above

53. An elderly male patient has evidence of a hard bony growth in the palate. This area will have to be removed prior to placement of an upper denture. The condition is known as a/an:
a. Torus mandibularis
b. Torus palatinus
c. Papilloma
d. Epulis

SUGGESTED READINGS

Boucher, C. O., editor: Current clinical dental terminology, ed. 2, Saint Louis, 1974, The C. V. Mosby Co.

Dunn, M. J., editor: Dental auxiliary practice, Baltimore, 1975, The Williams & Wilkins Co.

Provenza, D. V.: Fundamentals of oral histology and embryology, Philadelphia, 1972, J. B. Lippincott Co.

Richardson, R. E., and Barton, R. E.: The dental assistant, ed. 5, New York, 1978, McGraw-Hill Book Co.

Torres, H. O., and Ehrlich, A.: Modern dental assisting, Philadelphia, 1976, W. B. Saunders Co.

CHAPTER 19

Microbiology and sterilization

JOHN A. MOLINARI and MICHAEL J. PHILLIP

■ **What is microbiology?**

Microbiology is the study of unicellular organisms. Included in this diverse group are bacteria, fungi, protozoa, rickettsiae, chlamydiae, mycoplasmas, and viruses. The efforts and discoveries of a number of scientists were the beginnings of the science of microbiology. The achievements of these individuals opened new vistas in medicine and dentistry. The first person to see and describe microorganisms was Anton van Leeuwenhoek (1632-1723). He was a Dutch scientist who observed a world that could only be explored with a microscope. As a result of his efforts, he is called the father of bacteriology. Many scientists realized at that time that certain diseases were caused by bacteria, but this could not be proven until Robert Koch, a German physician (1843-1910), developed techniques for isolating and growing bacteria in pure culture. Willoughby D. Miller, an American dentist who worked in Koch's laboratory, postulated in 1881 that dental caries were caused both by chemical decomposition and the action of bacteria on the enamel and dentin. Miller is called the father of oral microbiology. Louis Pasteur (1822-1892), a French microbiologist, proved among other things that fermentation and putrefaction were caused by living microorganisms. He suggested a similarity between these processes and that of infectious diseases. Joseph Lister (1827-1912), an English surgeon, then applied Pasteur's discoveries to surgery, and Lister's work is the basis of present-day aseptic surgical technique.

■ **What are the characteristics of microorganisms?**

Cells are of two basic types: *procaryotic*, or

the simple cells of most microbes; and *eucaryotic*, the more complex cells of higher organisms. Table 19-1 compares the major features that distinguish each of these groups.

A microscope is required to study most types of microorganisms. Observation by this means reveals a variety of morphologic forms and subcellular components of microorganisms. The features noted for bacteria, mycoplasms, rickettsiae, chlamydiae, viruses, and fungi are summarized in Table 19-2. Fig. 19-1 provides a schematic representation of the structures in Table 19-2 by depicting the composition of a generalized bacterial cell.

Following are other relevant aspects of microorganisms.

Most bacteria lack chlorophyll.

Because a cell wall is absent, mycoplasmas are *pleomorphic* (can appear in a number of different morphologic shapes).

Rickettsiae and chlamydiae are obligate intracellular parasites and have a cell wall, cell membrane, and granular cytoplasm with a central nucleus.

Viruses are not cells in the defined sense, since the former are composed of a nucleic acid enclosed in a protein coat.

Fungi or mycotic organisms appear in tissues as characteristic threadlike bodies called *hyphae*. Aggregations of these filaments are called *mycelia*.

Bacteria must be provided with the proper environment for growth and reproduction. This involves supplying the bacteria with adequate nutritional requirements. The important nutritional elements are (1) *carbon*, needed for the synthesis of the organic compounds that make up protoplasm; (2) *nitrogen* and *sulfur*, needed

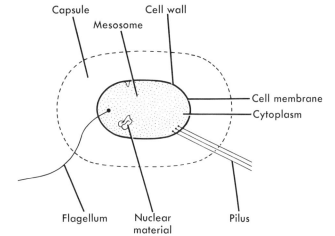

Fig. 19-1. Generalized bacterial cell.

Table 19-1. Comparison of procaryotic cells and eucaryotic cells

Characteristic	Procaryotic cells	Eucaryotic cells
Cell wall	Complex; with glycopeptide	Not as complex; no glycopeptide
Cell membrane	No sterols	Sterols
Mesosomes	Present	None
Nucleus	DNA; no membrane	DNA (complexed with histones); membrane
Cell division	Binary fission; budding	Mitosis; meiosis
Ribosomes	70S	80S
Chromosomes	Single	Multiple
Mitochondria	None	Present
Chloroplasts	None	Present
Chromatophores	Present in some organisms	None

Table 19-2. Morphologic differences between cell types*

Cell type	Cell wall	Nucleus	Cell membrane	Cytoplasm	Ribosomes	Flagella	Pili	Spores
Bacteria	Complex; with glycopeptide	Procaryotic	+	+	+	+	+	+
Mycoplasmas	−	Procaryotic	+	+	+	−	−	−
Rickettsiae	+	Procaryotic	+	+	+	−	−	−
Chlamydiae	+	Procaryotic	+	+	+	−	−	−
Viruses	−	−	−	−	−	−	−	−
Fungi	+	Eucaryotic	+	−	+	−	−	+

*Features noted for each cell types are identified by +. Features *not* characteristic of a cell type are identified by −.

for protein synthesis; and (3) *phosphorus,* required in the synthesis of adenosine triphosphate (ATP) and nicotinamide-adenine dinucleotide phosphate (NADP). Potassium (K^+), magnesium (Mg^{2+}), calcium (Ca^{2+}), and iron (Fe^{2+}) are also needed as enzyme activators. Most bacteria grow best at pH 7 and at a temperature between 30° C and 37° C; such bacteria are called *mesophiles.* Other bacteria grow optimally at temperatures between 15° C and 25° C; these are called *psychrophiles. Thermophiles* grow best at temperatures between 50° C and 60° C.

Bacteria also have varying requirements for oxygen. *Aerobic* organisms need molecular oxygen, whereas *anaerobic* organisms will not

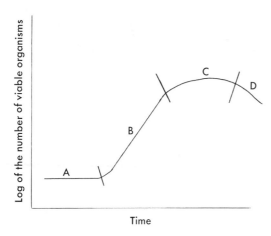

Fig. 19-2. Typical growth curve of bacteria.

grow in the presence of oxygen and may even be destroyed in aerobic environments. There are also other microorganisms that can thrive in the presence or absence of oxygen; these are called *facultatives*. Agar is the substance used to culture most bacteria. It is a polysaccharide obtained from marine algae, and it is an excellent solid medium for bacteria, since it is not degraded by bacterial action.

■ What are the phases of the life cycle of bacteria?

Bacteria placed in a suitable environment will reproduce. Microbial growth is measured by observing an increase in number. The time it takes for one bacterium to divide to form two bacteria is called the *generation time* for the specific species. If a bacterial species is inoculated into a broth (liquid) medium, a growth curve as shown in Fig. 19-2 can be plotted.

Portion *A* of the curve is called the *lag* phase. During this phase there is no actual reproduction, but the organisms are very active metabolically, synthesizing new protoplasm. *B* is the *log* phase in which there is a tremendous increase in the number of cells because of growth in an exponential manner. *C* is the *stationary* phase in which cells begin to die because of depletion of nutrients and accumulation of toxic materials. However, some cells still divide, and these balance those that die, so the number of viable cells remains constant. *D* is the decline or *death* phase in which most of the organisms die.

■ What is metabolism?

Metabolism is the sum total of chemical activities associated with living organisms. There are two types of metabolic reactions: *anabolic reactions* in which new materials are synthesized, and *catabolic reactions* in which organic compounds and other materials are broken down. Some important anabolic reactions in bacteria include (1) *bacterial photosynthesis,* performed by specific photosynthetic bacteria that convert inorganic or organic compounds into carbohydrates; (2) *protein synthesis;* (3) *lipid synthesis;* and (4) *murein synthesis* for cell wall formation. Important catabolic reactions include (1) *digestion,* or the conversion of complex water-insoluble foods into a simple water-soluble form; and (2) *respiration,* or the conversion of food stuffs into usable energy.

■ How do bacteria inherit their characteristics?

Bacteria inherit characteristics from parent cells, a trait common to all forms of life. Bacteria have a *genotype,* or the genetic makeup that governs visible characteristics or traits of the organism, and a *phenotype,* or morphologic and physiologic characteristics that are determined by the genotype. Sometimes the phenotype of an organism may exhibit a temporary change that may be environmental; such changes are called *modifications.* Organisms, however, may undergo permanent genetic changes that will be reflected in their phenotypes. There are four such phenomena: (1) *mutation,* or sudden heritable changes in a genotype; (2) *transformation,* or changes in a genotype mediated by soluble deoxyribonucleic acid (DNA) from another organism; (3) *conjugation,* or alterations in a genotype due to actual sexual union of two organisms; and (4) *transduction,* or changes in a genotype mediated by a bacterial virus.

■ How are bacterial infections controlled?

Chemotherapy is the chemical treatment of diseases. Antimicrobial treatment with antibiotics is one of the most common forms of chemotherapy. An *antibiotic* is a chemical substance produced by microorganisms; the substance can inhibit the growth of or can completely kill other microorganisms. There are two basic types of antibiotics: *bacteriostatic* which inhibit the growth of microorganisms, and *bactericidal* which actually kill microorganisms. The mode of action of bacteriostatic drugs is to inhibit protein synthesis. Bactericidal antibiotics act by (1) inhibiting cell wall synthesis, (2) interfering with the permeability of the cell membrane, and (3) inhibiting protein synthesis. Other drugs such as those in the sulfa group are competitive inhibitors, since they compete for the active center of enzymes in the biosynthesis of essential metabolites.

■ What measures can be taken to control microbial contamination?

The scope of oral procedures performed in the practice of dentistry ranges from simple polishing of enamel surfaces to extensive maxillofacial surgery. The control of microbial contamination during these patient contacts requires strict adherence to the principles of sterilization and disinfection and involves an initial comprehension of the following terms:

sterilization—the destruction of all forms of life with particular reference to microorganisms
disinfection—the destruction of most pathogenic microbes but not spores
asepsis—the absence of infection or infectious materials or agents
bactericidal—able to kill bacteria (extended where appropriate to virucidal, fungicidal, sporicidal, etc.)
bacteriostatic—able to arrest bacterial growth but not able to kill bacteria
sanitization—the reduction of the concentration of microorganisms to acceptable levels
cold sterilization—a misnomer commonly used for disinfection at room temperatures

It is obvious that the maintenance of asepsis in dental medicine is difficult to accomplish by the use of either physical or chemical methods, and yet it is of prime importance in the delivery of patient care. Thus, to implement proper techniques one must first be aware of the possible sources of cross-infection and contamination between patients and personnel. The following list gives potential sources of cross-infection and contamination in dental medicine.

Environment
  Dust
  Floor
  Walls
  Furniture
  Telephone
  Light switch
Equipment
  All instruments
  Air and water syringes
  Matrix bands
  Rubber dam
  Suction tubing
  Chair switches
  Light handles
  Needles and injectables
Personal
  Hair
  Skin
  Clothing
  Plaque
  Saliva

Control of these hazards of cross-infection and autogenous posttreatment infection is facilitated by use of appropriate *chemical disinfectants* and *physical methods of sterilization.* When a chemical agent is being considered for possible clinical use, the antimicrobial effectiveness (Table 19-3) and other relevant aspects of the substance (that is, penetration capacity, epithelial irritation properties, corrosion properties, and allergenicity) must be evaluated. The conditions for sterilization by specific physical modalities are given in Table 19-4. Final implementation should then reflect the highest standards of sterilization and disinfection.

■ How does the body respond to microbial invasion?

Immunity is a state of increased reactivity and specific protection against a substance that is most commonly induced by contact with the agent. A comprehension of this definition requires understanding of the basic nomenclature of immunology.

antigen—any substance capable of inducing an immune response
antibody (immunoglobulin)—protein molecules produced in response to certain antigens, which are specific for the substance

Table 19-3. Antimicrobial range of chemical disinfectants

Class of chemical agent	Gram-positive organisms	Gram-negative organisms	Bacterial spores	Mycobacterium tuberculosis	Hepatitis viruses
Phenols	Sensitive	Sensitive	Resistant	Resistant except to "lysol"	Resistant
Formaldehyde	Sensitive	Sensitive	Sensitive at temperatures >40° C	Sensitive	Resistant
Glutaraldehyde	Sensitive	Sensitive	Sensitive at temperatures >20° C	Sensitive	Resistant
Alcohols	Sensitive	Sensitive	Resistant	Sensitive	Resistant
Iodine compounds	Sensitive	Sensitive	Sensitive	Moderately resistant	Resistant
Chlorine compounds (hypochlorite)	Sensitive	Sensitive	Moderately resistant	Moderately resistant	Moderately resistant
Mercury compounds	Sensitive	Moderately sensitive	Resistant	Resistant	Resistant
Quaternary ammonium compounds	Sensitive	Less sensitive than other organisms	Resistant	Resistant	Resistant
Chlorhexidine	Sensitive	Sensitive	Resistant	Resistant	Resistant

Table 19-4. Conditions for sterilization by physical methods

Method	Temperature	Pressure	Time required per cycle
Steam autoclave	121° C/250 to 255° F	15 psi	15 to 30 minutes
Dry heat oven	160° C/320° F		2 hours
	170° C/340° F		1 hour
Unsaturated chemical vapor	131° C/270° F	20 psi	30 to 90 minutes
Ethylene oxide*	Room temperature 25° C/77° F		10 to 16 hours (depending on material)

*Ethylene oxide gas is actually classified as a chemical but is capable of sterilizing instruments and other contaminated objects. This feature distinguishes ethylene oxide from most other chemical disinfectants, and for that reason it is included in physical methods of sterilization.

Immunity may be manifested by *nonspecific* (innate) or *specific* (acquired) responses. The former mode of protection is not dependent on specific recognition by the host and is responsible for the initial resistance against many pathogenic microorganisms. The following outline details the nonspecific defense mechanisms (innate immunity).

 I. Mechanical barriers
   A. Intact skin and mucous membranes
   B. Fatty acids
   C. Natural flow of tears, saliva, and urine
   D. Nasal secretions, saliva, and sputum
   E. Mucus
 II. Temperature
   Temperature is an important factor in the sur-

vival and multiplication of microorganisms in the body.
 III. Oxygen concentration
   The presence or absence of oxygen in tissues affects the multiplication of certain pathogens.
 IV. Presence, absence, or imbalance of certain metabolites (role in the determination of pathogenicity)
   A. Para-aminobenzoic acid (PABA)
   B. Hormones
   C. Vitamins
 V. Bactericidal activity of tissue fluids
   A. Lacterin
   B. Lysozyme
   C. Certain basic polypeptides
   D. Spermine and spermidine
   E. Lipids, organic acids, and carbon dioxide
 VI. Properdin system

Table 19-5. Properties of humoral and cell-mediated immune responses*

Property	Humoral immunity	Cellular immunity
Microbial pathogens	Pyogenic and encapsulated bacteria (staphylococci, streptococci, gonococci, pneumococci)	Intracellular parasites; chronic infections *(Mycobacterium tuberculosis,* most viruses, protozoa, and fungi)
Microbial toxins		
Exotoxins	+	–
Endotoxins	+	–
Active component	Antibody	Specifically sensitized lymphocytes (secretion of lymphokines)
Hypersensitivity reactions	Immediate	Delayed
Transplantation rejection reaction	Hyperacute and chronic rejection phenomena	Major mechanism for rejection of transplanted organs and tissues

*A property observed as present in an immune response is identified by +. If a property is not part of an immune response, this fact is noted by –.

This system protects man and animals from a wide variety of microorganisms.

VII. Phagocytic system
  A. Phagocytosis
  B. The inflammatory response
VIII. Destruction and indifference to toxin
  "Nonpathogenicity" may be, in part, due to destruction or indifference of certain microbial toxins.
  IX. Role of normal flora
  Production of antibiotic substances by the normal flora of our bodies is thought to be a powerful, but normally unrecognized, mechanism of defense.
  X. Genetic differences
  A. Blacks—sickle cell anemia
  B. American Indians and Eskimos—tuberculosis

These responses may be compared to the protective aspects of the specific host defense systems, *humoral* and *cellular immunity* (Table 19-5). All three of these components—innate, humoral, and cellular immunity—must function properly for effective protection of the host.

In the control of the numerous infectious diseases mediated by humoral immunity, the characteristics of the classes of antibodies involved must be considered as primary factors. For example, certain immunoglobulins are most effective under specific environmental conditions (that is, IgG is responsible for most systemic immunity, whereas local immunity of mucosal surfaces is primarily mediated by secretory IgA). An understanding of the biologic prop-

erties of the different immunoglobulins is thus important when comprehending the scope and diversified activity of the humoral immune mechanisms (Table 19-6).

A type of specific immunologic reaction may develop within an individual that may be detrimental. These *hypersensitive,* or *allergic, reactions* are defined as altered immune responses that cause harm and/or tissue damage to the host but do not appear in all members of the species. These adverse reactions may be mild or life threatening in their severity and are potential hazards during patient treatment. The classes of hypresentivitiy responses may be divided according to the presence (immediate) or absence (delayed) of specific antibodies against the antigen involved *(allergen).* Thus, *immediate hypersensitivity* is a type of humoral immunity, whereas *delayed reactions* are manifestations of cellular responses. Table 19-7 presents the characteristic reactions and features of both.

■ **What medical problems are caused by disease-producing microorganisms?**

One important aspect of microorganisms is that they infect and cause disease. In the following outline microbial virulence and mechanisms of pathogenicity are detailed.

  I. Antiphagocytic factors
  Capsules—*Streptococcus pneumoniae; Hemophilus influenzae*
  II. Enzymes increasing spread through tissues ("spreading factors")

Table 19-6. Selected properties and functions of human immunoglobulins

Class	Serum concentration (mg/ml)	Molecular weight	Half-life (days)	Biologic functions	Disease agents affected
IgG	8 to 14	150,000	23	Active placental transport Activates complement Responsible for protection against most extracellular infectious agents	Staphylococcus Streptococcus Pneumococcus Influenza
IgM	0.6 to 2.0	900,000	10	No placental transfer Activates complement Produced as early response to antigens	Major response to enteric bacteria Isohemmagglutinins Wasserman antibodies in syphilis
IgA	1 to 3	160,000 (monomer in serum) 400,000 (secretory IgA[s-IgA])	5.8	Most active as s-IgA in external secretions (saliva, mucous, tears, colostrum) No placental transfer Does not activate complement by classic pathway Secretory antibodies produced locally	Responsible for local immunity to a number of viral and bacterial infections (eg, poliovirus and *Vibrio cholerae*)
IgE	0.00004	190,000	2.3	No placental transfer Reaginic activity Involved in human anaphylaxis May have important protective role in respiratory tract and as defense against certain parasites	Possible protective correlation of IgE and eosinophilia in parasitic diseases (eg, *Toxocara, Fasciola,* and those caused by *Trichinella*)
IgD	0.03	180,000	2.8	Exact biologic function unknown	

Table 19-7. Comparison of immediate and delayed hypersensitivity responses

Feature	Immediate response	Delayed response
Time of onset	Can occur within a few minutes	Begins within several hours
Antibody	Present in serum	Absent in serum
Passive transfer of sensitivity	With serum	With lymphoid cells or their extracts
Histopathology	Little cellular infiltration; dilation of arterioles and capillaries accompanied by erythema and edema	Early lesion a neutrophilic inflammatory cellular response; after 2 to 3 days, predominant cell type is mononuclear
Clinical states*	Anaphylaxis; serum sickness; asthma; hay fever; Arthus reaction	Contact dermatitis (poison ivy, antibiotics, etc.); tuberculin reaction; responses to microorganisms (viruses, bacteria, protozoa, and fungi)
Treatment	Epinephrine; antihistaminics	Corticosteroids

*Allergic reactions to drugs and anesthetics administered orally or locally may be manifested as immediate or delayed hypersensitivities.

A. Lecithinase c—the alpha toxin of *Clostridium perfringens*
B. Proteinase and protease
   1. "Nonspecific"
   2. Collagenase produced by *Bacteroides melaninogenicus*
   3. Fibrinolysin produced by *Streptococcus pyogenes*
C. Polysaccharase
   1. Hyaluronidase produced by *Streptococcus pyogenes*
   2. Neuramidinase produced by influenza virus
D. Nuclease
   Deoxyribonuclease (streptodornase) produced by *Streptococcus pyogenes*
III. Enzyme increasing localization
   Coagulase produced by *Staphylococcus aureus*
IV. Toxins
   A. Endotoxins—the integral components of cell wall of the gram-negative bacteria *Escherichia coli, Neisseria gonorrhoeae, Salmonella typhi,* and *Bacteroides fragilis*
   B. Exotoxins—secreted primarily by specific gram-positive bacteria
      1. Botulism produced by *Clostridium botulinum*
      2. Tetanus produced by *Clostridium tetani*
      3. Diphtheria produced by *Corynebacterium diphtheriae*
      4. Anthrax produced by *Bacillus anthracis*
      5. Bacillary dysentery produced by *Shigella dysenteriae*
      6. Staphylococcal enterotoxin produced by *Staphylococcus aureus*
      7. Hemolysins
         a. Alpha hemolysin produced by streptococci
         b. Beta hemolysin produced by staphylococci
      8. Erythrogenic toxin produced by *Streptococcus pyogenes*

Although there may be many mechanisms of infection for different pathogens, the principles are the same for all infectious agents. Comprehension of these similarities involves distinguishing the different forms of host-microbial associations: (1) *parasitism* in which one organism exists and benefits at the expense of the other; (2) symbiosis in which both the host and the infecting agent are of mutual benefit to each other; and (3) *commensalism* in which one organism derives benefit by living near the other organism or on its surface without evidence of injury to that organism. With regard to parasitic agents, three different types of obligate parasites are demonstrable on the basis of their relationship with the host:

Extracellular parasites: microorganisms that exist outside of the host cells (eg, *Staphylococcus aureus*).

Intracellular parasites: microorganisms that require the internal environment of the host cell for their existence (eg, *Brucella abortus*).

Facultative parasites: microorganisms that are capable of living either inside or outside host cells (eg, *Mycobacterium tuberculosis*).

If the parasite in any of the aforementioned situations injures the host to a sufficient degree, disturbances will result either locally or systemically and will manifest themselves as *disease*. A successful parasitic microbe, therefore, tends to obtain what it can from its host while causing minimal tissue damage. If severe damage is caused, the host may become crippled or destroyed, and the parasite will lose its ecologic habitat.

It is obvious then that although a few microorganisms induce disease in the majority of individuals infected, most parasitic agents are comparatively innocuous under normal conditions. They either fail to cause disease or initiate illness in only a small percentage of their hosts. This fact becomes apparent when one considers the composition of the normal indigenous microflora of the various anatomic locations. The most important representative organisms normally present in adult head and neck tissues, that is, oral cavity, nasopharynx, oropharynx, and skin are presented in the following list.

Oral cavity
(provides multitude of growth environments)

Streptococcus mitis and other alpha-hemolytic streptococci
Streptococcus salivarius
Staphylococcus epidermidis
Staphylococcus aureus
Veillonella alcalescens
Lactobacilli
Actinomyces israelii
Enterobacteriaceae
Fusobacterium nucleatum

Candida albicans
Treponema dentium
Borrelia refringens
Bacteroides melaninogenicus
Bacteroides fragilis
Bacteroides oralis
Peptostreptococci

Nasopharynx
(primarily aerobic conditions)

Staphylococcus epidermidis
Staphylococcus aureus
Aerobic corynebacteria
Streptococcus pneumoniae
Neisseria catarrhalis
Haemophilus influenzae

Skin
(aerobic and anaerobic conditions)

Staphylococcus epidermidis
Propionibacterium acnes (anaerobic corynebacteria)
Staphylococcus aureus
Aerobic corynebacteria
Candida species, particularly *Candida paropsilosis*

Oropharynx
(primarily aerobic conditions)

Alpha and nonhemolytic streptococci
Aerobic corynebacteria
Staphylococcus aureus
Staphylococcus epidermidis
Streptococcus pneumoniae
Neisseria catarrhalis
Haemophilus influenzae
Haemophilus parainfluenzae
Streptococcus pyogenes
Neisseria meningitidis

This list illustrates the concept that most clinical infections occur as a result of the activity of the *endogenous normal flora* instead of as the result of *exogenous microorganisms* entering the body. The range of microbial types in this list also indicates that the human oral cavity offers the widest variety of ecologic environments. The mouth is an ideal incubator, and the different sites possess the necessary atmospheric, temperature, moisture, and nutritional requirements that allow microorganisms to grow at a rapid rate.

One scheme employed in investigating the disease-producing capabilities of both indig-

Table 19-8. Transmission of infectious disease

Mode of transmission	Representative diseases
Airborne	Tuberculosis, influenza, bacterial and viral pneumonia
Food and water	Typhoid fever, cholera, bacillary dysentery, amoebiasis, poliomyelitis, type A hepatitis, bacterial and viral food poisoning
Insects (zoonosis)	Malaria, plague, rickettsial infections
Venereal	Gonorrhea, syphilis, lymphogranuloma venereum, chancroid
Miscellaneous transmission (wounds, animal bites, ingestion of microbial toxins)	Type A hepatitis, tetanus, rabies, type B hepatitis

enous and exogenous agents is the classification of infectious diseases on the basis of the modes of microbial transmission during clinical outbreaks (Table 19-8). This description of modes of microbial transmission may be used as a guide when considering the representative common microbial infections that are described in Table 19-9.

■ **What dental-associated diseases are induced by oral bacteria?**

The aforementioned principles and concepts of infectious disease relating to host-parasite interactions are as applicable for dental disease as they are for the microbial infections shown in Table 19-9. These common oral diseases are defined as

Caries: actually several diseases caused by the interaction of resident bacteria in dental plaque, suitable environmental conditions, and the surfaces of teeth. The prominent types of carious lesions are *pit* and *fissure* caries, *smooth surface* caries, and *root surface* (cementum) caries.

Gingivitis: this condition is manifested by areas of gingival inflammation without discernable loss of bone.

Periodontitis: this is a disease state with extensive inflammation of the gingivae, develop-

Table 19-9. Clinical features of representative infectious diseases

Disease state	Primary location of lesions	Clinical appearance	Organism most frequently responsible
Boils, carbuncles, osteomyelitis	Skin	Pyogenic infections originating in hair follicles	*Staphylococcus aureus*
Bacterial pneumonia	Lungs	Inflammation of the lungs	*Streptococcus pneumoniae*
Scarlet fever	Mucous membranes of mouth and fauces	Generalized eruption of small, bright red macules	*Streptococcus pyogenes*
Diphtheria	Mucous membranes of throat	Inflammation and formation of fibrinous exudate	*Corynebacterium diphtheriae*
Syphilis	Genitalia and oral cavity	Chancre	*Treponema pallidum*
Gonorrhea	Mucous membranes	Catarrhal suppuration; urethritis	*Neisseria gonorrhoeae*
Tuberculosis	Lungs*	Sepsis; emaciation	*Mycobacterium tuberculosis*
Ringworm	Skin	Circular patches with red vesicular border and central scaling; pruritus	*Microsporum canis*
Athlete's foot†	Interdigital spaces of feet	Acute Itching; red vesicular border Chronic Itching; scaling; fissures	*Tinea rubrum*
Moniliasis (thrush)	Mucous membranes of oral cavity and vagina	Flaky, white patches	*Candida albicans*
Influenza	Mucous membranes of respiratory tract	Febrile anorexia and muscular headaches	Myxovirus
Mumps	Mucous membranes of respiratory tract	Swelling of parotid glands	Paramyxovirus
Poliomyelitis	Gastrointestinal tract; sometimes nervous tissue	Flaccid paralysis of muscles	Picornavirus
Rabies	Nervous tissue	Convulsions; disorientation; death	Rhabdovirus
Hepatitis	Liver		Hepatitis A virus, hepatitis B virus
Epidemic typhus	Vascular system	Patchy gangrene	*Rickettsia prowazekii*

*May affect any tissue or organ.
†May be associated with lesions of hands and nails.

ment of a pathologic gingival pocket, and resorption (loss) of bone around affected teeth.

Dental caries and periodontal diseases have been shown to be transmissible in experimental animal systems, and thus these oral syndromes fulfill an important criterion for infectious disease—they can be produced when appropriate bacteria are passaged to recipient animals. The situation for human disease appears to differ somewhat, that is, caries and periodontal diseases are considered to involve more of a shift in the local composition and activity of the microflora rather than a transferable infection as seen with animal studies.

It appears that the accumulation of *dental plaque* on either enamel surfaces or in the gingival sulcus predisposes oral tissues to the pathogenic problems noted with carious lesions and periodontal diseases. *Plaque* is defined as the aggregation of bacteria, salivary glycoproteins, and mineral salts that adhere to tooth surfaces. Most experimental evidence suggests that some of the plaque bacteria (1) are responsible for the production of acid which results in the induction of caries; and (2) release toxins, enzymes, and other antigens which are involved in the destruction of dental-supporting tissues, as observed in gingivitis and chronic periodontitis (Fig. 19-3). Although both host and parasitic responses are involved factors in these oral

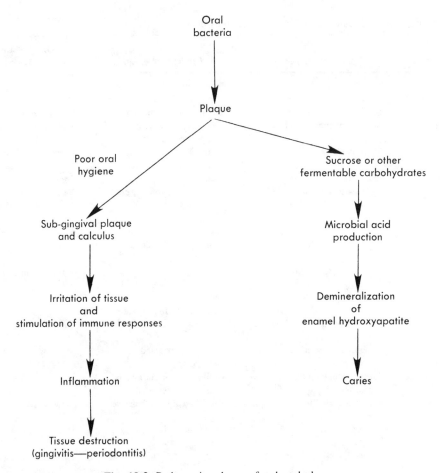

Fig. 19-3. Pathogenic schemes for dental plaque.

diseases and are quite complex, certain groups of microorganisms have been frequently implicated as possible etiologic agents. The following outline gives the predominant microorganisms cultured from diseased dental tissue.

Caries

Pit and fissure caries
    Streptococcus mutans
    Lactobacillus species
Smooth surface caries
    Streptococcus mutans
    Actinomyces viscosus
Root surface caries
    Actinomyces viscosus
    Actinomyces naeslundii
    Other filamentous organisms

Gingivitis

Actinomyces species
Streptococcus species
Rothia dentocariosa
Veillonella alcalescens
Camphylobacter sputorum

Periodontitis

Actinomyces species
Bacteroides melaninogenicus
Eikenella corrodens
Other gram-negative anaerobic rods

Thus the clinical manifestations of each of the dental diseases probably represent distinct pathologic processes induced by the interaction of the host with challenge by different bacterial species.

MULTIPLE-CHOICE QUESTIONS

1. Which of the following conditions for growth is affected by osmotic pressure?
   a. Ph
   b. Oxidation-reduction
   c. Available moisture
   d. Gas requirement

2. The structural integrity of a bacterial cell is determined by the:
   a. Osmotic pressure inside the cell
   b. Proteins in the cell membrane
   c. Polysaccharide in the cell wall
   d. Mucopeptide in the cell wall

3. If all of the bacterial cell wall is removed, the remainder of the bacterium is called:
   a. Leucoplast
   b. Plastid
   c. Protoplast
   d. Elioplast

4. Mesosomes:
   a. Are the functioning sites of the ribosomes
   b. May be the site of the cytochrome enzymes in bacteria
   c. Are only found in autotrophic bacteria
   d. Have similar functions to the lamellae

5. The function of bacterial ribonucleic acid (RNA) appears to be:
   a. Storage of genetic information
   b. Control of protein synthesis
   c. Storage of high-energy phosphate in diester linkage
   d. Oxidation-reduction reactions in the mesosomes of the cytoplasm

6. The transfer of genetic determinants in a cell-free, phage-free, deoxyribonucleic acid (DNA) preparation is:
   a. Mutation
   b. Adaptation
   c. Transduction
   d. Transformation

7. Which of the following organisms lack the enzyme catalase:
   a. Obligate aerobes
   b. Facultative aerobes
   c. Obligate anaerobes
   d. Gram-negative aerobic types
   e. Gram-positive aerobic types

8. The oxidation of foodstuffs with the liberation of energy is called:
   a. Aeration
   b. Digestion
   c. Respiration
   d. Autolysis
   e. Hydrolysis

9. The microorganism associated with the onset of dental caries in humans is:
   a. *Staphylococcus aureus*
   b. *Streptococcus mutans*
   c. *Candida albicans*
   d. Lactobacilli
   e. None of the above

10. Plaque in the oral cavity is composed of:
    a. Saliva glycoproteins
    b. Oral bacteria
    c. Both saliva glycoproteins and oral bacteria
    d. None of the above

11. Most pathogenic streptococci are classified as:
    a. Alpha hemolytic
    b. Beta hemolytic
    c. Gamma hemolytic
    d. Enterococci

12. Which disease is an intoxication caused by the ingestion of toxin:
    a. Botulism
    b. Tetanus (lockjaw)
    c. Gas gangrene
    d. Diphtheria

13. The organism that causes influenza is:
    a. *Bordetella pertussis*
    b. *Haemophilis influenzae*
    c. *Vibrio cholerae*
    d. None of the above

14. Your patient has an abscess of the jaw, and the causative agent is found in the pus as small yellow granules called *sulfur granules*. The infection is caused by:
    a. *Actinomyces israelli*
    b. *Rickettsia akari*
    c. Myxoviruses
    d. *Candida albicans*

15. Sterilization in the hot air oven requires a temperature of _____ for _____.

a. 100° C (212° F); 30 minutes
b. 100° C (212° F); 1 hour
c. 121° C (250° F); 15 minutes
d. 170° C (340° F); 1 hour

16. Mixing quaternary ammonium compounds with a soap yields:
   a. A synergistic compound
   b. An enzyme inhibitor
   c. An inert compound
   d. Both a synergistic compound and an enzyme inhibitor
   e. None of the above

17. Bactericidal is:
   a. The ability to kill bacteria
   b. The ability to inhibit growth of bacteria, but not the ability to kill them
   c. What most nonionic detergents are
   d. None of the above

18. Glutaraldehydes are effective against which of the following:
   a. Gram-positive bacteria
   b. Acid-fast bacilli
   c. Spores
   d. Gram-negative bacteria
   e. All of the above

19. Heat-stable dental instruments and materials are most efficiently sterilized by:
   a. Autoclave
   .b Filtration
   c. Dry heat
   d. Tyndallization

20. An antibody that will neutralize a toxin is a/an:
   a. Antibiotic
   b. Antitoxin
   c. Toxoid
   d. Vaccine

21. Pooled human gamma globulin represents _____ immunity.
   a. Natural active
   b. Natural passive
   c. Artificial active
   d. Artificial passive
   e. Innate

22. Immunity to microorganisms that colonize the interior of host cells (intracellular parasites) is accomplished by:

a. Cellular immunity
b. Humoral immunity
c. Antitoxin formation
d. Plasma cells
e. IgM synthesis

23. The causative organism of syphilis is morphologically described as a:
   a. Coccus
   b. Bacillus
   c. Spirochete
   d. Diplococcus
   e. Spore former

24. *Neisseria gonorrhoeae* has affinity for which of the following structures:
   a. Mucous membranes
   b. Nerve cells
   c. Smooth muscle fibers
   d. Cardiac muscles
   e. Both smooth muscle fibers and cardiac muscles

25. Iodophors are effective against all of the following except:
   a. Bacterial spores
   b. Gram-positive bacteria
   c. Hepatitis viruses
   d. Both bacterial spores and gram-positive bacteria
   e. Both gram-positive bacteria and hepatitis viruses

SUGGESTED READINGS

Gibbons, R. J., and van Houte, M. A.: Bacterial adherence in oral microbia ecology, Ann. Rev. Microbiol. **29:**19, 1975.

Mims, C. A.: The pathology of infectious disease, London, 1976, Academic Press, Inc.

Nolte, W. A.: Oral microbiology: with basic microbiology and immunology, ed. 3, St. Louis, 1977, The C. V. Mosby Co.

Smith, A. L.: Principles of microbiology, ed. 8, St. Louis, 1977, The C. V. Mosby Co.

Volk, W. A.: Essentials of medical microbiology, Philadelphia, 1978, J. B. Lippincott Co.

Wilson, G.: The normal flora of man: introduction, general considerations and importance. In Skinner, F. A., and Carr, J. G., editors: *The normal microbial flora of man*, London, 1974, Academic Press, Inc., pp 1-5.

Youmans, G. P., Paterson, P. Y., and Sommers, H. M.: The biologic and clinical basis of infectious diseases, Philadelphia, 1975, W. B. Saunders Co.

CHAPTER 20

Nutrition

FELICE LEVINE HIRSCH

■ **For a basic understanding of nutrition, define the terms "diet," "nutrition," "food," and "nutrients."**

Diet is the regimen of food intake made up of the sum of meals and between-meal snacks.

Nutrition is a science dealing with the study of nutrients and food and their effect on the nature and function of the organism.

Food is an edible substance made up of a variety of nutrients that nourish the body.

Nutrients are chemical constituents of food.

■ **There are six categories of nutrients. Name these categories.**

Carbohydrates
Fats
Proteins
Vitamins
Minerals
Water

■ **Identify the four main functions of carbohydrates.**

Carbohydrates provide energy, a protein-sparing action, and an antiketogenic effect, and they are necessary for proper functioning of the central nervous system.

■ **Identify and define the three major groups of carbohydrate foods.**

The three major groups of carbohydrate foods are monosaccharides, disaccharides, and polysaccharides.

Monosaccharides are simple sugars.

Glucose (dextrose): moderately sweet sugar found naturally in some foods but mainly created in the body from starch digestion; also found in honey and corn syrup

Fructose (levulose): sweetest of the simple sugars found in honey and fruits

Galactose: not found naturally in foods; produced in human digestion from lactose and is then broken down to aid in energy production

Disaccharides are double sugars made of two monosaccharides.

Sucrose (glucose + fructose): common table sugar; other sources are cane, beet sugar, brown sugar, molasses, maple syrup, carrot roots, and pineapple

Lactose (glucose + galactose): sugar in milk; least sweet of the disaccharides

Maltose (glucose + glucose): occurs in malt products and in germinating cereals; important in starch digestion

Polysaccharides are complex carbohydrates made up of many units of one monosaccharide.

Starch: made up of many glucose chains; the most important source of carbohydrate and accounts for about 50% of the total carbohydrate intake in the American diet; main sources include grains, potatoes and other root vegetables, and legumes

Cellulose: humans cannot digest this polysaccharide because they lack the necessary digestive enzymes; contributes bulk to the diet that aids in peristalsis and elimination; main sources include stems, leaves, vegetable seeds, grain coverings, and many fruits

Glycogen: animal starch; formed in the body from glucose and stored in small amounts in the liver and muscle tissue

■ **Another major fuel source in the body is fat (lipids). This nutrient constitutes about twice the energy value of carbohydrates.**

Fats are also divided into three main groups. Name and describe these groups.

Simple. These are the neutral fats, the chemical name being *triglyceride* which indicates a glycerol base with three fatty acids attached.

Compound. In this group are various combinations of fat with other components.

Derived. These are fat substances produced from fats and fat compounds.

■ **Differentiate between an unsaturated, a saturated, and a polyunsaturated fatty acid, and give an example of each.**

An *unsaturated fatty acid* does not have as much hydrogen as it can hold. Food fats composed mainly of unsaturated fatty acids are usually from plant sources, eg, vegetable oil.

A *saturated fatty acid* is filled with as much hydrogen as it can hold. This causes the food fats composed mainly of saturated fatty acids to present a hardened or solid appearance, eg, pure butter.

A *polyunsaturated fatty acid* has two or more places where fewer or no hydrogen atoms are attached. Food fats composed of polyunsaturated fatty acids present a cross between a liquid (unsaturated) and a solid (saturated) state, such as the vegetable shortening that is usually packaged in a can.

■ **Discuss the difference between an essential fatty acid and a nonessential fatty acid.**

Essential fatty acids are those that the body does not produce; therefore they must be obtained through the diet. *Nonessential fatty acids* are those that the body can produce; therefore they are unnecessary in the diet.

■ **In addition to their being a primary source of energy, identify the other functions of fats.**

Provide structural function
Protect and insulate the body
Prevent hunger pain and give a sense of fullness

■ **What is a protein.**

Proteins may be defined as organic substances that yield their constituent building blocks, amino acids, at digestion. Proteins are found in meat, milk, cheese, and eggs.

■ **What are the main functions of proteins?**

The primary function of proteins is to aid in the growth and maintenance of tissue. Proteins also supply amino acids for building other essential protein substances, contribute to energy metabolism, repair worn-out body tissues through anabolism (building up) that occurs after catabolism (breaking down) takes place, and play a large role in the body's resistance to disease.

■ **What is an amino acid?**

Amino acids are the individual building units of protein.

■ **Differentiate between a complete protein and an incomplete protein.**

Complete proteins and incomplete proteins are determined according to the amount of essential amino acids that protein foods possess. *Complete proteins* contain all the essential amino acids in sufficient quantity to supply the body's needs, whereas *incomplete proteins* are those deficient in one or more of the essential amino acids.

■ **Name the sources of both complete proteins and incomplete proteins.**

Complete proteins are of animal origin, for example, milk, cheese, meat, and eggs. Incomplete proteins are of plant origin, for example, grains, legumes, seeds, and nuts.

■ **How many amino acids are said to be essential, and how many are considered nonessential?**

There are eight *essential* amino acids and eleven *nonessential* amino acids. The amino acids manufactured by the body are called nonessential.

■ **What is a vitamin?**

A vitamin is a vital organic dietary substance that is necessary in small amounts for a particular metabolic function or for prevention of an associated deficiency disease. A vitamin cannot

Table 20-1. Fat-soluble vitamins

Vitamin	Functions	Sources	Results of deficiency
A	Promotes growth; maintains healthy eyes and skin; prevents infection by maintaining healthy mucous membranes	Fatty animal food, that is, butter, cream, whole milk, cream cheese, egg yolk, fish liver oils, green and yellow fruits and vegetables	Night blindness; susceptibility to disease; dry rough skin
D	Helps to regulate body's use of calcium and phosphorus; builds and maintains normal bones and teeth	Sunshine, fish liver oil, egg yolk, liver, some salt water fish, fortified dairy products	Rickets
E	Appears important to health of red blood cells, but no clinical evidence to confirm this importance; antioxidant used to retard spoilage; claims to be an antisterility vitamin, but demonstrated only in the rat, not in man	Wheat germ, wheat germ oils, germs of rice and other seeds, dark green leafy vegetables, nuts, legumes, egg yolk, fish, milk fat	Not confirmed at present
K	Necessary to normal blood clotting	Kale, spinach, cabbage, cauliflower, liver	Deficiency occurs in specific clinical situations, that is, hemorrhagic disease of the newborn, following biliary disease and surgery, after prolonged use of antibodies, and in intestinal diseases

be manufactured by the body; therefore it must be supplied in the diet.

■ **State the two classifications of vitamins and the vitamins in each group.**

Fat soluble: vitamins A, D, E, and K
Water soluble: vitamins C and B complex

■ **State the main function, source, and deficiency that may result from the lack of each vitamin in the fat-soluble group and each vitamin in the water-soluble group.**
(See Tables 20-1 and 20-2 for a description of these vitamins.)

■ **What are minerals?**

Minerals are inorganic elements that are widely distributed in nature; many have vital roles in metabolism.

■ **How are minerals classified, and what minerals belong in each classification?**

Minerals are classified as *major* and *minor*. The elements in each classification are indicated in the following list:

Major	Minor (trace)
Calcium	Iron
Phosphorus	Iodine
Sodium	Copper
Potassium	Manganese
Magnesium	Zinc
Chloride	Cobalt
Sulfur	Fluorine

■ **How are calcium and phosphorus related to vitamin D?**

Vitamin D aids in the absorption of calcium and phosphorus for the development of bones and teeth.

■ **Why is sodium necessary for body functions?**

Sodium maintains body neutrality, water balance, and osmosis and regulates muscle and nerve irritability.

■ **What are good sources of sodium?**

Common table salt, meat, poultry, fish, eggs, and milk are good sources of sodium.

■ **Even though iodine is a trace element, it**

Table 20-2. Water-soluble vitamins

Vitamin	Functions	Sources	Results of deficiency
C (ascorbic acid)	Cell activity; maintains strength of blood vessels; development of teeth; maintains healthy gingiva	Citrus fruits, strawberries, melons, tomatoes, green vegetables	Scurvy; tendency to bruise easily; susceptibility to infection; sore gingiva; hemorrhagic manifestations; anemia; abnormal formation of bones and teeth
B complex B_1 (thiamine)	Control agent in metabolism; maintains healthy appetite; aids in function of CNS	Wheat germ, lean pork, yeast, legumes, whole grains, enriched cereal products, liver and other organ meats	Beriberi (muscle weakness, gastrointestinal disturbances, and neuritis); depression
B_2 (riboflavin)	Growth and cellular metabolism; maintains healthy eyes, skin, and mouth; Oxidation	Yeast, liver, meat, fish, poultry, eggs, milk, enriched breads and cereals, green leafy vegetables	Cheilosis (condition in which lips become reddened, swollen, and cracks develop at the corners of the mouth); blurring of vision; intolerance to light; glossitis
Niacin (nicotinic acid)	Carbohydrate, fat, and protein metabolism; prevention of pellagra	Meats, poultry, fish, yeast, enriched bread and cereals, peanuts	Pellagra; glossitis; skin eruptions; nausea; diarrhea; nervous disorders; anorexia (loss of appetite)
B_6 (pyridoxine and pantothenic acid)	Essential for protein metabolism	Organ meats, peanuts, soybeans, whole grain cereals	Anemia; dermatitis; anorexia; nausea; kidney stones
B_9 (folic acid)	Growth and development of red blood cells	Dark green leafy vegetables, liver, kidney, asparagus	Anemia; sprue (gastrointestinal disease)
B_{12} (cobalamin)	Essential in formation of normal red blood cells, nerve function, and growth	Organ meats, eg, liver and kidneys and milk, cheese, eggs	Pernicious anemia; general nervous symptoms; amenorrhea; sore mouth and tongue

has a very important role. What role does it play in the body?

Iodine forms hormones in the thyroid gland; therefore it produces thyroxine in the thyroid gland that stimulates the cell oxidation required for growth.

■ **What is the most common clinical manifestation of iodine deficiency?**

The classic manifestation of iodine deficiency is goiter, which is an enlargement of the thyroid gland that results from lack of iodine.

■ **Name the minerals, and give an example(s) of sources for each mineral.**

Mineral	Source
Calcium	Milk, cheese
Phosphorus	Milk, cheese
Sodium	Salt, milk
Potassium	Meat, fruits
Chloride	Salt, meat

Mineral	Source
Magnesium	Dry beans, nuts
Sulfur	Protein foods
Iodine	Salt water fish, iodized salt
Iron	Liver
Copper	Muscle meats
Manganese	Blueberries
Zinc	Seafood
Cobalt	Supplied in Vitamin B_{12}
Fluorine	Fluoridated water

■ **List the duties of the interviewer during a nutritional counseling interview.**

Put the patient at ease.
Listen to the patient.
Do not interrupt the patient.
Maintain eye contact with the patient.
Communicate with the patient on the patient's level.
Make the patient responsible for all decisions.

■ **In aiding a patient to achieve optimum nutritional and dental health, what steps should be taken?**

Obtain a complete health history.
Explain the caries formula.

Carbohydrates + bacteria → Acids
Acids + susceptible tooth structure →
Demineralization → Decay

Explain the importance of eating food from each of the four basic food groups with the following daily recommended servings:

Meat	2 or more servings
Milk	2 or more servings
Fruit and vegetables	4 or more servings
Bread and cereal	4 or more servings

Collect a daily routine diet from the patient and apply the principles of the four basic food groups to an analysis of it.
Identify cariogenic foods in the patient's diet.
Request a revised diet from the patient, thus securing feedback.

■ **Define the terms "fortified foods" and "enriched foods."**

Fortified foods contain more nutrients than are present naturally, such as milk fortified with vitamins A and D. *Enriched foods* are processed foods to which those vitamins and minerals that were removed during milling are added, such as enriched breads and cereals with vitamins A and D. Standards for food enrichment were established by the Food and Drug Administration.

■ **Why are preservatives and additives placed in foods? Give examples of these substances.**

Preservatives and additives are used to keep foods fresh and maintain quality.

Monosodium glutamate is used to enhance flavor.
Butylated hydroxyanisole (BHA) and *butylated hydroxytoluene* (BHT) are antioxidants that act to prevent spoilage.
Calcium propionate is a mold inhibitor.
Lecithin (monoglycerides and diglycerides are emulsifiers) provide fine texture in bakery products.
Emulsifiers provide dairy products with a smooth creamy consistency.
Pectin and *vegetable gums* act as stabilizers and thickeners to maintain a smooth texture and give body to certain foods.

■ **How is the population protected in relation to the purchasing and safety of foods?**

The Food and Drug Administration (FDA) is the major governmental agency charged with the responsibility of maintaining the safety of food. This agency is part of the U.S. Department of Health, Education, and Welfare. The purpose of this agency is to ensure that food purchased is safe, pure, and wholesome. The FDA is responsible in three basic areas:

Agricultural chemicals. The FDA seeks to control the use of chemicals and prevent pesticide residues in food crops. The chemicals must have initial approval for use, and there is continued surveillance of use by strict monitoring and periodic sampling of the field produce.

Packaging of foods. The FDA sets standards of identity, standards of quality, and standards on the filling process of containers. Foods must be labeled without false information.

Food additives. The law states that no additive could be added to food unless, after careful review of the test data, the FDA agrees that the compound is safe at the intended levels of use.

MULTIPLE-CHOICE QUESTIONS

1. Nutrition is:
   a. An edible substance made up of a variety of nutrients that nourish the body
   b. A regimen of food intake made up of a sum of meals and between-meal snacks
   c. A science dealing with the chemical balance of food
   d. A science dealing with the study of the chemical constituents of food and edible substances and their effect on the nature and function of the organism

2. Simple sugars are referred to as monosaccharides. Which two are considered simple sugars?
   a. Sucrose and cellulose
   b. Lactose and galactose
   c. Levulose and dextrose
   d. Maltose and glucose

3. Which of the following is referred to as common table sugar?
   a. Lactose
   b. Fructose
   c. Maltose
   d. Sucrose

4. Even though the body cannot digest cellulose, why is this polysaccharide important to body functions?
   a. It aids in elimination of body waste.
   b. It helps the digestion of fats.
   c. It accounts for about 50% of the total carbohydrate intake in the American diet.
   d. It is stored in small amounts in the liver and muscle tissue.

5. The main difference between saturated, unsaturated, and polyunsaturated fatty acids is:
   a. How much hydrogen is held in the fatty acid chain
   b. The difference between a solid, liquid, and semisolid state
   c. Both of the above
   d. None of the above

6. The fatty acids that the body produces itself are called:
   a. Complete
   b. Incomplete
   c. Essential
   d. Nonessential

7. The primary function of a protein is to:
   a. Contribute to energy metabolism
   b. Play a large role in the body's resistance to disease
   c. Supply amino acids for building other essential protein substances
   d. Aid the growth and maintenance of tissue

8. Complete proteins are those that (1) contain all the essential amino acids in sufficient quantity to supply the body's needs, (2) are derived from foods of animal origin, and/or (3) contain 11 amino acids.
   a. 1 and 2
   b. 1 and 3
   c. 3
   d. 2

9. A deficiency in vitamin D can cause (1) poor growth of teeth, (2) rickets, (3) poor health of gums, and/or (4) poor absorption of calcium and phosphorus.
   a. 1 and 4
   b. 1, 3, and 4
   c. 2, 3, and 4
   d. 1, 2, and 4

10. A deficiency of vitamin A would be manifested by:
    a. Prolonged clotting time of the blood
    b. Sore gingiva
    c. Loss of appetite
    d. Night blindness

11. A deficiency of vitamin C can cause (1) hemorrhagic disease in newborns, (2) cheilosis, (3) anemia, (4) scurvy, and/or (5) weakness of blood vessels.
    a. 1, 4, and 5
    b. 4 and 5
    c. 2, 3, and 5
    d. All of the above

12. Vitamin B complex can cause (1) pellagra, (2) cheilosis, (3) beriberi, and/or (4) anemia.
    a. 1, 3, and 4
    b. 1 and 3
    c. 2 and 4
    d. All of the above

13. One of the main functions of carbohydrates is:
    a. Energy storage

b. Energy metabolism
c. Energy source
d. Energy-sparing action
14. Besides that of being a primary source of energy, what is another function of fats?
    a. Aid growth and maintenance of tissue
    b. Protect and insulate the body
    c. Contribute to energy metabolism
    d. Repair worn-out body tissues through anabolism, which occurs after catabolism has taken place
15. Proteins are defined as:
    a. Amino acids
    b. Inorganic substances
    c. Organic substances
    d. Inert substances
16. A true sign that one is deficient in the trace mineral iodine is:
    a. Speckled palate
    b. Goiter
    c. Glossitis
    d. Red rash on the head and neck
17. A patient is seen for an initial nutritional counseling session. What information must first be obtained from the patient?
    a. A daily diet
    b. A complete health history
    c. A prescribed diet
    d. The caries formula
18. A sample diet from the patient includes:

Breakfast
6 ounces orange juice
2 slices white toast
1 egg
1 cup coffee

Lunch
1 tuna fish sandwich
1 diet beverage
3 carrots
2 slices tomato

Dinner
1 8-ounce steak
1 cup peas and carrots
1 medium baked potato
1 dinner roll
1 small green tossed salad with oil and vinegar dressing
1 serving fresh pineapple

The patient appears to have a well-balanced meal, but the diet is deficient in which one of the basic four food groups?
    a. Meat
    b. Milk
    c. Fruit and vegetable
    d. Bread and cereal

19. What would be a good noncariogenic substitute for snack food?
    a. Coke
    b. Donuts
    c. Pretzels
    d. Caramel popcorn
20. When a food is called "fortified" it refers to the:
    a. Addition of substances that were lost during processing
    b. Addition of vitamins A and D
    c. Addition of vitamin C to fruit punch
    d. Addition of more nutrients to foods than are found naturally
21. Standards for enrichment of foods is governed by what agency?
    a. Food and Drug Administration (FDA)
    b. American Dental Association (ADA)
    c. National Food and Drug Administration (NFDA)
    d. Federal Trade Commission (FTC)
22. Preservatives and additives are put into our foods to (1) prevent spoilage, (2) enhance flavor, (3) keep foods fresh and maintain quality, (4) provide fine texture, and/or (5) provide smooth and creamy consistency.
    a. 1, 2, and 4
    b. 3, 4, and 5
    c. 1 and 5
    d. All of the above
23. The Food and Drug Administration's (FDA) main purpose is to:
    a. Protect the public in relation to the purchasing and safety of foods
    b. Educate the public to read labels
    c. Test food additives
    d. Seek control of chemicals that are used in agriculture

SUGGESTED READINGS

Nizel, A. E.: Nutrition in preventive dentistry: science and practice, Philadelphia, 1972, W. B. Saunders Co.
Townsend, C. E.: Nutrition and diet modifications, Albany, N.Y., 1972, Delmar Publishers.
The Upjohn Co.: Vitamin manual, Kalamazoo, Mich., 1965, The Upjohn Co.
Williams, S. R.: Essentials of nutrition and diet therapy, ed. 2, St. Louis, 1978, The C. V. Mosby Co.

CHAPTER 21

Pharmacology

SUSAN HARPER VAN STEENHOUSE

■ **Define pharmacology.**

Pharmacology is the science that deals with the study of the properties of chemical substances to be used as drugs. Drugs, in turn, are those chemical compounds, or elements, used in the treatment of disease.

■ **What is chemotherapy?**

Chemotherapy pertains to the use of chemical substances in treatment of specific diseases. A particular drug is selected that is known to have a specific and toxic (poisoning) effect on the disease-producing microorganism without causing undue toxicity to the patient.

■ **From what sources are drugs derived?**

Drugs used for medicinal purposes may be obtained from *natural* or *synthetic* sources. Natural sources include plant, animal, or mineral substances or their chemical alterations. Those man-made drugs produced in the laboratory from nonnatural sources are termed *synthetics*.

■ **What information from the patient's health history should be reviewed before drugs are prescribed?**

The health history is a factual record of the patient's past and present medical status, and before a drug is prescribed, the following information should be reviewed:

Conditions that required or are presently requiring medical consultation

Conditions, past and present, for which medication has been prescribed

Drugs presently being taken—prescription and nonprescription medication

Drugs or substances to which the patient may be allergic or to which the patient may have experienced unusual reactions

■ **What is a drug prescription?**

A prescription is a written and occasionally spoken order from a licensed practitioner to a pharmacist directing the dispensing of a specific drug to a specified patient.

■ **Is a written prescription necessary for all drugs?**

Not always. However, a written prescription is required for any Schedule II substance that is considered to have a high potential for abuse as in the case of some of the opium derivatives such as methadone, meperidine, and dihydromorphinone (Dilaudid); some of the amphetamines such as dextroamphetamine (Dexedrine) and amphetamine (Benzedrine); and barbiturates such as secobarbital, (Seconal) and pentobarbital (Nembutol).

There are occasions when verbal prescriptions are more expedient and allowable, that is for schedule III, IV, and V drugs. Often a dentist must prescribe from outside the office, or the patient is not present. In such cases the dentist may prescribe by telephone that information which would otherwise be in a written prescription.

■ **How might Schedule III, IV, and V substances be differentiated?**

Substances classified as Schedule III include depressant drugs such as some of the intermediate-acting barbiturates and those mixtures of drugs containing limited quantities of narcotics such as in codeine-containing preparations acetaminophen (Tylenol) and Empirin W/ Codeine No. 1, 2, 3, and 4).

Schedule IV drugs are substances that have less potential for abuse than Schedule III drugs but that may still produce a limited psychologic and physical dependence. Examples include some of the less abused sedative-hypnotics, that is, phenobarbital and chloral hydrate and anti-anxiety agents such as diazepam (Valium).

Those agents listed as Schedule V drugs have still less potential for abuse than Schedule III and IV substances.

■ What is a DEA registration number, and why is this number required on a prescription form?

In order to prescribe, purchase, and administer controlled substances, the dentist must register with the Drug Enforcement Administration (DEA) that is under the auspices of the U.S. Department of Justice. On acceptance of the registration a DEA number is assigned that when placed on a prescription allows the dentist, under specific regulations, to prescribe controlled substances if the practitioner is personally attending to the patient's treatment.

The DEA number has recently replaced the Bureau of Narcotics and Dangerous Drugs (BNDD) registry number.

■ How is the drug prescription written?

A prescription is written on a particular form with the following components in a definite sequence (see Fig. 21-1):

Headings: this section contains the prescriber's name and address with space available for writing in the patient's name, address, age, and date of the prescription.

Superscription: the symbol *Rx* is the Latin abbreviation for recipe. Rx is the order for the pharmacist to dispense the prescribed drug.

Inscription: this is the body of the prescription and contains the name, dosage, form, and strength of the drug. Drugs may be designated by generic name or brand name.

Subscription: this section contains directions to the pharmacist regarding the quantity of the drug to be dispensed.

Signature: this is the instruction for patient use of the medication and is also called the *label.* Directions should be carefully worded and written on the drug label for the patient's information.

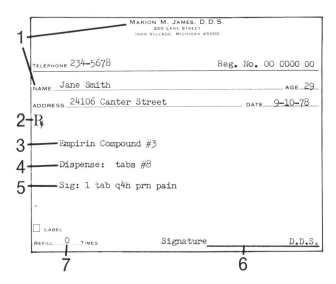

Fig. 21-1. The written prescription and its parts. *1,* Headings (prescriber and patient); *2,* superscription; *3,* inscription; *4,* subscription; *5,* signature; *6,* prescriber's signature; *7,* refill information.

Prescriber's signature: drug prescriptions require the signature of the licensed practitioner. The prescription for controlled substances is required to contain a DEA number as well.

Refill information: this item designates the number of times a drug prescription may be refilled by the patient.

■ What do the abbreviations of Latin words used in prescription writing mean?

The abbreviations of Latin words commonly used for completing a drug prescription are given in Table 21-1. Dental assistants should be familiar with these terms so that they can aid the dentist in prescription writing.

■ Under what conditions can a prescription be refilled?

The terms of the Durham-Humphrey Act specify that prescription drugs may not be refilled except when the practitioner indicates the number of prescription refills. If the medication is a Schedule II drug, the prescription may not be refilled without a new prescription.

Schedule III and IV controlled substances require a written or an oral prescription and may not be refilled more than 6 months after the prescription date or refilled more than five times without a renewed prescription.

If a prescriber does not wish for a patient to be issued any refills the abbreviation *nr* (no repeat) should be placed on the prescription form. When no refill information is given, the pharmacist may call the prescriber to inquire as to how to handle the matter.

■ Who may write a drug prescription?

The dental assistant may write a prescription as directed by the dentist, but by law the dentist must place the signature on the form. A careful check of the prescription should be made by the dentist to be sure the correct drug name and dosage have been written.

■ Compare brand name and generic name as they relate to drug dispensing.

A drug brand name is also known as its *proprietary* name. Brand name drugs are preparations that are protected from competition by secrecy, patent, or copyright. By comparison, the generic name of a drug is its general or chemical name, for example

Brand name: V-Cillin-K
Generic name: potassium phenoxymethyl penicillin

The practitioner may order a drug either by generic name or by brand name. If the generic name is used, the pharmacist may select from several available brands of the drug.

■ What federal agencies deal with drugs and the protection of the consumer?

The Federal Food and Drug Administration (FDA) of the U.S. Department of Health, Education, and Welfare (DHEW) is responsible for the protection of the public in the purchase and use of drugs, cosmetics, and other related substances. All manufacturers of new drugs and cosmetics must provide evidence to the FDA that the product is safe for humans if used as it is intended.

The Drug Enforcement Administration (DEA) of the U.S. Department of Justice is responsible for monitoring the manufacture, distribution, and dispensation of controlled substances and narcotic drugs. The DEA has outlined specific regulations to health practitioners for dispensing and prescribing these agents.

Table 21-1. Common Latin abbreviations used in prescription writing

Latin abbreviation	Definition
ac	before meals
pc	after meals
hs	at bedtime
prn	when needed
qh	every hour
q 4 h	every 4 hours
bid	two times a day
tid	three times a day
qid	four times a day
nr	do not repeat; no refill
ss	one half
m	mix
stat	immediately

Controlled substances cannot legally be prescribed by a practitioner without a DEA registration number.

■ **What is the U.S.P.?**

The U.S.P. stands for *The United States Pharmacopeia,* which is recognized as an official drug standard. This publication is revised and issued every 5 years. The U.S.P. lists commonly used drugs, their sources, appearances, properties, and related specifications. Recognized drugs bear the U.S.P. insignia on their label.

■ **What is the National Formulary?**

The National Formulary (N.F.) is another official drug standard containing the histories of drugs that are not listed in the U.S.P. In addition, the N.F. includes standard drug mixtures.

■ **Which publications are most useful as drug references?**

The *Physicians' Desk Reference* (PDR) is probably the most widely used reference by health practitioners. It provides information and identification of drugs, along with their brand and generic names.

The American Dental Association compiles a valuable publication called *Accepted Dental Therapeutics* (ADT) which is revised and issued every 2 years. It is a therapeutics handbook of recognized and accepted drugs for use in dental treatment.

■ **List and describe methods for administering drugs for dental treatment.**

Drugs used in dentistry can be administered for local or systemic effects by the following methods:

Parenteral—injection of drugs
  Intramuscular—injection into muscle (IM)
  Intravenous—injection into a vein (IV)
  Subcutaneous—injection just below the skin
Oral—administered by mouth in the form of pills, tablets, capsules, or liquids
Inhalation—breathing of a gaseous substance

Topical—application of drugs to the surface of the skin or mucosa
Sublingual—placement of a drug under the tongue

■ **How are drug dosages modified for children?**

There are formulas for computing drug dosages for children or adult patients who are extremely small in size.

Clark's rule computes dosage based on the weight of a patient, and *Young's rule* calculates the dosage based on the patient's age. Recent concepts of drug therapy indicate that weight, or body surface area, has more relevance to drug dosage determinations than does age.

Manufacturer's package inserts are included with drug products and provide important information on the dosage of the drug.

■ **List four types of adverse effects that can be caused by drugs, and describe each type of effect.**

Side effect. This is an unintended nuisance response to drugs, eg, stomach upset and diarrhea with antibiotic therapy.

Drug interaction. This kind of response results from the simultaneous action of more than one drug, eg, alcohol and tranquilizers, both CNS depressants, when taken simultaneously are potentially life threatening if the CNS depression is excessive.

Hypersensitivity. This is an allergic reaction to a drug. Allergic reactions are variable, ranging from mild skin irritation (urticaria) to anaphylaxis with the possibility of death.

Idiosyncrasy. This is an abnormal response, or a response that is opposite to the expected drug action, eg, CNS stimulation from a barbiturate (sedative) rather than the expected depressive effect.

It is important to update the health history during subsequent patient visits to record any new and pertinent medical information including reactions and sensitivities to drugs.

■ **Should drugs dispensed to or prescribed for a patient be recorded?**

Accurate, complete patient records are integral facets of successful and safe dental care. All drugs, dispensed or prescribed, should be recorded on the patient's chart, and this record should include the drug name, dosage, date given, and any unusual reactions to the drug.

■ **What is an analgesic drug?**

Analgesic drugs are useful for relieving pain and do not cause the loss of consciousness. Analgesics are one of the most widely used groups of drugs in dentistry. They are frequently classified or grouped as mild, moderate, or strong, based on the intensity of pain the drug will relieve.

■ **What drugs might be prescribed for mild to moderate dental pain?**

Mild analgesics are used in cases of low intensity pain such as pain with a headache or mild neuralgia. Acetylsalicylic acid, aspirin, is an example of this type of analgesic drug. Acetaminophen (such as Tylenol and Percogesic) are alternative analgesics often prescribed for patients who indicate hypersensitivity to aspirin.

In addition to its analgesic properties, aspirin demonstrates antipyretic (fever-reducing) and antiinflammatory effects.

■ **What does the abbreviation A.P.C. refer to?**

An A.P.C. is a mild analgesic drug compounded of aspirin, phenacetin, and caffeine. Caffeine has a property that alleviates the tension related to certain types of headaches.

Several of the narcotic analgesics are combined with A.P.C. for added pain relief.

■ **What are strong analgesics?**

Strong analgesics are divided into two groups: narcotic and nonnarcotic. *Narcotic analgesics* have the potential to produce morphine-like dependence and are classified as Schedule II, controlled substances. *Nonnarcotic analgesics* are compounds not subject to the provisions of the Controlled Substances Act because they are not considered to be habit forming. An example would be pentazocine (Talwin), which is used for acute and chronic pain of strong intensity.

■ **Are there analgesics that can be obtained without a prescription?**

Agents such as aspirin and its compounds (A.P.C., Empirin Compound, Bayer, and Excedrin) or acetaminophen and its compounds (such as Tylenol, Datril, Vanquish, and Percogesic) may be purchased as "over-the-counter" drugs (without prescription) for mild pain relief.

■ **What is a narcotic drug?**

Narcotic drugs are primarily used to achieve analgesia (pain relief). Sedation and hypnosis (sleep induction) are other possible effects of narcotic drugs.

These agents can be opium derivatives, or can be produced synthetically. Narcotic analgesics have an addicting potential and are governed by the Controlled Substances Act. Examples of these drugs are codeine, morphine, methadone, dilaudid, oxycodone (Percodan), and meperidine (Demerol).

■ **Describe drug addiction.**

The World Health Organization defines drug addiction as a state of periodic or chronic intoxication produced by the repeated use of a substance. Addiction is characterized in a person as a compulsive need to continue the use of a substance in order to obtain a desired feeling. With prolonged use of a drug, a tolerance may develop that makes the person require increased dosages to maintain the desired feeling. Consequently, physical and psychologic dependence can extend to actual life-threatening situations.

■ **What are antianxiety agents?**

Antianxiety drugs are commonly called *tranquilizers* and have a depressant effect on the central nervous system. These agents may be used to suppress mild to moderate preoperative anxiety or apprehension. Examples are chlordiazepoxide (Librium), diazepam (Valium), hydroxyzine pamoate (Vistaril), and promethazine (Phenergan). Since the duration of these drugs may extend beyond the appointment, it is necessary to inform the patient or guardian of the length of time of the drug's effect and that someone should assist the patient home.

■ **What is sedative-hypnotic?**

Sedative-hypnotics can be either barbiturate or nonbarbiturate drugs. They produce a quieting effect to allay nervous excitement or induce sleep. Examples of barbiturate sedative-hypnotics are

Phenobarbital—long acting
Butabarbital—intermediate acting
Secobarbital (Seconal)—short acting
Pentobarbital (Nembutal)—short acting

Examples of nonbarbiturate sedative-hypnotics are chloral hydrate and ethinamate (Valmid).

■ **Is there any difference between a sedative and a hypnotic?**

Drugs which are said to be sedatives can, generally, also act as hypnotics. The state of CNS depression desired is dependent on the dosage prescribed with the hypnotic states generally occurring with a greater dosage.

■ **Why is nitrous oxide used?**

Nitrous oxide is a psychosedation inhalation agent administered during operative procedures to produce a quiet, or tranquil, state to allay apprehension. There has been a resurgence of interest in this gaseous mixture in dentistry because of its relative ease of use and safety. The drug effect has a fast onset and can be quickly eliminated with the administration of 100% oxygen.

■ **Who is credited as being the first practitioner to use general anesthesia?**

Dr. Horace Wells in 1844 used nitrous oxide to allay pain while extracting a tooth.

■ **Define general anesthesia.**

General anesthesia is a state of complete loss of sensation as well as consciousness. General anesthesia may be accomplished by an intravenous injection of a drug or through inhalation of gases that ultimately reach the brain by way of the circulatory system. General anesthetics have limited use in general dentistry.

■ **Define local anesthesia.**

Local anesthesia is the loss of sensation to a localized area. It is the most common means of reducing pain during minor dental surgical and restorative procedures. Local anesthesia is accomplished by injection of a drug into the proximity of the nerve system (innervation) of the area to be treated or by the application of a topical agent.

■ **What agents are available as local anesthetics?**

There are two chemical categories of local anesthetic drugs: the ester group and the amide group. Lidocaine (Xylocaine), mepivacaine (Carbocaine), and prilocaine (Citanest) are agents in the amide group and constitute the most commonly used local anesthetics in dentistry. Anesthetic drugs of the ester group include procaine (Novocaine), tetracaine (Pontocaine), and propoxycaine (Ravocaine).

If a patient is thought to be allergic to one of these drug groups, an agent from the other category should be selected since cross-sensitization is generally not exhibited.

■ **Why is a vasoconstrictor combined with a local anesthetic drug?**

A vasoconstrictor prevents rapid absorption of the anesthetic drug and prolongs the effect of anesthesia. By slowing the drug uptake into the circulatory system at the site of injection, toxic reactions are less likely to occur. Epinephrine and neo-cobefrin are vasoconstrictors used in local anesthetics.

■ **Explain the use of topical anesthetic agents.**

These solutions or ointments are used prior to anesthetic injections as well as for the temporary relief of ulcerated and injured areas and for the treatment of alveolar osteitis (dry socket). When applied to mucosal tissues, these agents produce temporary, superficial anesthesia.

■ **What is an antiepileptic drug?**

Antiepileptic drugs are drugs used in the treatment of convulsions and seizures in patients with epilepsy, cerebral palsy, and cerebrovascular accident. A commonly used anti-epileptic drug is phenytoin (Dilantin).

■ What is the intraoral effect associated with phenytoin therapy?

Thirty to sixty percent of the patients being treated with phenytoin are subject to an overgrowth of gingival tissue known as *gingival hyperplasia.* It is not completely understood why gingival hyperplasia occurs in some patients and not in others or why it occurs only in areas where natural teeth exist. Edentulous areas seem not to be affected. One theory suggests that local irritants such as plaque or calculus may be integral factors in its occurrence.

■ What drugs are used in the treatment of drug hypersensitivity?

Antihistaminics, such as diphenhydramine (Benadryl), may be used to treat minor types of allergic reactions in which urticaria or itching is the primary sign. For acute reactions such as anaphylactic shock, epinephrine is the initial drug of choice in the regimen for emergency treatment.

Oxygen, corticosteroids, or antihistaminics may be included in the regimen of treatment depending on the development of the reaction.

■ What is an antibiotic?

Antibiotics are agents used to destroy or inhibit the growth of disease-causing microorganisms. They may be extracted naturally from certain microorganisms, or they may be synthetically manufactured. Examples of antibiotics are penicillin and tetracycline.

■ When is an antibiotic prescribed?

An antibiotic may be used when there are systemic signs and symptoms of infection. Another use of antibiotics is for prophylactic premedication in the treatment of a patient with valvular damage or valvular prosthesis when an induced bacteremia might initiate subacute bacterial endocarditis (SBE). The antibiotic is used as a preventive agent against SBE. Patients with a history of rheumatic fever and heart murmur should always be considered for this treatment.

■ What is the antibiotic of choice in dentistry?

Penicillin is the antibiotic of choice in dentistry, since most infections in and around the oral cavity respond well to it. Erythromycin is often substituted when a patient has a known allergy to penicillin.

■ What is meant by "broad spectrum antibiotics"?

Broad spectrum antibiotics are antibiotics having effectiveness against a wide range of microorganisms. Penicillin is a good example of a broad spectrum antibiotic, and this suggests one reason why it is often the drug of choice for infection of unknown bacterial origin.

■ What side effect of tetracycline is significant to tooth development?

Tetracycline is generally not as effective as penicillin or erythromycin for dental infections, but it does have various medical uses. It must be dispensed with caution to a patient beyond the fourth month of pregnancy and to infants and children, since these are periods of tooth development. Tetracycline absorbed into tooth structure during development can produce a discoloration, "tetracycline staining," as well as areas of poorly developed enamel.

■ What antibiotic drugs are used for fungal infections?

Nystatin (Mycostatin), an antifungal agent, is the drug of choice used for the treatment of moniliasis (thrush).

■ Name some preparations that are used to control bleeding of postextraction sites.

Gelfoam, Oxycel, Novacell, and Surgicel are common brand names of absorbable hemostatic preparations. These substances aid in the production and formation of an artificial clot.

■ Why can patients be instructed to "bite on a tea bag" if there is slight, continued bleeding after oral surgery?

Tannic acid is present in tea and can be an effective astringent. This agent works by precipitating tissue protein to initiate hemostasis.

■ **How is epinephrine used for hemostasis?**

Cotton pledgets soaked with 0.1% epinephrine applied to the bleeding site will act on the vessels to cause vasoconstriction and reduced bleeding. With infiltration injection, local anesthetics that include a vasoconstrictor can reduce soft tissue bleeding during operative procedures in a similar manner.

■ **What topical astringent agent can be used as an alternative to epinephrine?**

Hemodent, a brand name for an astringent mixture of aluminum chloride, is useful in reducing gingival bleeding and providing topical anesthesia.

A cord impregnated with an astringent agent and placed into the gingival sulcus can produce gingival retraction for taking final impressions as in crown and bridge procedures.

It is purported that there are no serious systemic reactions to aluminum chloride such as may be experienced with the use of epinephrine.

■ **What precautions must be taken with patients who are receiving anticoagulant therapy?**

Here again the health history plays an important part in the evaluation of a patient to be treated. Anticoagulant drugs, blood thinners, are prescribed to patients for certain cardiovascular diseases to delay the coagulation of blood. Because these drugs disrupt the normal process of blood clotting, prolonged bleeding may result from surgical procedures. Patients receiving anticoagulant therapy will be taking such drugs as heparin, dicumarol, or warfarin (Coumadin). Prior to any dental surgery, prophylaxis, scaling, or gingival curettage the physician should be consulted as to how to handle the patient.

■ **How is methantheline used in dental treatment?**

Methantheline (Banthine) is an anticholinergic drug that suppresses salivary and bronchial secretions. Many orthodontic and restorative procedures are more easily carried out when the flow of intraoral secretions is temporarily depressed. Examples of other anticholinergic drugs are atropine, belladonna, and propantheline (Pro-Banthine).

■ **What preparations relieve the pain associated with dry socket?**

Alveolar osteitis, dry socket, produces a painful condition that is rarely relieved by systemic analgesics. An effective pain obtundent is a combination of topical anesthetic, antiseptic, and analgesic drugs impregnated into strip gauze used as a packing. There are various combinations of agents available including guaiacol, benzocaine, eugenol, glycerin, and iodine.

■ **What are oxidizing agents?**

Oxidizing agents include hydrogen peroxide and carbamide peroxide (Gly-oxide), the latter of which is of value for cleansing suppurating wounds and inflamed mucous membranes. These agents develop a gas that tends to loosen deposits and debris, and they should be used only in open wounds so that the gas is allowed to escape freely. Oxidizing agents are also useful as a mouthwash for the treatment of Vincent's stomatitis (trench mouth).

MULTIPLE-CHOICE QUESTIONS

1. The method of drug administration that produces the fastest onset of effects is:
   a. Intravenous
   b. Sublingual
   c. Subcutaneous
   d. Inhalation

2. Prior to selecting and prescribing any drug for a patient, what must be done?
   a. Allergy tests should be performed.
   b. Blood count should be taken.
   c. Accurate medical history should be compiled.

d. Weight and height measurements should be taken.
3. An order for the preparation and dispensation of a pharmaceutical substance is called a:
   a. Recipe
   b. Work order
   c. Prescription
   d. Label
4. The Latin abbreviation *qid* is defined as:
   a. For 4 days
   b. Every fourth day
   c. Every 4 hours
   d. Four times a day
5. The Latin abbreviation *nr* when placed on a prescription indicates that the substance is:
   a. A nonnarcotic
   b. To be taken when necessary
   c. Not refillable
   d. Governed by the Drug Enforcement Administration
6. The *body* of the prescription contains which kind of information:
   a. Patient's name and address
   b. Number and amount of drug
   c. Practitioner's name and registry number
   d. Drug name and strength
7. A 98 pound 25-year-old patient requires medication for pain. What one consideration would be used for modifying the dosage for this patient?
   a. Age
   b. Weight
   c. Race
   d. Sex
8. Which of the following drugs *require(s)* a written prescription:
   a. Methadone
   b. Morphine
   c. Empirin Compound
   d. Diazepam (Valium)
   e. Both methadone and morphine
   f. Both methadone and Empirin Compound
   g. None of the above
9. The proprietary name of a drug is known as the:
   a. Brand name

b. Generic name
   c. Chemical name
   d. Classification name
10. Which of the following is the generic name of a drug?
    a. Valium
    b. Propantheline bromide
    c. V-Cillin-K
    d. Percogesic
11. Which of the following contain the official drug standards:
    a. Bureau of Narcotics and Dangerous Drugs and *Journal of the American Dental Association*
    b. *National Formulary* and *Journal of the American Dental Association*
    c. *National Formulary* and *United States Pharmacopeia*
    d. Bureau of Narcotics and Dangerous Drugs and *United States Pharmacopeia*
12. A publication that lists and describes accepted drugs for dental treatment is:
    a. *Journal of the American Dental Association*
    b. *Physicians' Desk Reference*
    c. *Accepted Dental Therapeutics*
    d. *Dental Survey*
13. Nitrous oxide is administered by which of the following methods:
    a. Intravenous
    b. Oral
    c. Inhalation
    d. Sublingual
14. A patient taking aspirin can experience stomach irritation. This effect is called:
    a. Drug interaction
    b. Side effect
    c. Idiosyncrasy
    d. Anaphylaxis
15. The drug that can be used in counteracting anaphylactic shock is:
    a. Diazepam (Valium)
    b. Secobarbital (Seconal)
    c. Epinephrine
    d. Lidocaine (Xylocaine)
16. Barbiturates may be sedative or hypnotic depending on:
    a. Mode of administration
    b. How the drug is excreted

c. Amount of dosage

d. Absorption rate

17. Which of the following are characteristics of an antibiotic:

a. Is produced by other microorganisms, destroys or inhibits bacterial growth, and inhibits viral growth

b. Is produced by other microorganisms, destroys or inhibits bacterial growth, and is useful in treating infection

c. All of the above

18. What federal agency protects the safety and welfare of the consumer in relation to pharmaceutical substances?

a. Federal Safety Commission

b. Food and Drug Administration

c. World Health Organization

d. American Medical Association

19. Which federal agency regulates the dispensing and prescribing of narcotic drugs?

a. Food and Drug Administration

b. *The United States Pharmacopeia*

c. Drug Enforcement Administration

d. Drug Formulary

20. Which publication would provide drug identification indices?

a. *Accepted Dental Therapeutics*

b. *Drug Digest*

c. *Journal of the American Medical Association*

d. *Physicians' Desk Reference*

21. What adverse effect could be produced by the simultaneous administration of alcohol and diazepam (Valium)?

a. Side effect

b. Idiosyncrasy

c. Allergic response

d. Interaction

22. Prophylactic antibiotic therapy is indicated prior to oral surgery for a patient with the medical history of:

a. Hemophilia

b. Rheumatic fever

c. Hypertension

d. Herpetic stomatitis

23. Epinephrine is added to a local anesthetic solution to:

a. Speed the absorption rate into the circulatory system

b. Prevent syncope

c. Decrease dry toxicity

d. Prolong the anesthetic effect

24. Which one of the following is an example of a local anesthetic:

a. Lidocaine hydrochloride

b. Thiopental sodium

c. Heparin

d. Epinephrine

25. Which antibiotic is the drug of choice for treatment of dental infections?

a. One of the sulfa group

b. Nystatin

c. Tetracycline

d. Penicillin

26. Hemostatic agents function to:

a. Allay apprehension

b. Reduce bleeding

c. Thin the blood

d. Prevent hypertension

27. A patient receiving anticoagulant therapy poses a problem related to:

a. Hemorrhage

b. Anxiety

c. Hypertension

d. Depression

28. Drugs that reduce fever are referred to as:

a. Antihistaminics

b. Corticosteroids

c. Antipyretics

d. Antiemetics

29. A substance used in the dental office to reduce anxiety during the treatment procedure is:

a. Lidocaine

b. Aspirin

c. A.P.C.

d. Nitrous oxide

30. An epileptic patient would most likely be taking which of the following drugs?

a. Secobarbital (Seconal)

b. Methantheline bromide (Banthine)

c. Insulin

d. Phenytoin (Dilantin)

31. A patient complains of mild postextraction pain. Which analgesic would most likely be prescribed?

a. Morphine

b. Codeine

c. Aspirin

d. Oxycodone (Percodan)

32. Which one of the following is an important aspect of the health history that should be considered prior to applying a topical pharmaceutical agent?
    a. Age of the patient
    b. Weight of the patient
    c. Directions from the manufacturer
    d. Patient's allergies to drugs

33. A patient is in the dental office for deep scaling and polishing of the teeth. The health history reveals that warfarin (Coumadin) is being taken for phlebitis. Warfarin is an:
    a. Anticonvulsant
    b. Antipyretic
    c. Anticoagulant
    d. Antiepileptic

34. Prophylactic antibiotics should be prescribed, unless there is an evident contraindication, for any patient who has a history of:
    a. Hemophilia
    b. Subacute bacterial endocarditis
    c. Epilepsy
    d. Diabetes

35. An anticholinergic drug can be used to reduce:
    a. Vomiting
    b. Nausea
    c. Secretions
    d. Inflammation

36. Which of the following drugs produces hemostasis by causing constriction of the blood vessels?
    a. Gelfoam
    b. Tannic acid
    c. Epinephrine
    d. Diphenhydramine (Benadryl)

37. A male patient is going to have full orthodontic appliances placed during his 1-hour appointment. The dentist asks him to take a pill 2 hours before the appointment to reduce the salivary flow. What would this drug be?
    a. Phenylephrine (Novahistine)
    b. Methantheline (Banthine)
    c. Cortisone
    d. Methadone

38. During cavity preparation a pulp exposure occurs. Which medication would most likely be placed in an attempt to stimulate the production of secondary dentin for natural pulp protection?
    a. Eugenol
    b. Parachlorophenol
    c. Clove oil
    d. Calcium hydroxide

39. The method of administering nitroglycerin is:
    a. Sublingual
    b. Intravenous
    c. Topical
    d. Oral

40. For what condition is nitroglycerin prescribed?
    a. Hypertension
    b. Angina pectoris
    c. Allergy
    d. Diabetes

41. Which of these drugs is a sedative-hypnotic?
    a. Aspirin
    b. Diazepam (Valium)
    c. Phenobarbital
    d. Methantheline (Banthine)

42. Aluminum chloride (Hemodent) is useful to:
    a. Prolong local anesthesia
    b. Produce secondary dentin
    c. Reduce pain
    d. Reduce blood flow

43. Physical or psychologic dependence on a drug is called:
    a. Tolerance
    b. Abuse
    c. Addiction
    d. Hypersensitivity

44. Barbiturates are:
    a. Anesthetics
    b. Sedatives
    c. Tranquilizers
    d. Stimulants

45. What drug is usually associated with an overgrowth of gingival tissue?
    a. Phenytoin (Dilantin)
    b. Morphine
    c. Cortisone
    d. Dihydromorphine (Dilaudid)

46. An agent used in endodontic treatment for cleansing root canals is:
   a. Calcium hydroxide
   b. Iodine
   c. Hydrogen peroxide
   d. Sodium hypochlorite

47. An agent used on the mucosal surface for topical antisepsis is:
   a. Parachlorophenol
   b. Mercocresols (Mercresin)
   c. Hydrogen peroxide
   d. Lidocaine (Xylocaine ointment)

SUGGESTED READINGS

American Dental Association Council on Dental Therapeutics: Accepted dental therapeutics, ed. 37, Chicago, 1977, The American Dental Association.

Cowan, F. F.: Pharmacology for the dental hygienist, Philadelphia, 1978, Lea & Febiger.

Dunn, M. J., Booth, D. F., and Clancy, M.: Dental auxiliary practice—pharmacology, pain control, sterile technique and oral surgery, Module 5, Baltimore, 1975, The Williams & Wilkins Co.

Dunn, M. J.: Drug evaluation in dentistry, J. Am. Dent. Assist. Assoc. **47:**33, 1978.

Kutscher, A. H., et al.: Pharmacology for the dental hygienist, Philadelphia, 1967, Lea & Febiger.

Richardson, R. E., and Barton, R. E.: The dental assistant, ed. 5, New York, 1978, McGraw-Hill Book Co.

CHAPTER 22

Dental radiography

MARIAN R. ALGARDA

■ **When, by whom, and under what circumstances were x rays discovered?**

On November 8, 1895 Wilhelm Konrad Roentgen, a physicist, discovered x rays. While experimenting with cathode rays from a Crookes tube (vacuum tube), Roentgen noticed that a heretofore unknown radiation penetrated the thick black paper and caused a fluorescent screen to glow. When objects were placed between the screen and the tube, their shadows were seen on the screen. Further experiments verified the existence of a new ray (x ray) that was invisible and capable of penetrating opaque substances whose images could be recorded on a photographic plate.

■ **What are some of the characteristics of x rays?**

Among the important properties of x rays are the following: (1) the ability to penetrate opaque substances; (2) the ability to affect silver halide salts on films in the same manner as light does; (3) the ability to stimulate or destroy tissue by ionization; (4) they travel at a constant speed, the speed of light, 186,000 miles per second; (5) they cause fluorescence; (6) they are high energy waves; (7) they travel as electromagnetic waves or energy; (8) they have no mass; and (9) they travel in a straight line and are invisible.

■ **How do x rays relate to the electromagnetic spectrum?**

X rays are part of the electromagnetic spectrum. The various members of the spectrum arranged according to wavelength include: radio, heat or infrared, visible light, ultraviolet light, x rays, gamma rays, and cosmic rays.

Although radio waves are measured in meters, x rays are measured in angstrom units. An angstrom unit is one ten-billionth of a meter.

The differences in energy and therefore penetrating power in any kind of electromagnetic radiation are directly related to wavelength—the shorter the wavelength, the higher the energy and the penetrating power.

The practical aspect of this as it relates to x-ray technique is that the higher the kilovoltage, the shorter the x-ray wavelength, hence, the greater the penetrating power.

■ **What is ionization?**

Ionization is the production of ions (or ion pairs) by the removal of electrons from the atoms of the matter that are struck by the x rays. Ionization occurs whenever x rays penetrate matter.

■ **What is electric current?**

Electric current is the flow of electrons from one point to another or through a conductor. This flow is measured in amperes.

■ **What is direct current?**

Direct current (DC) is current flowing in one direction, that is, from positive to negative. Direct current can be interrupted at certain set intervals.

■ **What is alternating current?**

Alternating current (AC) is current that flows first in one direction and then reverses itself and flows in the opposite direction. The combination of one forward and reverse flow constitutes a cycle.

202

■ **What is an ampere?**

An ampere (amp) is a unit of *current flow* through a circuit. The unit of current flow is a measure of the quantity of electrons.

■ **What is a volt?**

A volt (V) is a unit of electric *pressure* that forces the electromotive force.

■ **What is a kilovolt?**

A kilovolt (kV) equals 1000 volts.

■ **What is a watt?**

A watt (W) is the unit of electric work as measured by a wattmeter. It is determined by multiplying the voltage by the amperage.

■ **What is an ohm?**

An ohm (Ω) is the unit of electric *resistance*. One volt will force 1 ampere of current thru 1 ohm of resistance.

■ **What is an electron?**

An electron is a small negatively charged component of the atom.

■ **What is an anode?**

An anode is a positively charged electrode. In the x-ray tube the anode is positively charged from 65 to 90 kV, is made of copper (for good heat dissipation), and contains the tungsten target where x rays are produced.

■ **What is the cathode?**

The cathode is the negatively charged electrode in the x-ray tube consisting of a tungsten filament wire that is surrounded by the focusing cup.

■ **What is kilovoltage?**

Kilovoltage is usually designated as kilovolt peak (kVp). It is a measure of the force between the negative cathode and the positive anode and controls the energy of the electrons striking the tungsten target. Kilovoltage controls the penetrating ability of the x rays.

■ **What is milliamperage?**

Milliamperage (mA) is the measurement of the quantity or the number of electrons passing from cathode to anode per second. As the number of these electrons is increased, more x rays are produced at the target. Note that the milliamperage determines only the strength of the x-ray beam; it has nothing to do with the penetrating power of the beam.

■ **What is the maximum permissible dose (MPD) for occupationally exposed persons?**

The MPD is the quantity of radiation to which a person may be exposed without danger. The National Committee on Radiation Protection restricts the maximum permissible dose for occupationally exposed workers to 0.1 roentgen equivalent man (rem) in any 1 week, 3 rem in any 13-week period, and 5 rem in any 1 year.

■ **What is the MPD formula for total accumulated dose for occupationally exposed persons?**

The formula for total accumulated dose for occupationally exposed persons is MPD = 5 rem $\times$ (N-18). N is the age in years. This formula subtracts 18 from the worker's age because persons 18 years and younger are not supposed to work around x rays.

■ **Define rad (radiation-absorbed dose).**

The rad is a measurement devised to express the quantity of radiation absorbed by soft tissue. With x rays, 1 roentgen (R) of exposure will usually produce about 1 rad of absorbed dose in soft tissue.

■ **Define rem (roentgen equivalent man)**

A rem is a measurement unit to provide the estimated amount of energy absorbed in tissue that is biologically equivalent in man to one R of gamma rays or x rays.

■ **What is an erythema dose?**

Erythema is a temporary reddening of the skin. An erythema dose is the amount of radiation necessary to produce erythema.

■ **What is a lead diaphragm, and what is its purpose in the x-ray cone?**

The lead diaphragm is a metal disk 0.16 cm

(1/16 inch) thick of lead with a hole in the center. Its purpose is to collimate or limit the size of the beam of radiation. The diameter recommended is one that does not exceed 6.88 cm (2.75 inches) at the cone tip.

■ **What is the purpose of aluminum filtration?**

The purpose of aluminum filtration is to selectively absorb the longer wavelengths of less penetrating radiation. (Actually the useless radiation would be totally absorbed by the patient and would not contribute to the radiographic picture.)

■ **What is inherent filtration?**

Inherent filtration is that filtration which is built into the x-ray machine and is the result of the various construction materials in the path of the beam, that is, the glass wall of the x-ray tube, oil surrounding the tube, and the permanent tube seal.

■ **What is added filtration?**

Added filtration is usually an aluminum disk of such thickness as to bring the aluminum equivalent filtration to a total of 1.5 mm to 2.5 mm aluminum depending on the kilovoltage.

■ **What is total filtration?**

Total filtration is the sum of inherent and added filtration. The lowest requirement for total filtration is 2.5 mm of aluminum for all x-ray machines operating at greater than 70 kV. For those machines operating at less than 70 kV, only 1.5 mm of aluminum filtration is required.

■ **What is primary radiation?**

Primary radiation is radiation coming directly from the target of the x-ray tube. It is the useful beam.

■ **What is secondary radiation?**

Secondary radiation is produced whenever x rays strike matter. When x rays pass through the tissues of the face during dental x-ray procedures, secondary x rays are produced.

Scattered radiation is primary radiation that has been deviated in direction during passage through a substance.

■ **What is leakage radiation?**

Leakage radiation may come from the wall of the tube housing or may come from around the cone.

■ **What are the three important conditions necessary for the production of x rays?**

A source of electrons (heated filament)
A means of accelerating the high-speed electrons between one third and one half the speed of light (a high positive potential)
A means of stopping these high-speed electrons suddenly (tungsten target)

■ **What is meant by the focal spot of an x-ray tube?**

The focal spot is the small area on the tungsten target to which the electrons are directed. A small focal point permits sharper detail on the radiograph.

■ **What is meant by thermionic emission?**

Thermionic emission is the "boiling off" of electrons at the hot filament wire of the cathode.

■ **When are x rays produced?**

X rays are produced any time that high speed electrons are stopped suddenly.

■ **Explain the importance of the transformers in the x-ray machine.**

Step down transformer: This transformer steps the incoming line voltage down from 110 or 220 V to approximately 3 to 5 V necessary for the filament wire current.

Step up transformer: This transformer steps up the incoming line voltage to the x-ray machine from 110 or 220 V to 50,000 to 100,000 V or 50 kV to 100 kV. This high voltage is necessary to propel at a high speed the electrons from the negative cathode to the positive anode.

Autotransformer: Variations in the incoming line voltage are regulated by this transformer.

■ **What are somatic cells?**

Somatic cells are all cells of the body except those of the reproductive organs.

■ **What are genetic cells?**

Genetic cells contain the genes and are concerned with reproduction. Genetic effects from x rays may not appear for several generations.

■ **List some of the ways the operator may protect the patient from excessive radiation.**

Use the proper collimation.
Use proper aluminum filtration.
Use high-speed films.
Use protective lead aprons.
Use long, lead-lined open-end cones.
Use film-holding devices that block extraneous radiation.
Use care in x-ray technique and processing procedures.

■ **List some of the ways operators of x-ray machines can protect themselves.**

Keep out of the primary beam.
Stand at least 6 feet from the x-ray tube and patient during exposure and behind a lead shielded wall.
Never hold a film during an exposure.
Never hold the cone or x-ray tube housing during exposure.
Subscribe to a personnel monitoring (film badge) service.

■ **What is a film badge?**

A film badge is a special light-tight film covered by a copper-stripped wedge filter. The badge is worn by the operator for a month after which it is processed at the commercial lab. Film badge service will aid in determining the amount of radiation received by the operator, and the service will make a periodic report to the operator.

■ **What is the purpose of an intensifying screen?**

An intensifying screen is a device used to augment the effect of the x ray and thus shorten the time of exposure. It consists of a thin pliable base that is coated with minute crystals of calcium tungstate which, when acted on by x rays, emits a blue fluorescence, to which photographic and x-ray film are extremely sensitive. The light aids the action of the x rays, accounting for up to 90% of the darkening of the film.

■ **What is the composition of an x-ray film?**

The film itself has a firm but flexible base made of acetate or polyester. An emulsion of silver halide crystals mixed with gelatin is spread in a thin layer over both sides of the base.

■ **What is the purpose of the lead foil backing in an x-ray film packet?**

The lead foil prevents backscatter, which is fogging caused by secondary radiation created in the tissues behind the film.

■ **What are the three basic types of intraoral views?**

The most frequently used intraoral view is the *periapical* which shows the entire tooth and surrounding structures on the film. Another type is the *interproximal* view (bite-wing) taken primarily to detect interproximal caries. The *occlusal* view is necessary to observe the entire maxilla or mandible.

■ **Under what circumstances would an extraoral film be necessary?**

Extraoral films are placed outside the mouth and are needed for large areas of pathologic involvement, fractures of facial bones, temporomandibular joint exposures, head plates, and patients who cannot open their mouth. Common extraoral film sizes are 12.5 × 17.5 cm, 20 × 25 cm, and 25 × 30 cm (5 × 7 inches, 8 × 10 inches, and 10 × 12 inches).

■ **What is panoramic radiography?**

The term *panoramic radiography* refers to a technique that produces a single extraoral film showing the patient's complete upper and lower jaws. In using all of the panoramic machines, positioning the patient's head and maintaining that position during the exposure is extremely important; otherwise the desired dental structures may not be in focus.

■ **In cone angulation what causes elongation and foreshortening errors?**

Cone angulation that is too vertical results in foreshortening. Cone angulation with too little vertical results in elongation. Other factors causing elongation or foreshortening are improper positioning of the patient's head or improper film placement.

■ What causes overlapping?

Improper horizontal angulation causes overlapping. In a dental x-ray film, when the central ray is not directed through the contact points and is not parallel to the interproximal surfaces, overlap of the interproximal surfaces will occur.

■ What causes cone cutting?

If the central ray is not directed at the center of the film, cone cutting will result.

■ What is the purpose of the raised dot on the x-ray film?

The raised dot makes it possible to tell right from left when mounting x-ray films. When films are mounted with the raised portion of the dot facing you, you are mounting by the facial method. In a full-mouth series of mounted radiographs, the left side of the mount becomes the patient's right side.

■ Name nine cell types in order of their radiosensitivity.

1. Early embryo cells
2. Genetic cells
3. Blood cells
4. Epithelial cells
5. Connective tissue cells
6. Tubular cells of the kidneys
7. Bone cells
8. Nerve cells (brain cells)
9. Muscle cells

■ In what position is the patient's head placed for x-ray films of the maxillary teeth and for bite-wing exposures?

The patient's head should be positioned so that the occlusal plane is parallel to the floor, and the midsagittal plane is perpendicular to the floor.

■ In what position is the patient's head placed for x-ray films of all mandibular teeth?

The head is tilted back slightly so that when the mouth is open, the occlusal plane of the mandible is parallel to the floor, and the mid-

sagittal plane of the head is perpendicular to the floor.

■ What is the ala-tragus line?

The ala-tragus line is a line from the tragus of the ear to the ala of the nose. For maxillary films the central ray is directed through this line as it transverses the apices of the maxillary teeth.

■ Explain the bisection-of-angle x-ray technique?

With the bisection-of-angle technique the central ray is directed perpendicular to an imaginary line that bisects the plane of the film and the long axis of the tooth. The film is placed against the anatomic structures and the teeth. The target-film distance is 8 inches.

■ What are occlusal views?

Occlusal views are intraoral radiographs taken with the film placed in the occlusal plane. The radiation is directed from above for the maxillary view and from below for the mandibular view.

Interpretation of a combination of occlusal and periapical views makes it possible to pinpoint the position of impacted teeth, cysts, supernumerary teeth, fractures, foreign bodies, and other abnormalities.

■ What is a lateral jaw radiograph?

A lateral jaw radiograph is an extraoral film exposure that shows either the right or left side of the maxillae in profile.

The body and ramus of the mandible, including the teeth from the cuspid to the third molar, are visualized with little superimposition from other structures. The beam of radiation must be directed from the opposite side from just below and behind the angle of the mandible.

■ How may a regular size (No 2) film be placed to radiograph the difficult mandibular third molar area?

A periapical-size film may be placed over the third molar area in the occlusal plane. It is allowed to ride up on the ramus until the anterior edge of the film is at the middle of the occlusal surface of the lower first molar. The patient's head is tilted backward so that it is possible to direct the central ray upward through the angle of the mandible at approximately 45 degrees.

■ **What type of exposures are generally used for children up to age six?**

For children up to age six, routine exposures might be an anterior occlusal film of each arch and a posterior bite-wing film of each side. An alternate method might be to make a Panorex exposure and the posterior bite-wing films.

■ **Why would it be necessary to x-ray an edentulous patient?**

Edentulous areas are x-rayed to rule out the possibility of impacted teeth, retained roots, cysts, and other pathologic conditions present within the bone.

■ **How is the vertical angulation adjusted when x-raying edentulous patients or children?**

When x-raying edentulous patients or children the vertical angulation is increased 5 to 10 degrees.

■ **Describe the technique used for root canal examination of multirooted teeth.**

When x-raying the upper first premolar, direct the central ray somewhat mesiodistally. This will overlap the crowns but will show the buccal and lingual roots with their canals separately. For the upper and lower molars, besides the routine periapical films, two additional films should be made. One view directs the x rays mesiodistally, and the other directs the x rays distomesially. For the lower molars two other exposures should be made, one with the x rays directed distomesially or at a 90-degree angle to the sagittal plane and the other with the x rays directed mesiodistally.

■ **What is the difference between a radiopaque and radiolucent landmark?**

Objects that absorb x rays are classified as radiopaque and appear white on a radiograph. Objects that are radiolucent do not absorb x rays and appear black on the film.

■ **Give some examples of radiopaque and radiolucent landmarks?**

Radiopaque objects and landmarks are gold crowns, metal fillings, teeth, bony projections such as the zygomatic process or molar bone, the external oblique line, and the coronoid process. Radiolucent objects and landmarks are silicate restorations, pulp canals, foramen, maxillary sinus areas, mandibular canal, and carious lesions.

■ **Identify anatomic landmarks in the maxillary and mandibular arches.**

The anatomic landmarks in both arches, including a tracing showing numbered landmarks is shown in Fig. 22-1.

■ **What factors are always involved in the taking of a radiograph of diagnostic quality?**

Position of patient's head
Placement of film
Milliamperage and voltage
Target-film distance
Angulation of the cone
Time of exposure
Processing of film

■ **List the ingredients in the developer solution, and give the purpose of each ingredient.**

Hydroquinone—reducing agent
Elon—reducing agent
Sodium sulfite—preservative
Potassium bromide—restrainer
Sodium carbonate—activator
Distilled water—solvent (vehicle)

■ **List the ingredients in the fixer solution, and give the purpose of each ingredient.**

Sodium thiosulfate (hypo)—clearing agent
Sodium sulfite—preservative
Potassium aluminum—hardener
Acetic acid or sulfuric acid—acidifier
Distilled water—solvent (vehicle)

■ **What is the purpose of the developer?**

The developing solution affects only those silver grains that have been exposed to the x rays. It reduces these grains by taking out the halide element and leaving only the metallic silver. The latent image becomes a real image at this time.

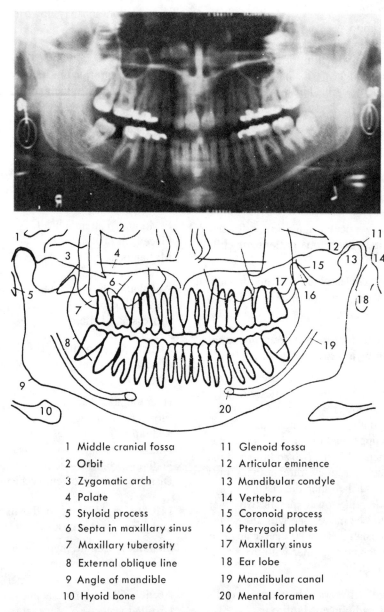

1 Middle cranial fossa	11 Glenoid fossa
2 Orbit	12 Articular eminence
3 Zygomatic arch	13 Mandibular condyle
4 Palate	14 Vertebra
5 Styloid process	15 Coronoid process
6 Septa in maxillary sinus	16 Pterygoid plates
7 Maxillary tuberosity	17 Maxillary sinus
8 External oblique line	18 Ear lobe
9 Angle of mandible	19 Mandibular canal
10 Hyoid bone	20 Mental foramen

Fig. 22-1. Panoramic radiograph and tracing showing numbered anatomic landmarks. (Courtesy General Electric Co., Milwaukee.) (From Frommer, H. H.: Radiology for dental auxiliaries, ed. 2, St. Louis, 1978, The C. V. Mosby Co.)

■ **What is the purpose of the fixer?**

The fixer dissolves the highly insoluble silver halide salts remaining in the emulsion, thereby clearing the image brought out by the developer.

■ **What is the purpose of a safelight? List two types of safelight filters used in the darkroom.**

A safelight is used for illumination in the darkroom during film processing. Two types of safelight filters are the Wratten 6B, which gives an orange-red light and uses a 7½-watt light bulb, and the Morelight filter ML-2, which has a brighter orange light and is used with a 15-watt light bulb. Although the former can be used for all films, the latter can only be used for processing intraoral film.

■ **List some of the errors in processing and the causes of these errors.**

Very light radiographs
Old (oxidized) developer
Insufficient time in developer
Underexposure
Cold developer
Reversed film placement
Decreased voltage or milliamperage
Very dark radiographs
Overexposure
Overdevelopment
Warm developing solution
Increased voltage or milliamperage
Unsafe illumination in darkroom
Blurred radiographs
Movement of film, patient, or tube
Double exposure
Distorted radiographs
Excessive bending of film
Elongation or foreshortening
Streaked, stained radiographs
Inadequate fixing and washing
Splashing developer or fixer before processing
Partial images
Cone cutting
Part of film not immersed in developer
Fogged radiographs
Old film
Stray radiation
Defective safelight
Light leaks in darkroom

■ **Identify anatomic landmarks and common errors on actual radiographs.**

For the purpose of review, the following radiographs (Figs. 22-2 to 22-29) are being illustrated with appropriate legends. It is suggested that a person preparing for an examination study several sets of radiographs and look for each of these landmarks and/or errors in them.

Text continued on p. 223.

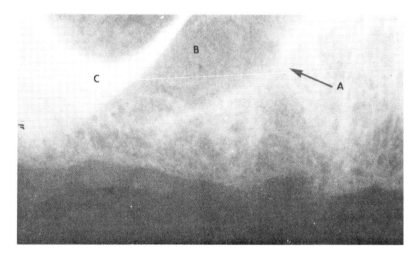

Fig. 22-2. Edentulous maxillary bicuspid area: *A,* anterior border of maxillary sinus; *B,* maxillary sinus; *C,* zygomatic arch. (From Frommer, H. H.: Radiology for dental auxiliaries, ed. 2, St. Louis, 1978, The C. V. Mosby Co.)

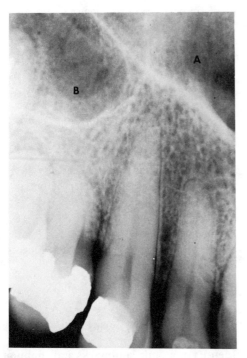

Fig. 22-3. Maxillary cuspid area: *A,* nasal cavity; *B,* maxillary sinus. (From Frommer, H. H.: Radiology for dental auxiliaries, ed. 2, St. Louis, 1978, The C. V. Mosby Co.)

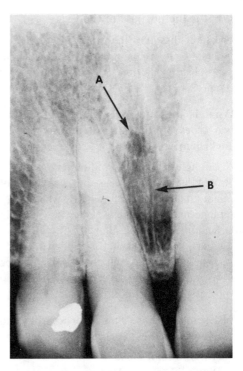

Fig. 22-4. Maxillary central incisor region: *A,* anterior palatine foramen; *B,* median suture. (From Frommer, H. H.: Radiology for dental auxiliaries, ed. 2, St. Louis, 1978, The C. V. Mosby Co.)

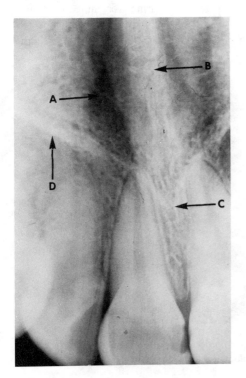

Fig. 22-5. Maxillary central incisor region: *A,* nasal cavity; *B,* median nasal septum; *C,* anterior nasal spine; *D,* floor of nose. (From Frommer, H. H.: Radiology for dental auxiliaries, ed. 2, St. Louis, 1978, The C. V. Mosby Co.)

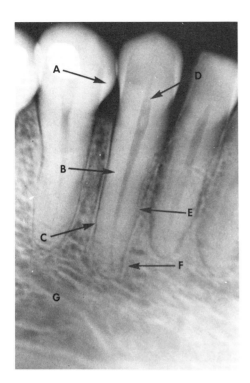

Fig. 22-6. Normal radiographic tooth anatomy: *A,* enamel; *B,* dentin; *C,* periodontal membrane; *D,* pulp chamber; *E,* cementum; *F,* lamina dura; *G,* alveolar bone. (From Frommer, H. H.: Radiology for dental auxiliaries, ed. 2, St. Louis, 1978, The C. V. Mosby Co.)

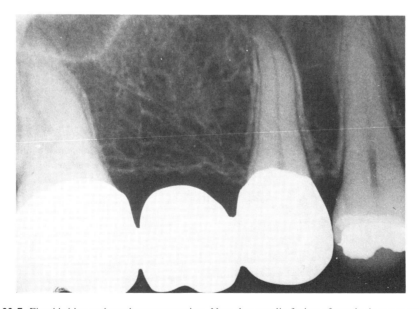

Fig. 22-7. Fixed bridge and amalgam restoration. Note that acrylic facing of pontic does not appear on radiograph. Also note difference in radiopacities between amalgam and its cement base. (From Frommer, H. H.: Radiology for dental auxiliaries, ed. 2, St. Louis, 1978, The C. V. Mosby Co.)

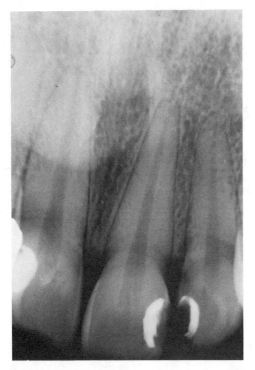

Fig. 22-8. Anterior synthetic restoration with cement bases. (From Frommer, H. H.: Radiology for dental auxiliaries, ed. 2, St. Louis, 1978, The C. V. Mosby Co.)

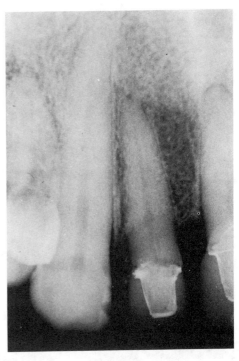

Fig. 22-9. Porcelain jackets. Note radiopacity of zinc oxyphosphate cement used. (From Frommer, H. H.: Radiology for dental auxiliaries, ed. 2, St. Louis, 1978, The C. V. Mosby Co.)

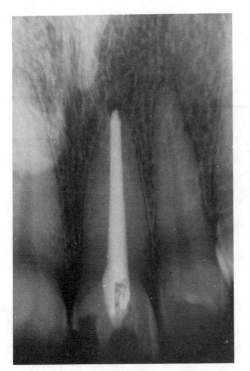

Fig. 22-10. Gutta-percha endodontic filling in maxillary central incisor. (From Frommer, H. H.: Radiology for dental auxiliaries, ed. 2, St. Louis, 1978, The C. V. Mosby Co.)

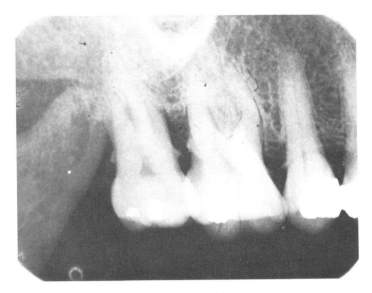

Fig. 22-11. Maxillary molar region. Note radiopaque U-shaped shadow of zygomatic arch. Note also coronoid process distal to the second molar. (From Frommer, H. H.: Radiology for dental auxiliaries, ed. 2, St. Louis, 1978, The C. V. Mosby Co.)

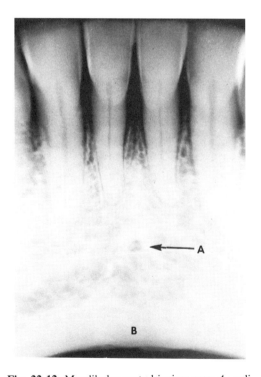

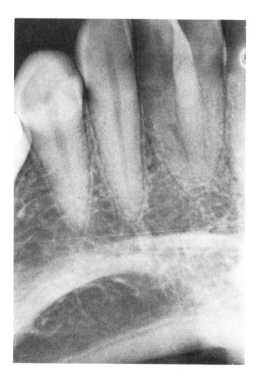

Fig. 22-12. Mandibular central incisor area: *A*, radiopaque genial tubercles with lingual foramen in center; *B*, inferior border of mandible. (From Frommer, H. H.: Radiology for dental auxiliaries, ed. 2, St. Louis, 1978, The C. V. Mosby Co.)

Fig. 22-13. Mental ridge in mandibular incisor cuspid region. (From Frommer, H. H.: Radiology for dental auxiliaries, ed. 2, St. Louis, 1978, The C. V. Mosby Co.)

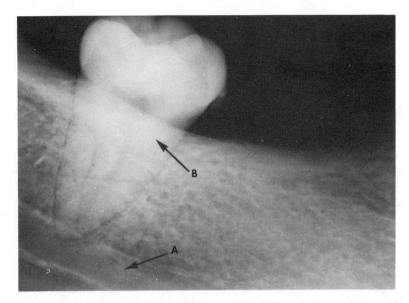

Fig. 22-14. Mandibular molar area: *A*, mandibular canal; *B*, radiopacity on tooth caused by super-imposition of oblique ridges. (From Frommer, H. H.: Radiology for dental auxiliaries, ed. 2, St. Louis, 1978, The C. V. Mosby Co.)

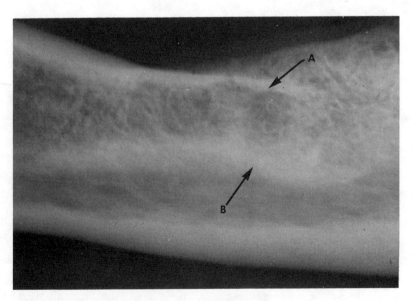

Fig. 22-15. Edentulous mandibular molar area: *A*, external oblique ridge; *B*, internal oblique ridge, and upward slope of crest of alveolar ridge as it goes distally. (From Frommer, H. H.: Radiology for dental auxiliaries, ed. 2, St. Louis, 1978, The C. V. Mosby Co.)

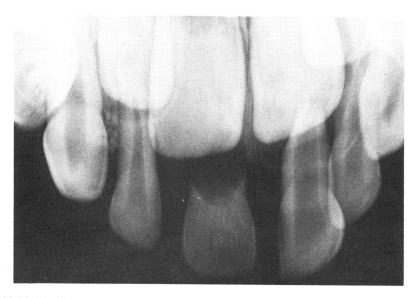

Fig. 22-16. Maxillary central incisor area in child. Permanent teeth are seen in bone. Note root resorption of deciduous central incisor due to eruptive force. (From Frommer, H. H.: Radiology for dental auxiliaries, ed. 2, St. Louis, 1978, The C. V. Mosby Co.)

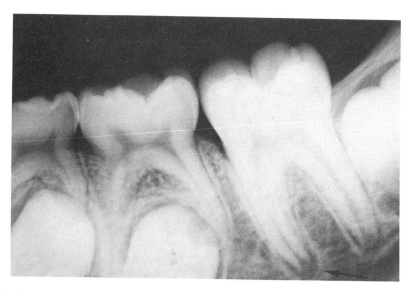

Fig. 22-17. Mandibular mixed dentition. Note incomplete root formation on first molar and developing tooth bud of second molar. (From Frommer, H. H.: Radiology for dental auxiliaries, ed. 2, St. Louis, 1978, The C. V. Mosby Co.)

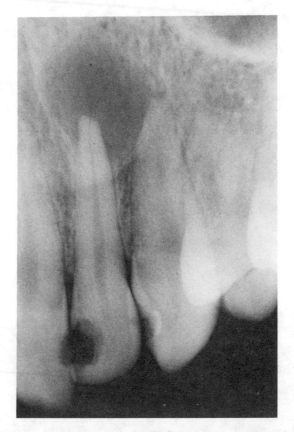

Fig. 22-18. Periapical cyst of maxillary lateral incisor. (From Frommer, H. H.: Radiology for dental auxiliaries, ed. 2, St. Louis, 1978, The C. V. Mosby Co.)

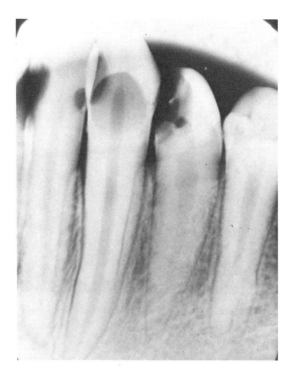

Fig. 22-19. Cone cut. The clear, unexposed area resulted because the beam of radiation did not completely cover the film (in addition, this film was not placed sufficiently deep in the floor of the mouth to receive the shadow of the cuspid apex). (From Wuehrmann, A. H., and Manson-Hing, L. R.: Dental radiology, ed. 4, St. Louis, 1977, The C. V. Mosby Co.)

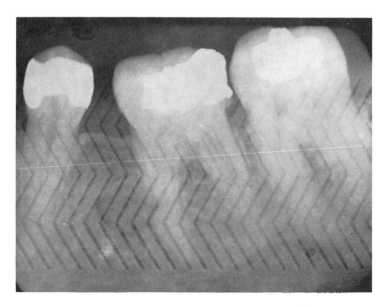

Fig. 22-20. Film exposed through nonexposure side. A light radiograph having a herringbone or some other characteristic pattern results when the film is placed with the nonexposure side toward the teeth. (From Wuehrmann, A. H., and Manson-Hing, L. R.: Dental radiology, ed. 4, St. Louis, 1977, The C. V. Mosby Co.)

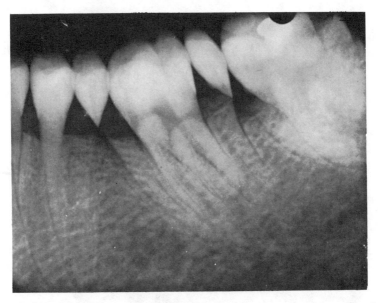

Fig. 22-21. Double image. Excessive density and two images result when a film is exposed twice. (From Wuehrmann, A. H., and Manson-Hing, L. R.: Dental radiology, ed. 4, St. Louis, 1977, The C. V. Mosby Co.)

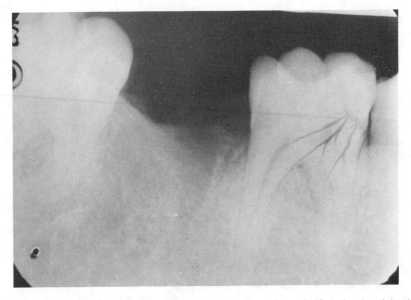

Fig. 22-22. Static electricity. Multiple black linear streaks can result if static electricity is produced when films are forcefully unwrapped or if the film is flexed to make it less stiff. (From Wuehrmann, A. H., and Manson-Hing, L. R.: Dental radiology, ed. 4, St. Louis, 1977, The C. V. Mosby Co.)

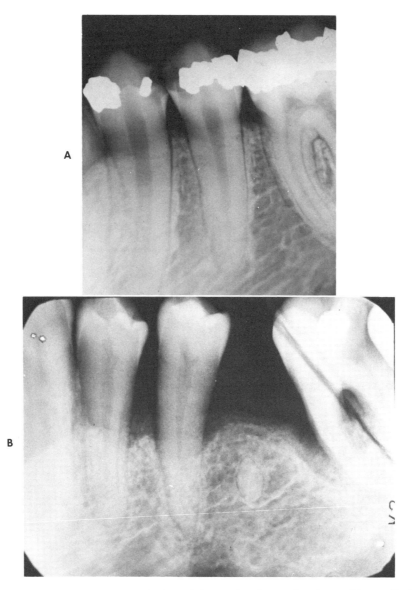

Fig. 22-23. Curved and bent films. **A,** Curved film produced a streaky, distorted image. **B,** A black lines occurs where the film is bent. (From Wuehrmann, A. H., and Manson-Hing, L. R.: Dental radiology, ed. 4, St. Louis, 1977, The C. V. Mosby Co.)

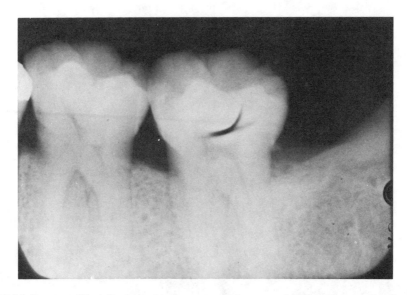

Fig. 22-24. Pressure. Black lines result when pressure is put on the film. Fingernails often cause such pressure marks (this film was also not placed sufficiently deep in the mouth to receive the tooth shadow completely). (From Wuehrmann, A. H., and Manson-Hing, L. R.: Dental radiology, ed. 4, St. Louis, 1977, The C. V. Mosby Co.)

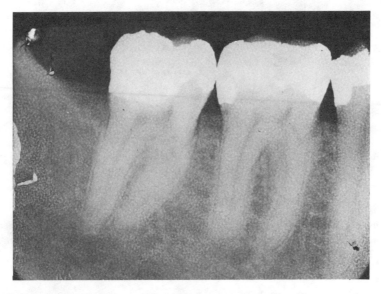

Fig. 22-25. Reticulation. The film emulsion often cracks when subjected to great changes in temperature between the different processing solutions. The temperature variation must go from warm to cold. (From Wuehrmann, A. H., and Manson-Hing, L. R.: Dental radiology, ed. 4, St. Louis, 1977, The C. V. Mosby Co.)

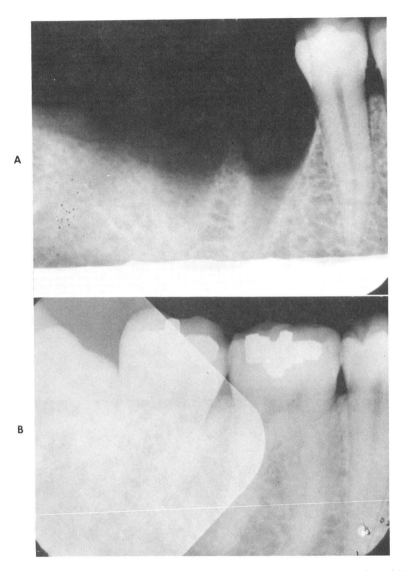

Fig. 22-26. Undeveloped clear areas. **A,** Clear area caused by incomplete immersion of film in the developer. **B,** Clear area caused by films sticking to each other while in the developer. A similar appearing area can occur if the film sticks to the side of the tank. (From Wuehrmann, A. H., and Manson-Hing, L. R.: Dental radiology, ed. 4, St. Louis, 1977, The C. V. Mosby Co.)

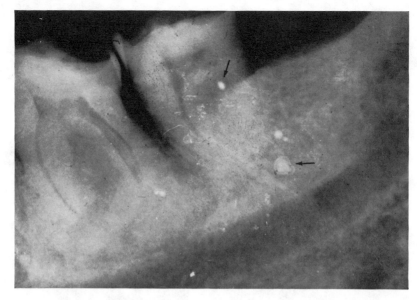

Fig. 22-27. Undeveloped areas. Accumulation of dust, air bubbles, or drops of fixer on the film surface can prevent proper development. White dots or marks result. (From Wuehrmann, A. H., and Manson-Hing, L. R.: Dental radiology, ed. 4, St. Louis, 1977, The C. V. Mosby Co.)

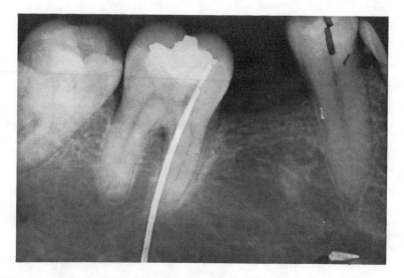

Fig. 22-28. Scratched films White lines result if the emulsion is scratched off the film base. Careful examination of the surface of the film will differentiate these lines from other white or clear lines. (From Wuehrmann, A. H., and Manson-Hing, L. R.: Dental radiology, ed. 4, St. Louis, 1977, The C. V. Mosby Co.)

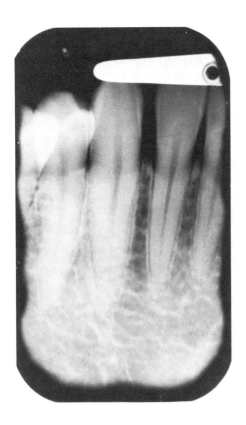

Fig. 22-29. Wet and leaking packets. Black, exposed borders are due to light entering a poorly sealed film wrapper. White smudges, when present, can be due to wet paper in the packet sticking to the emulsion during developing. (From Wuehrmann, A. H., and Manson-Hing, L. R.: Dental radiology, ed. 4, St. Louis, 1977, The C. V. Mosby Co.)

MULTIPLE-CHOICE QUESTIONS

1. Who of the following is the physicist who experimented with the Crookes's vacuum tube and ultimately discovered x rays in 1895?
   a. Sir William Crookes
   b. Edmund Kells
   c. Wilhelm Roentgen
   d. Dr. W. G. Morton
2. The anode is the positively charged component in the x-ray tube. Its function is to:
   a. Allow electrons to boil off of it
   b. Conduct heat away from the target
   c. Attract negatively charged electrons
   d. Measure the amount of electrons
3. An operator of x-ray equipment receives 0.1 rem of radiation for a period of 1 week. We could assume from this information that the operator had received:
   a. An erythema dose
   b. The maximum permissible dose

   c. The minimum primary radiation
   d. Whole body radiation
4. The dentist's new x-ray machine has inherent filtration of 2 mm of aluminum. The dentist is operating the x-ray machine above 70 kVp for diagnostic x-ray films. Which of the following amounts of added filtration will be necessary to meet the minimum total filtration required?
   a. 1.5 mm aluminum
   b. 0.5 mm aluminum
   c. 2.5 mm aluminum
   d. 2.0 mm aluminum
5. The operator of x-ray equipment should be protected against which of the following types of radiation?
   a. Primary
   b. Secondary
   c. Leakage
   d. All of the above

6. Which of the following tissues are most affected by ionizing radiation?
   a. Nerve tissue and adult bone
   b. Reproductive cells and blood-forming cells
   c. Skin and muscle tissue
   d. Glandular tissue and alimentary epithelium

7. Which of the following devices controls the temperature of the tungsten filament?
   a. kVp meter
   b. Electronic timer
   c. Collimator
   d. Milliamperage control or selector switch

8. For the production of x rays, all of the following conditions must exist *except:*
   a. A limited number of electrons
   b. Sudden stoppage of electrons
   c. A source of electrons
   d. A concentration of high-speed electrons

9. For maximum penetration of x rays, which of the following combinations would you select?
   a. 90 kV/10 mA
   b. 85 kV/5 mA
   c. 65 kV/15 mA
   d. 10 kV/65 mA

10. Many aids for film placement are available. Which of the following could be used?
    a. SAR II and XCP
    b. XCP and bite block
    c. SAR II, XCP, and bite block
    d. SAR II, XCP, bite block, and forceps

11. The dental assistant is asked to change from the 8-inch short cone to the 16-inch long cone technique. At twice the distance the intensity of the x rays is now only:
    a. One half as great
    b. One fourth as great
    c. One sixth as great
    d. One eighth as great

12. Which type of radiograph would you normally expose if the dentist suspects an apical abscess?
    a. A bite-wing film
    b. A periapical film
    c. An extraoral film
    d. An occlusal film

13. The imaginary line from the nose to the ear used as a maxillary reference is known as the:
    a. Midsagittal line
    b. Occlusal line
    c. Ala-tragus line
    d. External oblique line

14. A patient with an extremely narrow maxillary arch presents placement problems in x-raying the premolar areas. In the bisection technique, which of the following placements would help solve this problem?
    a. Use the parallel technique for this film.
    b. Use cross section film placement.
    c. Force film into the midline of the palate and increase vertical angulation.
    d. Lay the film on a flat plane in contact with the opposite side of palate to increase vertical angulation.

15. During exposure you notice that the patient had released contact with the film on a mandibular premolar. What could the operator expect to see on this processed film?
    a. A blurred image
    b. A foreshortened image
    c. A partial image
    d. Both a blurred image and a foreshortened image

16. The radiographic image on a maxillary x-ray film is longer than the actual tooth size. An error in angulation was made by:
    a. Increasing the horizontal angulation
    b. Decreasing the vertical angulation
    c. Increasing the vertical angulation
    d. None of the above

17. A radiograph of the mandibular cuspid reveals a distorted blurred area on the lower corner section of the film. The top or upper section of the film has a clear detailed image of the teeth. What caused the distorted image?
    a. Insufficient vertical angulation
    b. Excessive film bending
    c. Increased vertical angulation
    d. Film movement

18. A patient suspected of having a salivary stone blocking Wharton's duct requires an x-ray film. Which of the following projections would best reveal this salivary stone?
    a. Maxillary posterior extraoral
    b. Panorex view

c. Mandibular periapical

d. Mandibular cross section occlusal

19. A maxillary molar film reveals a triangular radiopaque landmark on the lower corner of the film. The landmark visible in this x-ray film is the:
    a. Maxillary tuberosity
    b. Maxillary sinus
    c. Coronoid process of mandible
    d. Hamular process

20. A Panorex film in which one side of the film is lighter than the other and distortion is present in the molar area indicates that:
    a. The patient's head was not tipped down at a 5-degree angle.
    b. The wrong caliper adjustment scale was read.
    c. A cotton roll was not placed between maxillary and mandibular incisors.
    d. The patient's chin was not positioned symmetrically.

21. Under normal processing conditions, the fixer solution acts on
    a. The film gelatin
    b. The film gelatin, polyester base, and unexposed silver halide grains
    c. The film gelatin and unexposed silver halide grains
    d. The film gelatin and ionized silver bromide grains

22. A processed film reveals some small circular shaped white spots indicating incomplete development. The error on the film during processing was caused by:
    a. Exposure to visible light and incomplete fixing
    b. Films not agitated in developer and trapped air bubbles on film
    c. Incomplete fixing and films not agitated in developer
    d. Exposure to visible light and trapped air bubbles on film

23. You have mounted a full-mouth series of radiographs using the buccal method of mounting. The maxillary molar films on the left side of the mount were cone cut on the distal half of the film. Which of the following corrections in technique should be made on a retake of this film?
    a. Move the film mesially, and move the tube head mesially.
    b. Move the tube head mesially, and, move the film distally.
    c. Move the tube head mesially, and direct the central ray toward the center of the film.
    d. Move the film distally, and direct the central ray toward the center of the film.

SUGGESTED READINGS

Brown, G. E., Renne, R. L., and Bontrager, K. L.: Dental radiography, Denver, 1976, Multimedia Publishing, Inc.

De Lyre, W. R.: Essentials of dental radiographs for dental assistants and dental hygienists, Englewood Cliffs, N.J., 1975, Prentice-Hall, Inc.

Frommer, H. H.: Radiology for dental auxiliaries, ed. 2, St. Louis, 1978, The C. V. Mosby Co.

O'Brien, R. C.: Dental radiology, ed. 3, Philadelphia, 1977, W. B. Saunders Co.

McCall, J. O., and Wald, S. S.: Clinical dental roentgenology, ed. 4, Philadelphia, 1965, W. B. Saunders Co.

Richardson, R. E., and Barton, R. E.: The dental assistant, ed. 5, New York, 1978, McGraw-Hill Book Co.

Wainwright, W. W.: Dental radiology, New York, 1965, McGraw-Hill Book Co.

Wuehrmann, A. H., and Manson-Hing, L. R.: Dental radiology, ed. 4, St. Louis, 1977, The C. V. Mosby Co.

CHAPTER 23

Dental materials

ROBERT G. CRAIG

■ **Why and how are fluoride gels used, and what is their general composition?**

Clinical studies have shown that fluoride ions applied to the surface of teeth are effective in reducing the incidence of dental caries. One convenient method of applying fluoride ions is the application of acidulated fluoride-phosphate gels.

The gels are usually applied to clean and saliva-free teeth in trays after a dental prophylaxis. The gel is placed in the mandibular and maxillary trays which are then placed in position, and pressure is applied by squeezing the buccal and lingual parts of the tray so that the gel is forced between the teeth. The patient is told to bite lightly on the trays for 4 minutes, the trays are removed, and the patient is instructed not to eat for 30 minutes.

A typical fluoride gel contains 2% sodium fluoride, 0.3% hydrogen fluoride, and 1% orthophosphoric acid plus thickening, flavoring, and coloring agents in water.

■ **Why should athletic mouth protectors be worn in contact sports, and is there a difference in the effectiveness of the various types?**

Oral injuries account for at least 50% of the injuries in contact sports such as football and hockey.

Studies have shown that the three types of mouth protectors (stock-type, mouth-formed, and custom-made) from a practical viewpoint are equally effective in reducing oral injuries; however, players prefer the custom-made type because of comfort, retention, and low speech impairment during use.

■ **Describe the general procedures for fabricating a custom-made mouth protector.**

An alginate impression is made of the maxillary arch with any removable appliances absent, and a gypsum model without a palate is prepared in this impression. A flexible thermoplastic sheet, 14 cm square and 3 mm thick (5½ inches square and ⅛ inch thick), is heated in boiling water for about 20 seconds. The softened sheet is draped over the gypsum model and adapted with wet fingers or pulled down over the model with a vacuum as shown in Fig. 23-1. When the material has cooled, it is trimmed with scissors as shown in Fig. 23-2. The cut edges can be smoothed by being heated with an alcohol torch and can then be adapted to the model with moist fingers.

■ **What is the basis for the use of pit and fissure sealants?**

Pits and fissures in the occlusal surfaces of teeth result from the noncoalescence of enamel during the formation of the tooth and may or may not extend to the dentinoenamel junction. Debris collects in these areas, and these sites have a high incidence of caries. Sealants are used in an attempt to fill the pits and fissures and thus to prevent dental caries in these areas.

■ **What clinical evidence is there to indicate the success of pit and fissure sealants?**

Although the results of carefully controlled clinical studies on first permanent molars vary, the retention of the sealant by teeth after 2 years was about 60% to 85%, and the effectiveness in preventing occlusal caries was about 70%. Lower success rates have been reported for sec-

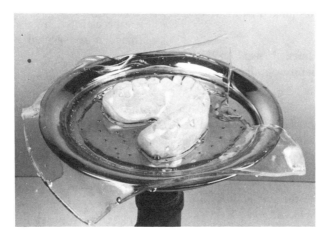

Fig. 23-1. Softened thermoplastic sheet has been adapted to the model with a vacuum. (From Craig, R. G., O'Brien, W. J., and Powers, J. M.: Dental materials: properties and manipulation, ed. 2, St. Louis, 1979, The C. V. Mosby Co.)

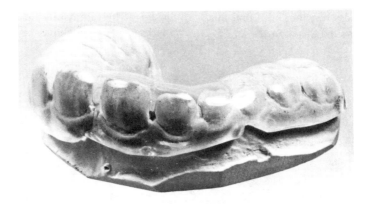

Fig. 23-2. Mouth protector has been trimmed with scissors, and edges are ready to be smoothed by heating with an alcohol torch. (From Craig, R. G., O'Brien, W. J., and Powers, J. M.: Dental materials: properties and manipulation, ed. 2, St. Louis, 1979, The C. V. Mosby Co.)

ond primary molars. These data justify the use of sealants on a selected basis as part of a preventive program.

■ **What is the principal type of material used as a pit and fissure sealant, and what is its general composition?**

The main component of pit and fissure sealants is a moderate molecular weight dimethacrylate usually identified as BIS-GMA. It is a viscous liquid, and it is made more fluid by dilution with lower molecular weight reactive organic molecules. Appropriate initiators and activators are used to cause setting at mouth temperature with or without exposure to an ultraviolet lamp. Most sealants do not contain any inorganic filler, but a few sealants contain as much as 40% of a glass filler.

■ **How are the sealants supplied?**

Sealants that set as a result of acceleration by exposure to ultraviolet light are usually supplied as a single liquid in a squeeze bottle or tube.

Sealants that set as a result of initiation by a chemical are supplied as two liquids. One liquid contains diluted BIS-GMA and an initiator, and the second tube contains diluted BIS-GMA and an accelerator.

■ **What type of treatment is used on the pit and fissure area before application of the sealant?**

The teeth are cleaned with pumice and the occlusal surfaces of the teeth to be treated are etched for 1 minute with acid solutions, often 37% to 50% phosphoric acid, thoroughly washed with water, and carefully dried with air.

■ **What is the basis for the acid etching of the occlusal enamel surfaces?**

The sealant does not chemically bond to enamel and must be retained by the shape of the pit or fissure or by penetration into the crevices produced by etching the enamel as shown in Fig. 23-3. The etching provides mechanical retention and reduces penetration of oral fluids between the sealant and the enamel.

■ **Compare the manipulation of sealants that are accelerated by a chemical with those that are accelerated by ultraviolet light.**

In the first instance, equal volumes of the two liquids are dispensed onto a mixing pad or small disk and are thoroughly mixed with a spatula for 10 to 15 seconds. The mixed material may be applied to the etched pit and fissure area with a small brush or with an applicator supplied by the manufacturer. Sealant should not be applied to unetched areas. Application should be done promptly, since the viscosity of the sealant increases as the reaction progresses, and its ability to penetrate the pits and fissures and etched areas decreases rapidly as indicated by setting times of about 1 minute.

For the ultraviolet light–accelerated sealant the liquid is applied to the etched occlusal surface. After the completion of the application, the tip of the ultraviolet light source is positioned about 2 mm above the occlusal surface,

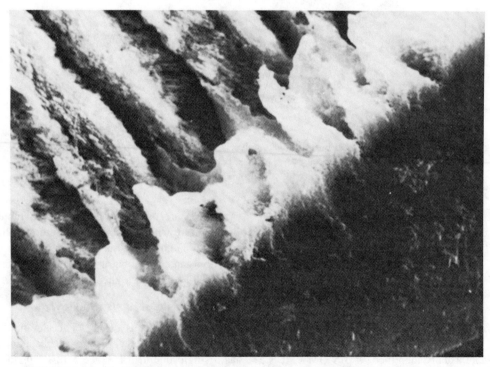

Fig. 23-3. Tags of sealant that have penetrated into areas of enamel that have been attacked by the etchant. (From Dennison, J. B.: Restorative materials for direct application. In Craig, R. G., editor: Dental materials: a problem-oriented approach, St. Louis, 1978, The C. V. Mosby Co.)

and the sealant is exposed to ultraviolet light for 20 seconds.

■ **When the sealant is lost from the tooth over a period of time, how is reapplication accomplished?**

The same procedure is used as with an untreated tooth—the area is cleansed, etched, washed, and dried. The occlusal surface is then ready for application of the sealant.

■ **What are the indications and contraindications for the use of pit and fissure sealants?**

Sealants are indicated when (1) the patient maintains good oral hygiene, (2) when pit and fissures exist, (3) as soon as possible after the teeth have erupted and it is possible to maintain a dry field, and (4) where occlusal morphology provides adequate retention for the sealant. Sealants are not indicated in patients in older age groups when unrestored teeth have displayed resistance to caries or in patients in younger age groups that have shown resistance to caries in the primary dentition. Teeth with flat cuspal inclines, wide fissures, and no accessory grooves are poor candidates for treatment. Also, the teeth of patients with very poor oral hygiene are poor choices for treatment with sealants.

■ **What is the main function of a dentrifice, and what is its general composition?**

The main function of a dentifrice is to clean and polish the surfaces of the tooth. Dentifrices contain abrasives, detergents, flavoring, sweeteners, binders, and water. Some products contain therapeutic agents such as fluoride.

■ **What does the abrasivity index of a dentifrice mean?**

The abrasivity index, AI, is the amount of dentin removed from teeth by a water slurry of the dentifrice compared with the amount removed by a standard abrasive. Low values for the abrasivity index indicate low amounts of dentin removed by the dentifrice when compared to the standard. For example, Listerine, Colgate with MFP, regular Crest, and Vote have AIs of 26, 51, 95, and 134, respectively.

■ **What four types of cohesive gold are used in the dental office, and how do they differ from each other?**

The four types of cohesive gold are (1) fibrous gold foil, (2) electrolytic (mat) gold, (3) powdered gold, and (4) powdered gold-calcium alloy. Fibrous gold foil is supplied in sheets about 0.0006 mm and 10 cm square, or the foil may have been rolled into cylinders from which increments of the desired size may be cut. Electrolytic gold is pure gold powder prepared by electrodeposition and sintered; it may be contained between strips of gold foil for ease of handling. Powdered gold is prepared by atomizing liquid gold or chemically precipitating gold; the powder is wrapped in small envelopes of gold foil. Powdered gold-calcium alloy is supplied like electrodeposited gold, but it contains a small amount of calcium to improve clinical manipulation of the gold.

■ **Why are cohesive golds annealed before being used?**

As supplied these golds are noncohesive, and increments cannot be condensed to a single piece. They are noncohesive because of intentional or unintentional surface contamination. Annealing the gold for a short time at 300° C removes the contaminants and allows increments to be bonded together in the cavity preparation to form a gold foil restoration.

■ **How and why is cohesive gold condensed into the cavity preparation?**

A small increment of the cohesive annealed gold is placed in the cavity preparation, and force is applied to it so that voids are eliminated and it bonds to other increments of gold. Force can be applied using a hand mallet and a gold foil condenser or by using a mechanically driven or electrically driven condenser. The cohesive gold is condensed to adapt it to the cavity preparation, to eliminate voids and thus produce a nonporous restoration, and to improve the properties of the gold by work hardening.

■ **In what forms is dental amalgam supplied?**

Dental amalgam is supplied as two components, the amalgam alloy and mercury. The amalgam alloy is supplied as a powder, the particles of which may be irregularly shaped filings, graded spherical particles, or mixtures of these. The amalgam alloy powder may have been compacted into a tablet. The alloy and mercury may be supplied in separate containers, or they may have been placed in separate portions of a disposable mixing capsule.

■ **What are the main components in the amalgam alloy?**

The main components in the amalgam alloy are silver, tin, and copper. Regular-type alloys might contain 69% silver, 27% tin, and 3% copper, whereas high-copper types could contain 40% to 60% silver, 25% to 30% tin, and 12% to 30% copper.

■ **By what name is the mixing of alloy and mercury called, and how is the mixing accomplished?**

The term used to describe the mixing of alloy and mercury is *trituration*. Trituration is usually accomplished using a mechanical mixer

called an *amalgamator*. The appropriate amounts of alloy and mercury are either dispensed into a mixing capsule, or a predispensed capsule containing the appropriate amounts of alloy and mercury is selected.

In the first instance, depending on whether the alloy is in the form of a tablet or powder, a pestle of proper size and weight may also be placed in the capsule. The capsule is screwed shut and placed on the holder of an amalgamator, several examples of which are shown in Fig. 23-4. The correct time of trituration is set on the timer, and the amalgamator is started. Trituration is accomplished because the capsule rotates in an eccentric path that moves the capsule in a back and forth motion.

When using the predispensed capsules, the mercury is squeezed into the alloy just before trituration by compressing the capsule along the long axis.

■ **How can you tell if the amalgam alloy and mercury have been properly triturated?**

An overtriturated mix is excessively wet appearing and may be hard to remove from the

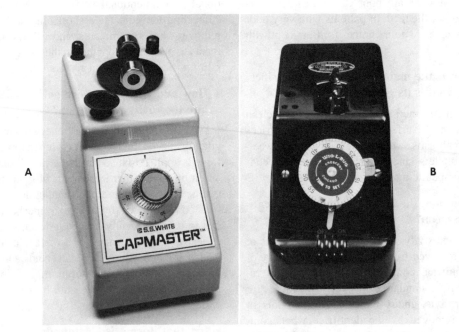

Fig. 23-4. A, high-speed, and, **B,** moderate speed mechanical amalgamators. (From Dennison, J. B.: Restorative materials for direct application. In Craig, R. G., editor: Dental materials: a problem-oriented approach, St. Louis, 1978, The C. V. Mosby Co.)

capsule. An undertriturated mix is dry and dull in appearance, tends to crumble, and appears as if not enough mercury were used. A correctly triturated mix will appear shiny and can be removed in a single mass from the capsule.

■ **If a mix of amalgam alloy and mercury is undermixed, what factors could have caused the problem?**

If a mix of amalgam alloy and mercury is undermixed, the following factors should be checked:

1. Are the mercury and alloy dispensers clean so that the correct alloy–mercury ratio is obtained?
2. Is the correct pestle being used?
3. Is the proper trituration time being selected?
4. If a variable speed amalgamator is being used, is the speed setting correct?
5. Is the line voltage in the building low and causing the amalgamator to run slower?

■ **Is there any danger in handling mercury in a dental office?**

Improper handling of mercury can be a health hazard. If improperly used, liquid mercury can be absorbed through the skin, and mercury vapor or airborne droplets can be inhaled. Mercury should not be handled by the fingers or the palm of the hand. Mercury spills should be cleaned up promptly using accepted procedures, and unused set amalgam should be stored under water in a sealed bottle. Worn capsules should be discarded, since mercury can leak out during trituration. Also screw-type capsules are preferred to minimize any escape of mercury during trituration.

■ **In what forms are composites supplied for use in the dental office?**

The most common form of composite is two pastes, usually identified as catalyst and base, that are mixed in equal quantities. They are commonly available in about four different shades to match typical colors of teeth. Composites are also available from some manufacturers as a powder and a liquid. These two forms set as a result of an initiator in one part

and a chemical accelerator in the other part of the system.

Composites are also available as a single paste in which the setting reaction is accelerated by exposure to ultraviolet light.

■ **What is the most common composition of dental composites?**

Composites consist of about 50% by volume of a BIS-GMA polymer similar to that used in sealants and 50% by volume of treated inorganic filler such as quartz or glass. The chemically accelerated type contain an initiator in the catalyst paste (or powder in the power-liquid type) and an accelerator in the base paste (or liquid in the power-liquid type). The ultraviolet light–accelerated composites contain an initiator and an ultraviolet light absorber.

■ **How are the various types of composites dispensed?**

Prior to dispensing the pastes in a two-paste system, the pastes in the jars should be stirred with a disposable plastic or wooden spatula, since settling of the inorganic particles may have occurred. One end of the spatula should be used for the catalyst paste and the other end for the base paste since cross-contamination should be avoided. Equal portions of the two pastes should be dispensed on a treated paper mixing pad in amounts that will provide a small excess of mixed material for the particular cavity preparation.

Dispensing of the powder-liquid system is done using a scoop and a dropper bottle supplied by the manufacturer. The powder-liquid type is also available in predispensed capsules with the powder in the lower part of the capsule and the liquid in a sealed diaphragm in the top of the capsule. Just before mixing the capsule is compressed to squeeze the liquid into the powder.

■ **After dispensing the composite how are the components mixed?**

The two pastes are mixed with a plastic or wooden spatula on the mixing pad for 20 to 30 seconds. A metal spatula should be avoided, since the filler particles are abrasive, and wear particles from the spatula can alter the color of the mixed composite. Mixing should be done with a folding action designed to avoid incorporation of air bubbles and must be done quickly, since the mix should be inserted 1 to 1½ minutes after the start of mixing. Of course, no mixing is required for the single paste system to be used with ultraviolet light, and the material does not set until exposed to the ultraviolet lamp.

The powder-liquid types usually require 1 scoop of powder to 1 drop of liquid and are mixed in the same way as for the two-paste systems except that care should be taken to incorporate all the liquid into the powder, or the working and setting time will be adversely affected.

The predispensed powder-liquid type is mixed on a mechanical amalgamator, and a plastic pestle is present in the capsule. If a high-speed mixer is used, 10 to 15 seconds is adequate time for mixing; and if a low-speed mixer is used, 30 seconds for mixing is usually recommended.

■ **How is the mixed composite placed into the cavity preparation?**

The paste may be placed into a syringe and injected, or it may be packed into the preparation using a variety of plastic instruments (shown in Fig. 23-5, *A*) to which the mix does not readily stick. If the injection method is to be used, a moderate viscosity mix must be obtained. This is placed in the plastic tip of the syringe, the rubber cone is inserted, and both are placed in the syringe (see Fig. 23-5, *B*). The syringe must be assembled and the injection started 1 to 1½ minutes after the start of mixing, since the composite sets in 4 to 5 minutes.

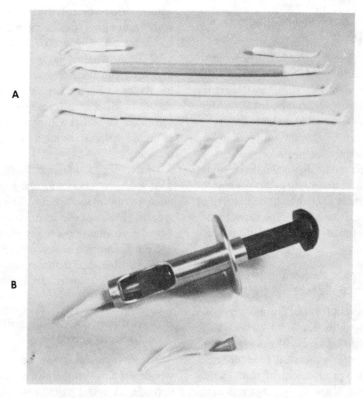

Fig. 23-5. A, Instruments for placement of composites, and, **B,** a syringe for inspecting composites. (From Craig, R. G., O'Brien, W. J., and Powers, J. M.: Dental materials: properties and manipulation, ed. 2, St. Louis, 1979, The C. V. Mosby Co.)

■ **What is the usual procedure for finishing composites?**

Finishing to a glossy surface like gold or amalgam is not possible, since the composite is a combination of a hard filler and a soft plastic. As a result the best finish is that produced by the plastic matrix strip. However, since some overcontouring is common, some finishing usually must be done. The most successful finishing is done by using coarse abrasives for gross removal and finer abrasives for final finishing.

Recently composites with about 30% submicron filler particles that yield smoother finished surfaces have been introduced. However, these composites do not resist abrasive wear as well as the standard composites.

■ **How should the package of composites be stored?**

The shelf life of composites is extended by storing them in the refrigerator but not in the freezing compartment. Unopened packages should be removed and allowed to come to room temperature before use. The composites to be used with the ultraviolet lamp also should not be dispensed before they are needed

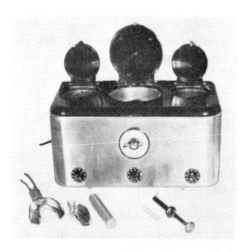

Fig. 23-6. Agar hydrocolloid conditioner with three controlled-temperature water baths. Water-cooled trays, a tube of tray agar, a stick of syringe agar, and a syringe are shown in the foreground. (From Craig, R. G., and Peyton, F. A., editors: Restorative dental materials, ed. 5, St. Louis, 1975, The C. V. Mosby Co.)

and should not be exposed to ultraviolet light until after insertion into the cavity preparation.

■ **What armamentarium is needed to take an agar impression?**

The items needed to take an agar impression are shown in Fig. 23-6. These include (1) an agar hydrocolloid conditioner with three controlled-temperature water baths, (2) a selection of water-cooled impression trays, (3) a tube of agar tray material, (4) a stick or cartridge of agar syringe material, and (5) an agar syringe.

■ **How is the agar tray material prepared for taking an impression?**

A tube of the tray material is placed in one of the water baths at 100° C for 10 to 15 minutes; this converts the agar gel into a fluid sol. It is then transferred to a second water bath held at 60° to 66° C where it will remain fluid all day. When an impression is to be taken, it is squeezed into a water-cooled impression tray and further cooled to 43° to 46° C for 2 minutes in the third controlled-water bath. The outer layer of agar impression material in the tray is scraped off, and the cooling water hoses are connected. The tray is then ready for insertion without danger of the agar burning the oral tissues. After placement by the dentist, water at 13° C is circulated through the tray until the agar impression gels.

■ **How is the agar syringe material prepared for taking an impression?**

A stick or cartridge of syringe material is placed in the syringe, heated in the boiling water bath, and placed in the second bath in the same way as the tray agar. When it is time for the material to be injected, the syringe is removed from the storage bath and agar is injected into the tooth preparation without further cooling. The thin strand of material is cooled sufficiently during injection so that the temperature does not harm the dental tissues. After injection of the syringe material, the tray material frequently is placed as before and an agar syringe-tray combination impression is obtained.

■ **After the agar impression has been removed from the mouth, what procedures**

are done before a gypsum model or cast is poured?

The agar impression is rinsed with cool water to remove any saliva or blood, the bulk of the excess water is removed by shaking, and the remainder is removed by a gentle stream of air without dehydration of the surface. This final condition can be recognized when the surface of the agar loses its glossy appearance.

■ **When should a gypsum model or cast be made from the agar impression, and why is the timing important?**

The gypsum model or cast should be prepared as soon as possible, since if too long a time elapses the agar impression material will dehydrate and shrink resulting in an inaccurate model or cast.

■ **What are the differences in the various gypsum products available for pouring models or casts?**

The four common gypsum products are listed in Table 23-1 along with the amount of water used to mix with 100 g of powder and the compressive strength of the set material in the wet condition. Different amounts of water are required to produce mixes of reasonable consistency for pouring into impressions. Model plaster requires the most and improved stone the least water for a given weight of powder. The larger the amount of water needed, the lower the compressive strength and the lower the resistance to abrasion. Also the cost increases from model plaster to improved stone.

■ **In what form are alginate impression materials supplied, and how are they dispensed?**

Alginate is supplied as a powder in bulk in a hermetically sealed metal can or in predispensed foil sealed packets.

The bulk powder is dispensed with a scoop supplied by the manufacturer. The powder should be fluffed up before dispensing for each mix, the powder should not be packed into the scoop, and only level scoops should be used. The manufacturer also supplies liquid measuring vials marked at levels to be used with various numbers of scoops. The vials are also sup-

Table 23-1. Gypsum product materials, mixing proportions, and wet compressive strength

Material	Milliliters of water/ 100 g powder	Compressive strength (psi [MN/m²])
Model plaster	45	1800 (12.4)
Orthodontic plaster	37	2400 (16.6)
Dental stone	30	3000 (20.7)
Improved stone	22 to 24	6000 (41.4)

plied by the manufacturer to be used with the preweighed packages.

■ **What mixing equipment and technique are used with alginate impression materials?**

The only equipment needed is a rubber bowl and an alginate spatula.

The desired amount of water is poured into the rubber bowl, and the correct amount of powder is added. The powder is wetted by the water with a stirring action. This is followed by vigorous mixing by squeezing the alginate between the blade of the spatula and the side of the bowl using a stropping action. Mixing should be done for 1 minute for regular-set and for 40 seconds for fast-set materials. This method of mixing should produce a smooth creamy mix.

■ **What are the setting times of alginate impression materials, and what effect do the water temperature and powder:water ratio have on the setting times?**

The setting time of regular-set materials is about 3 to 4 minutes and the setting time for fast-set materials is about 1½ minutes.

Increasing the temperature of the mix water shortens the setting time of alginate impression materials as does increasing the amount of alginate powder with respect to water.

■ **List the items needed for mixing polysulfide rubber impression materials.**

A heavy quality paper mixing pad and a stiff-bladed tapered spatula are required for mixing polysulfide rubber impression materials.

■ **What viscosity types of polysulfide impression materials are available?**

Four viscosities are available: light or syringe, regular, heavy or tray, and putty.

■ How are polysulfides supplied, and how are they dispensed?

With the exception of the putty, polysulfides are supplied as two pastes in tubes identified usually as base and accelerator or catalyst. The putty is supplied in two jars.

Dispensing of the pastes is done by extruding equal lengths of base and accelerator in separate ropes onto the paper mixing pad being careful that the ropes have the same diameter as the orifices of the tubes. The manufacturer supplies special scoops for dispensing the putty.

■ How are polysulfide materials mixed?

The base and accelerator pastes are initially mixed with a stirring action using the end of the spatula. Mixing is continued using broad strokes with the flat portion of the blade. After about 10 seconds most of the material is wiped off the blade onto the pad, and then the blade is wiped clean with a paper towel. Mixing is completed again using broad strokes until no streaking is observed. Mixing should be completed in 45 seconds. The putty type is mixed by mulling the two with the hands until free from streaks.

■ What factors affect the setting time of polysulfide impression material?

Increases in temperature and humidity will speed up the setting reaction and shorten the setting time. Increases in catalyst paste with respect to base paste shorten the setting time, but this effect is not critical unless the catalyst paste is increased 20% or more.

■ How is an impression tray or a syringe filled?

Filling of the impression tray with the mixed polysulfide paste is done by spreading out the mix with very broad strokes to break most of the bubbles in the mix, collecting the mix by scraping the narrow part of the blade against the pad, and scraping the material off the blade with the end of the impression tray so that it flows from one end of the tray to the other and no voids are trapped between the material and the tray.

The syringe is loaded with syringe material by collecting the mix into a pile and pushing the end of the syringe minus the plunger into the mix until it is sufficiently filled. The outside portion of the end of the syringe is wiped free from material, the plunger is attached, and then the plunger is depressed until material begins to extrude out the tip.

■ How can you be sure the polysulfide impression will remain attached to the tray on removal of the impression from the mouth?

Impression trays may be perforated, and the material that extrudes through these small holes locks the impression to the tray. A nonperforated tray may be used if an adhesive is applied to the inside of the tray and allowed to dry before being used. The adhesives consist of rubber in a solvent, and after application the solvent must be allowed to evaporate before the tray is used.

■ How are the polysulfide rubber impressions treated after removal and how should they be stored?

The polysulfide rubber impressions are thoroughly rinsed with water to remove saliva and dried with a mild stream of air. The polysulfide rubber does not dehydrate, so no problems exist as with the drying of hydrocolloid impressions. The impression should always be supported by the tray, since even small forces on the impression material, such as the impression being placed for a time on the table top with the impression material down, can cause permanent flow and an inaccurate impression. Although the polysulfide impressions do not dehydrate, gypsum models should be poured within 1 hour, since setting shrinkage continues long after the setting time has been reached.

■ What viscosities of silicones are available, and how are they supplied?

Silicone impression materials are available in light, regular, heavy, and putty viscosities. The first three are usually supplied as a base paste in a tube and a catalyst which may be supplied as a paste in a tube or a liquid in a dropping bottle. The putty is supplied as base in a jar with the catalyst as a liquid in a dropping bottle or a paste in a jar.

■ How are the silicone materials dispensed?

When supplied as two pastes, equal lengths of the pastes are extruded onto a paper mixing pad. When supplied as a paste and a liquid the appropriate amount of paste is extruded onto the paper pad, and the correct number of drops of catalyst are added per inch of paste, usually 1 drop per inch.

The manufacturers supply scoops to dispense the putty materials. If the catalyst is liquid, the manufacturer specifies the number of drops per scoop of putty.

■ How are silicone impression materials manipulated?

The two-paste and the paste-liquid materials are mixed in the same manner as polysulfides. The catalyst and base are of contrasting colors, and complete mixing is indicated by freedom from streaks.

If the silicone is a putty-liquid catalyst system, the putty is dispensed onto the paper pad with the scoop, and the surface is cross-hatched with the spatula. The correct number of drops of catalyst liquid are placed in the cross-hatched area, and mixing is started with the spatula. After the liquid has been incorporated into the putty, completion of the mixing can be done by mulling in the hand. Care should be taken with the mixing, since the catalyst can cause skin irritation.

If the silicone is a two-putty system, the correct scoops are used to dispense the catalyst and base, and mixing is done by hand until the mix is free from streaks.

The remaining procedures for manipulating silicones are the same as for polysulfide impression materials. It should be recognized that, in general, silicone impression materials set faster than polysulfides, and thus less working time is available for mixing and loading the syringe and tray. The faster setting time is partly compensated for by the improved ease of mixing of the silicones compared with mixing of the polysulfides.

■ What factors shorten the setting time of silicone impression materials?

Increases in temperature and humidity will shorten the setting time, and since the setting time is shorter than for polysulfides, these changes are more critical. Increases in catalyst will usually shorten the setting time, but for at least one two-paste system the reverse takes place because the catalyst paste is of lower viscosity than the base paste.

■ In what viscosities are polyether impression materials supplied?

Polyethers are supplied only in the regular viscosity type. A thinner is supplied that can be used to lower the viscosity.

■ How are polyether materials supplied, dispensed, and mixed?

Polyethers are supplied as a base and a catalyst paste in contrasting colors. The thinner is also supplied as a paste in a tube.

Equal lengths of base and catalyst are extruded onto a paper mixing pad and are mixed like polysulfides and silicones. The working time is about 2½ minutes, and rapid manipulation is essential.

If the thinner is used, satisfactory results have been obtained using equal lengths of base, catalyst, and thinner paste. This amount of thinner approximately doubles the working time without harming the other properties of the material.

Mixing is accomplished in the same manner as for the other rubber impression materials. The polyethers should not be stored in water, but normal contact with saliva and rinsing with water does not cause problems with accuracy. The tissue surface, however, does at times have a blanched appearance. Thorough mixing of polyethers is essential, since contact of the tissues with the catalyst have caused reactions of the mucosa.

■ How can the setting time of polyether impressions be lengthened?

The setting time of polyether impressions is lengthened by increasing the use of the thinner with equal lengths of thinner, base, and catalyst being the most common proportions. Decreasing the amount of catalyst paste also will lengthen the setting time, but use of the thinner is preferred.

In what forms is dental compound supplied?

Dental compound is supplied as dental impression compound and tray compound. The impression compound is supplied in sticks of various sizes and cones, while the tray compound is in the shape of rectangles or the dental arch.

What is the difference between impression compound and tray compound, and what are their applications?

The composition of impression compound is designed so that it softens at a lower temperature than tray compound, flows better at 7° C above mouth temperature than tray compound, and thus records surface detail better. At mouth temperature impression compound is sufficiently rigid so that minimal distortion occurs on removal of the impression.

Impression compound is used to check the cavity preparation for undercuts, since it will fracture on removal from an undercut area rather than be deformed. It also can be used to record impressions of prepared teeth for inlays and crowns where no undercuts are present. Tray compound is used to obtain a preliminary impression for a complete denture. This preliminary impression will hold a thin layer of a final impression material, such as zinc oxide–eugenol.

How is impression compound manipulated?

To take a check impression, the end of a stick or cone is heated in a flame until thoroughly softened and is pressed into the cavity preparation and held there firmly until it thoroughly cools. The compound is removed, and the impression is examined for fractures that might indicate undercuts. The compound is thermoplastic and also a poor conductor of heat; therefore care must be taken during heating so that the inside of the stick or cone becomes softened, and care must be taken during cooling to ensure that the impression is rigid inside as well as outside.

To take a final impression in compound, the compound is retained in a copper band that has been selected and adapted to the particular tooth. The softened compound in the band is pressed into the impression area and held firmly until cool. Water spray at about 18° C may be used to hasten cooling.

Describe the handling of tray compound.

Tray compound is softened in a special thermostatically controlled water bath at about 45° C. The water bath contains a gauze holder that prevents the compound sticking to the bottom of the bath. The heated compound may be supported by an aluminum tray and a preliminary edentulous impression taken. A final impression can be taken in zinc oxide–eugenol.

What kind of models may be obtained from compound impressions?

Impression compound can be copper plated and yield a model with a metal surface, or a gypsum material may be used.

Are there substitutes for tray compound and a zinc oxide–eugenol impression?

Yes. A custom-made acrylic tray may be made, and the final impression can be taken in polysulfide rubber.

In what form is zinc oxide–eugenol impression material supplied?

The most common form of zinc oxide–eugenol impression material is as two pastes. Zinc oxide–eugenol is also supplied as a powder and as a liquid. Both a fast-set and a slow-set liquid are available.

How is the two-paste system dispensed and mixed?

Equal lengths of the two pastes of contrasting colors are extruded onto an oil-resistant paper mixing pad. The material is mixed for 30 to 45 seconds with the same spatula used for rubber impression materials using broad strokes in a sweeping motion.

How is the powder-liquid type zinc oxide–eugenol dispensed and mixed?

One teaspoon of liquid to 2 teaspoons of powder are dispensed onto an oil-resistant paper mixing pad, and the stiff-bladed spatula used for the two-paste system is used. It is mixed to a smooth creamy consistency.

■ **What factors affect the setting time of zinc oxide–eugenol impression materials?**

Zinc oxide–eugenol impression materials are highly sensitive to moisture and set rapidly when the humidity is high. Increases in temperature also shorten the setting time. The fast-setting liquid is used when it is cold and dry, and the slow-setting liquid is used when it is moist and hot.

■ **After mixing how is zinc oxide–eugenol impression material manipulated?**

The mix is spread in a thin layer over the dry tissue-bearing surface of the compound or acrylic tray, and the tray with the zinc oxide–eugenol impression material is placed in the mouth.

■ **In what form is zinc phosphate cement supplied, and what items are needed for mixing the cement?**

Zinc phosphate cement is supplied in two bottles. One contains a specially prepared zinc oxide powder and the other a buffered solution of phosphoric acid in water. The powder is dispensed with a special plastic stick with a large and a small depression at opposite ends. The cement is mixed on a thick glass mixing slab with a thin-bladed stainless steel spatula.

■ **How is zinc phosphate cement dispensed and mixed?**

The powder is packed into the appropriate end of the dispensing stick by pressing it to the bottom of the bottle containing the powder; the excess is removed with the spatula. Tapping the stick with the spatula over the glass mixing slab releases the powder. This procedure is repeated until the appropriate amount of powder has been dispensed. The powder is divided into portions, usually fifths, and one of these portions is divided into two increments. The appropriate amount of liquid is placed on the slab with the aid of the dropping bottle.

One of the two smaller increments is mixed with the liquid using broad strokes of the spatula and a large area of the slab, and mixing is continued for 15 seconds. The second small increment and then the larger portions are mixed in the same manner at 15-second intervals, resulting in a total mixing time of 90 seconds. The last large portion may be added in smaller amounts until the correct consistency is obtained; the residue is discarded. If the mix is too thin after adding all of the last portion, extra powder is added until the proper consistency is obtained. This consistency is described as the *inlay, cementing,* or *primary* consistency.

If the material is to be used as a base in a cavity preparation rather than as a cement, additional powder is now added until a puttylike consistency is reached.

■ **How can the mix be checked to determine if the inlay or base consistency has been reached?**

The inlay mix at 90 seconds should string out for about 2 cm (¾ inch) when it is touched with the spatula and the spatula is raised.

The base consistency should be puttylike and capable of being rolled into a small rope with the flat blade of the spatula without sticking to it.

■ **What factors affect the working time of zinc phosphate cement?**

Increases in temperature will shorten the working time. The temperature of the room and the mixing slab affect the working time as well as does the area of slab over which the cement is mixed. This last effect arises from the heat of reaction of the powder and liquid which is not dissipated if the mixing area is small.

Incorporation of water into the mix will shorten the working time, other things being equal. The liquid is hygroscopic and can pick up moisture from the air if it is humid and lose water if it is dry. If the glass slab is cooled intentionally to provide a longer working time and moisture condenses on the slab because it was cooled below the dew point, the working time is altered. If the glass slab was frozen, the reduction in temperature is more important than the moisture incorporated, and the working time is lengthened. If the slab is just slightly below the dew point, then the moisture added to the mix is more important than the reduction in temperature, and the working time is shortened.

Increasing the amount of powder with respect to liquid will shorten the working time.

■ Why is it important to reach the inlay consistency after 90 seconds of mixing?

The objective is to incorporate the maximum amount of powder for a given amount of liquid and yet reach the proper viscosity at 90 seconds. More rapid incorporation of powder increases the temperature of the mix; slower incorporation allows less powder to be added, and a lower strength cement is obtained.

■ Why should the cement be used just after the completion of mixing?

The viscosity of zinc phosphate cements increases rapidly with time and if cementation of a gold restoration is delayed, complete seating of the restoration may be difficult or impossible because of excessive film thickness of the cement layer caused by the increased viscosity.

■ What types and modifications of zinc oxide–eugenol cement are available and what are their applications?

Two-paste zinc oxide–eugenol cements are used as cavity liners. Powder-liquid or paste types of zinc oxide–eugenol cement are used as temporary cement for restorations and a resin-modified type is available for temporary restorations and a resin-modified type is available for temporary restorations and permanent cementation of crowns and bridges. Ethoxybenzoic acid (EBA)-modified zinc oxide–eugenol cements containing fillers are available for permanent cementation of restorations. The strength of the zinc oxide–eugenol materials increases from their application as liners to temporary restorations to permanent cements.

■ How are the zinc oxide–eugenol materials used for liners dispensed and manipulated?

Equal quantities of the base and accelerator from two separate tubes are expressed onto the paper mixing pad supplied by the manufacturer. The two portions are thoroughly mixed for

about 15 seconds, and the mix is then ready for application.

■ How are the zinc oxide–eugenol materials used as temporary or permanent cements dispensed and mixed?

If a two-paste system is used, equal quantities are expressed onto a mixing pad and mixed with a cement spatula. If a powder-liquid system is used, a powder dispenser and a dropping bottle are supplied by the manufacturer. The components may be dispensed onto a mixing pad or a glass slab. All of the powder is mixed into the liquid initially with a patting, pressing, or folding action. After incorporating the powder, spatulation is continued with moderately wide strokes until a smooth mix of the correct consistency is obtained. It may appear at first that all of the powder cannot be mixed with the liquid, but the viscosity of the mix decreases as mixing is continued.

■ What are the critical factors affecting the working time of the zinc oxide–eugenol materials?

The most important factor is moisture or humidity. The setting reaction is accelerated by water and as a result the mixed material may have a rather long working time on the pad, but will set promptly when placed in the mouth where water is present.

Temperature has some effect on shortening the setting time, but the effect is not as pronounced as with zinc phosphate cements. Little heat is liberated during the reaction, and thus the powder can be added to the liquid all at once without altering the working time.

Increasing the amount of powder with respect to liquid will shorten the setting time.

■ In what form are zinc polyacrylate cements supplied?

Zinc polyacrylate cements are supplied as a powder and as a liquid; the powder is mainly a specially treated zinc oxide, and the liquid is a water solution of polyacrylic acid. Some manufacturers supply two liquids with different concentrations of polyacrylic acid for making an inlay and a base consistency mix.

■ **How are the zinc polyacrylate materials dispensed and mixed?**

The powder is dispensed with a scoop or a plastic dispensing stick, and the liquid is dispensed with a dropping bottle.

The appropriate proportions are dispensed onto a special disposable mixing pad supplied by the manufacturer. A commonly used proportion is three parts powder to one part liquid or one and a half parts powder to 1 part liquid by weight.

The cap on the liquid bottle should be replaced after dispensing so that the concentration will not change. Also the liquid should be dispensed just before using so water does not evaporate before mixing.

The powder and liquid are mixed with a cement spatula for about 30 seconds until a smooth creamy consistency is obtained.

■ **How does the consistency of zinc polyacrylate cement compare with zinc phosphate cement, and how is the working time estimated?**

The consistency of mixed zinc polyacrylate cement appears to be higher than zinc phosphate cement, although the viscosity is only slightly higher. The working time is about 3 minutes, and it loses its glossy appearance and becomes stringy at this time.

■ **How does the viscosity of zinc polyacrylate cement increase within the working time compared to that of zinc phosphate cement?**

The viscosity of zinc polyacrylate just after mixing is slightly higher than that of zinc phosphate cement, but 1 minute after mixing the viscosity of zinc phosphate cement is substantially higher than that of zinc polyacrylate cement.

■ **How does an increase in temperature affect the working time and viscosity of zinc polyacrylate cement?**

Temperature increases shorten the working time and increase the viscosity, although temperature is less effective with zinc polyacrylate cement compared to zinc phosphate cement.

■ **What types of materials are used for temporary restorations?**

As previously mentioned, modified zinc oxide–eugenol cements are used. In addition, prefabricated aluminum and polycarbonate crowns are available and custom-made acrylic polymer crowns and bridges can be constructed in the dental office. The acrylic material is available as a powder and a liquid that are mixed together; when the material reaches a doughlike condition, it can be formed into a temporary restoration by a variety of methods. The aluminum, polycarbonate, and acrylic restorations are cemented into place using a temporary cement.

■ **What types of materials are available for chairside denture relines?**

Temporary soft or hard reline materials are available. The temporary soft materials consist of a powder and a liquid with the powder being an acrylic polymer and the liquid being either an alcohol or an acrylic monomer with a softening agent (plasticizer). The powder and liquid are mixed usually for 1 minute in a disposable paper cup and then allowed to stand about 1 minute or until the proper viscosity is attained. The material is then spread on the prepared tissue-bearing surface of the denture which is properly positioned in the mouth by the dentist.

The soft temporary materials usually become harder with time in the mouth and are replaced at frequent intervals, every 3 or 4 days, during the healing of the tissue-bearing surface.

The hard relines are used usually to temporarily correct a poorly fitting denture during the construction of a new denture.

MULTIPLE CHOICE QUESTIONS

1. Which of the following statements apply to fluoride gels?
   a. The gel is kept in contact with the teeth for 30 seconds.
   b. The patient is instructed not to eat for 3 hours after the application.
   c. The gel contains 20% sodium fluoride.
   d. The gel contains 1% orthophosphoric acid.

2. Clinical studies with pit and fissure sealants have established which of the following statements?
   a. The retention of sealant by first permanent molars was 95% after 2 years.
   b. The effectiveness of the sealant in preventing occlusal caries in first permanent molars was about 70% after 2 years.
   c. Higher success rates were found for second primary molars than for first permanent molars.
   d. The results of the studies justify the routine use of sealants in a preventive program.

3. Preparing the teeth for application of a sealant involves which of the following steps?
   a. The teeth are cleaned with pumice followed by a fluoride treatment with a gel.
   b. The teeth are etched with a phosphoric acid solution for at least 3 minutes.
   c. After treatment with the acid etchant care must be taken not to disturb the surface by rinsing.
   d. None of the above steps are involved.
   e. All of the above steps are involved.

4. Why is acid etching of enamel necessary prior to application of pit and fissure sealants?
   a. It cleanses the tooth enamel.
   b. It forms a phosphate on the surface of enamel and improves the chemical bond to the sealant.
   c. It provides mechanical retention of the sealant to the enamel.
   d. It cleans the surface of enamel so that chemical attachment of the sealant occurs.

5. Manipulation of a chemically accelerated pit and fissure sealant involves which of the following steps?
   a. Two parts of base are dispensed to one part of catalyst.
   b. Mixing is accomplished in 10 to 15 seconds.
   c. A glass mixing slab must be used.
   d. Application to the pits and fissures can be done in a leisurely fashion, since setting is initiated by ultraviolet light.

6. Pit and fissure sealants are usually indicated when:
   a. Poor oral hygiene exists.
   b. Teeth have flat cuspal inclines and wide fissures.
   c. It is not possible to maintain a dry field.
   d. The teeth have recently erupted.

7. The abrasivity index of a dentifrice is a term that measures:
   a. The amount of dentin removed by a water slurry of the dentifrice compared to amount of dentin removed by a standard abrasive
   b. The amount of dentin removed by a water slurry of the dentifrice compared to the amount of enamel removed by the same dentifrice
   c. The amount of enamel removed by the dentifrice compared to the most abrasive dentifrice
   d. The amount of enamel removed by the dentifrice compared to the amount of enamel removed by a standard abrasive.

8. Cohesive golds are annealed before insertion to:
   a. Remove contaminants
   b. Harden them
   c. Make them noncohesive
   d. Heat-treat them

9. The mixing of amalgam alloy with mercury is called:
   a. Trituration
   b. Amalgamation
   c. Condensation
   d. Mulling

10. A mechanically mixed combination of

amalgam alloy and mercury that has been overmixed:
a. Is dry and crumbly
b. Is dull in appearance
c. Is released from the capsule in a single mass
d. Is wet looking

11. An undermixed mass of amalgam could result from which of the following factors?
a. Too much mercury in the mix
b. Too heavy a pestle used
c. Too high a mixing speed on the amalgamator
d. Low line voltage to the amalgamator

12. Which of the following statements are true with respect to the handling of mercury in the dental office?
a. Liquid mercury cannot be absorbed through the skin.
b. Mercury vapor is a health hazard.
c. Mercury is contaminated so readily that a spill on the floor presents no special problem.
d. Friction-type amalgam capsules are as satisfactory as the screw-type capsules in preventing escape of mercury during mixing.

13. In the dispensing of a two-paste composite:
a. One end of the spatula should be used for the base and the other end for the catalyst paste.
b. Equal or unequal portions of the base and catalyst paste are used depending on the working time desired.
c. A plastic or wooden spatula should not be used, since the pastes are abrasive.
d. None of the above
e. All of the above

14. Which of the following statements apply to the manipulation of a two-paste composite?
a. Mixing should be accomplished in 20 to 30 seconds.
b. Mixing should be done with a stirring action.
c. The mix should be placed in a syringe so that insertion can start at 4 to 5 minutes.
d. The mixed composite is inserted with abrasive resistant metal instruments.

15. Final finishing of composites is done with:
a. Polishing agents
b. Fine abrasives
c. Rouge
d. Silex and tin oxide

16. The shelf life of composites can be extended by storage:
a. In the freezing compartment of the refrigerator
b. Of the unopened package at room temperature in a dry area
b. In a warm, dry area to keep the pastes fluid
d. In the refrigerator portion of the refrigerator

17. Manipulation of tray-type agar hydrocolloid impression material includes which of the following steps?
a. Agar gel in a tube is converted into a sol by placing it in boiling water for 10 to 15 minutes.
b. After conversion to a sol it is stored in a controlled temperature water bath at 80° C until ready for use.
c. After being placed in a water-cooled impression tray it is cooled to 60° to 66° C for 2 minutes in a controlled temperature water bath.
d. After the impression material is placed in the mouth, water at 5° C is circulated through the tray to aid in gelation of the agar.

18. Which of the following statements apply to the manipulation of gypsum products?
a. The water is placed in the rubber mixing bowl after the powder is measured into it.
b. Spatulation is done with a whipping action.
c. Hand spatulation is carried out at about three revolutions per second for 20 seconds.
d. The hand-spatulated mix is vibrated to aid in the removal of air bubbles.

19. The setting time of gypsum products is lengthened by:
a. Moderate increases in the temperature of the mix water
b. Increasing the amount of powder in the mix

c. Contamination of the mix with set material from a previous mix

d. Using old material

20. Which statements apply to dispensing and mixing alginate impression material?
    a. The bulk powder should be packed into the scoop to ensure the correct powder-water ratio.
    b. The water should be dispensed into the mixing bowl before addition of the powder.
    c. The entire mixing should be done with a vigorous stirring action.
    d. Mixing should be carried out for 30 seconds for a regular setting time alginate.

21. The setting time of alginate is:
    a. Lengthened by increasing the temperature
    b. Lengthened by increasing the amount of alginate
    c. About 3 to 4 minutes for regular-set materials
    d. Less than 1 minute for fast-set products

22. The setting time of polysulfide impression material will be shortened if:
    a. The humidity decreases.
    b. The temperature increases.
    c. Five percent more than the recommended amount of accelerator is used.
    d. None of the above

23. Which of the following statements apply to silicone impression materials?
    a. They set faster than polysulfide impression materials.
    b. Their setting time is increased by increases in humidity.
    c. Their setting time is increased by increases in temperature.
    d. They are more viscous than polysulfide impression materials.
    e. All of the above

24. Polyether impression materials:
    a. Are supplied in a light, regular, and heavy viscosity
    b. Are supplied with a thinner to be used with the heavy viscosity material
    c. Have a short working time of about 2½ minutes

d. Can be stored indefinitely in water unlike hydrocolloids and experience no significant dimensional change

25. Which statements apply to dental impression compound?
    a. It has higher flow 7° C above mouth temperature than tray compound.
    b. It is a thermoplastic material.
    c. It is rigid and solid at mouth temperature.
    d. It can be used to record a check impression or a final impression of an area with no undercuts.
    e. All of the above
    f. None of the above

26. Zinc ozide–eugenol impression material:
    a. Is available as either a two-paste or a powder-liquid system
    b. Has a setting time that is greatly affected by water or moisture
    c. Limits the selection of the model material to a gypsum product
    d. Has a mixing time of 30 to 45 seconds
    e. All of the above
    f. None of the above

27. Which of the following statements apply to zinc phosphate cement?
    a. It is supplied as a powder which is mainly zinc oxide and a liquid which is a buffered water solution of phosphoric acid.
    b. The powder is dispensed with a plastic scoop.
    c. It is mixed on a waxed paper pad.
    d. All of the above

28. During the mixing of zinc phosphate cement which of the following measures are followed?
    a. Most of the powder and liquid are incorporated at one time, and the viscosity is adjusted with small amounts of powder.
    b. Mixing is done over a wide area of the slab to dissipate the heat of reaction.
    c. The correct consistency should be reached after 45 seconds of mixing.
    d. Cooling the slab to just above the dew point will shorten the working time of the mixed cement.

29. The correct inlay consistency for zinc phosphate cement:
    a. Is puttylike
    b. Will not stick to the spatula
    c. Will form a 2 cm (¾ inch) string when touched with the spatula
    d. Will be dull in appearance
30. When comparing the viscosities of zinc phosphate and zinc polyacrylate cements, the viscosity of the zinc phosphate is less:
    a. Just after mixing
    b. 2 minutes after mixing
    c. Affected by temperature
    d. All of the above
    e. None of the above
31. What is (are) the objective(s) in mixing a zinc phosphate cement of the inlay consistency?
    a. To incorporate the greatest amount of powder at the correct consistency
    b. To prepare a mix that will permit complete seating of the restoration
    c. To produce a set cement with enough strength to retain the restoration
    d. All of the above
    e. None of the above
32. Which of the following zinc oxide–eugenol cements has the highest strength?
    a. Resin-modified
    b. Two-paste cavity liner
    c. Powder-liquid type for temporary restorations
    d. Ethoxybenzoic acid–modified with fillers
33. In the dispensing and mixing of zinc oxide–eugenol liners:
    a. Two parts of base are used per part of accelerator.
    b. Two parts of accelerator are used per part of base.
    c. The two portions are mixed in about 15 seconds.
    d. None of the above statements are true.
34. Which of the following factors is the most important in altering the setting time of zinc oxide–eugenol cement?

a. Moisture or humidity
b. Temperature
c. Powder:liquid ratio
d. Mixing time

35. Zinc polyacrylate cements have which of the following qualities?
    a. The liquid is a water solution of zinc polyacrylate.
    b. A common proportion is one and a half parts powder to one part liquid by weight.
    c. The liquid should be dispensed well in advance of mixing to be sure it reaches room temperature.
    d. The powder and liquid are spatulated for at least 1 minute before a smooth creamy mix is obtained.
36. Which of the following are used for temporary restorations?
    a. Prefabricated aluminum crowns
    b. Prefabricated polycarbonate crowns
    c. Custom-made acrylic crowns and bridges
    d. All of the above
    e. None of the above

SUGGESTED READINGS

Council on Dental Materials and Devices: Pit and fissure sealants, J. Am. Dent. Assoc. 93:134, 1976.
Craig, R. G.: A review of properties of rubber impression materials, Mich. Dent. Assoc. J. 59:254, 1977.
Craig, R. G., editor: Dental materials: a problem-oriented approach, St. Louis, 1978, The C. V. Mosby Co.
Craig, R. G., O'Brien, W. J., and Powers, J. M.: Dental materials: properties and manipulation, ed. 2, St. Louis, 1979, The C. V. Mosby Co.
Going, R. E., and Mitchem, J. C.: Cement for permanent luting: a summarizing review, J. Am. Dent. Assoc. 91:107, 1975.
Paffenbarger, G. C., and Rupp, N. W.: Composite restorative materials in dental practice: a review, Int. Dent. J. 24:1, 1974.
Wei, S. H.: Prevention of injuries to anterior teeth, Int. Dent. J. 24:30, 1974.
Whitehurst, V. E., Stookey, G. K., and Muhler, J. C.: Studies concerning the cleaning, polishing, and therapeutic properties of commercial prophylactic pastes, J. Oral Ther. Pharmacol. 4(3):181, 1968.

CHAPTER 24

Dental laboratory procedures

MARILYN A. WESTERHOFF

■ **Define the terms "mold," "impression, "cast," and "model."**

A *mold* is a form in which a substance is given shape.

An *impression* is a mold of a dental arch or a negative reproduction.

The terms *cast* and *model* are often used interchangeably in reference to the object formed or shaped from the mold or impression; thus cast and model mean a positive reproduction.

■ **Describe the steps necessary to prepare a hydrocolloid impression for pouring.**

Rinse the impression to remove all mucus, saliva, and debris.

If the impression requires a fixing or hardening solution, allow it to soak in the solution for the appropriate time.

Wrap the impression in a wet paper towel, and then place it in a humidor if it cannot be poured immediately. Take care to avoid imbibition by pouring the impression within 20 minutes.

■ **Explain the steps for the inverted method of pouring an impression.**

Use the correct water:powder ratio of the gypsum product to ensure proper physical and working properties of the material.

Mix the material in a clean rubber bowl, and place it on a vibrator to reduce trapped air.

Place the impression on the vibrator, and place a small amount of plaster or stone on the distal portion of one side of the impression.

Tilt the impression on the vibrator to vibrate the material into the indentations of the teeth, allowing the material to flow from one tooth indentation to the next until all are filled. Continue to place small increments of material in the same area until the impression is filled.

Add larger portions of material to the impression if necessary until the mucobuccal fold area is reached.

Heap a portion of the remaining material onto the surface to provide bulk for the base. Place the remaining material on a glass slab, and invert the impression onto the mass, keeping the tray parallel to the glass slab.

Smooth the sides of the base with a spatula, taking care to avoid embedding the tray.

■ **Explain the double-pour method.**

The double-poor method is identical to the inverted method described before with the exception of the final step, which leaves the top surface of the material to set in a rough undercut condition.

The base portion of the cast is made by heaping a second mix of material onto a glass slab. This material should be of a thicker mix than the consistency of the original pouring. If the original pour has reached the final set, it should be soaked in water for 5 minutes.

The tray is then inverted into the mass, and the sides of the second pour are smoothed with a spatula. Care should be taken to avoid pressure that could cause the initial pour to sink into the freshly mixed mass.

■ **How are casts separated from impressions?**

Excess gypsum material is removed from the tray so that the tray edges are free and visible. The anterior portion of the tray is loosened and slightly raised. When the cast is loose, the impression is lifted off with a straight pull.

■ **Describe the dispensing techniques used for gypsum materials.**

The water is placed into the rubber bowl, and the powder is sifted into it. This procedure reduces the incorporation of air into the mix.

■ **What means can be used to prevent the incorporation of air into the model?**

A bowl containing the powder-liquid mixture is vibrated to prevent air bubbles. The impression is also vibrated during the pouring process to eliminate the incorporation of air. Vacuum mixers are being widely used to completely eliminate porosity.

■ **What are the effects of spatulation on the setting time of gypsum products?**

As the duration and rapidity of spatulation is increased, the setting time of gypsum products decreases because the nuclei of crystallization are broken up and redistributed thereby making more hardening centers.

■ **Discuss the effects of spatulation on the setting expansion of gypsum materials.**

The setting expansion is increased by increasing time or rate of spatulation.

■ **Compare the physical changes that occur at the initial and final sets of gypsum materials.**

The first set that gypsum materials go through is called *initial set* and usually occurs within 5 to 15 minutes of the start of the mix. The cast will lose its shine and become warm to touch. The *final set* occurs 30 to 60 minutes later and is manifested by hardness of the material. A fingernail or knife mark cannot be made on the material, and the gypsum has cooled and feels dry to touch.

■ **What accelerators may be added to gypsum products to speed the setting mechanism?**

Potassium sulfate and small amounts of sodium chloride are commonly used as accelerators. Set gypsum ground up, as after model trimming, is an excellent accelerator.

■ **What chemicals can be used to increase the setting time of gypsum materials?**

Borax, sodium citrate, and acetates are used as retardants.

■ **How do blood and saliva affect the setting of gypsum products when left on the impression?**

Blood and saliva are retardants in the setting reaction of gypsum products.

■ **What is the maximum time to wait before separating an alginate impression?**

If the alginate is allowed to remain in contact with gypsum for more than 2 hours, the alginate begins to absorb excess water from the cast causing a chalky surface.

■ **What methods are used for softening impression compound?**

The three methods used for softening impression compound in order of preference are dry heat, water bath at 110° to 130° F, or open flame.

■ **What precautions must be taken if using a water bath to soften impression compound?**

Care must be taken not to knead the material too much. Ingredients can be leached out, thereby changing the properties of the material.

■ **What precautions must be taken if using open flame to soften impression compound?**

The material must be rotated in the flame. Moderate kneading helps the material to soften evenly. For safety of the oral tissues the material must be tempered in water.

■ **What is the time limitation for pouring the compound impression?**

Casts should be poured within 2 hours.

■ **How are casts separated from compound impressions?**

The safest method to separate casts from compound impressions is to immerse the poured impression in warm water. This allows easy removal without fracturing the cast.

■ **Describe the steps necessary to prepare a zinc oxide–eugenol impression for pouring.**

The zinc oxide–eugenol impression is rinsed with cool water to remove saliva and then carefully air-dried.

■ **What is the best method for separating a zinc oxide–eugenol poured impression?**

Immersion in 140° F water for approximately 10 minutes softens the impression material to allow easy separation.

■ **What methods are available for cleaning spatulas of zinc oxide–eugenol impression paste?**

Spatulas may be cleaned with orange oil solvent or xylene. Some manufacturers supply solvents for this purpose.

■ **When is the best time to pour a polysulfide impression?**

Recommendations on the best time to pour the impression vary from immediately to as long as 1 hour. To compensate for recovery from dimensional distortion caused by removal, the impression is often poured after a short wait.

■ **Define "boxing" as it applies to pouring techniques.**

The term *boxing* refers to a method of preparing the impression to receive plaster or stone. Boxing an impression is advantageous because it produces a dense cast, it provides a uniform land area, it establishes the depth of the mucobuccal fold, and it acts as a time-saver in model trimming. The boxing procedure includes the "beading" of the impression and the application of a side wall around it. In the mandibular impression it is necessary to block out the lingual area with a piece of wax.

■ **Identify the two parts of a cast.**

The cast is composed of two parts—the anatomic portion and the art portion. The *anatomic* portion represents two thirds of the cast and includes the anatomic landmarks represented in the impression. The *art* portion or remaining one third of the cast is the part constructed as the base. This latter portion is artistic and presents a symmetrical effect.

■ **Identify the characteristics of a well-trimmed set of diagnostic models.**

Many criteria exist for evaluating a well-trimmed set of models. The following list includes most of these characteristics:

The art portion equals one third of the total height, and the remaining two thirds is the anatomic portion.

The maxillary base is parallel to the occlusal plane, and the mandibular base is parallel to the maxillary base.

The maxillary anterior bevels equal each other, and the mandibular anterior bevel is rounded in a contour.

All vertical lines are parallel to each other.

Approximately 5 mm exists from the mucobuccal, mucolabial, and distal aspects of the posterior teeth and the beginning of the art portion.

The heels of the models are between ½ to ¾ inch and are equal to each other.

The sides of the models are equal to each other.

The angles of mandibular and maxillary models are symmetrical.

The angles on the maxillary model terminate at the midline of the centrals and cuspids.

The models are free of voids and bubbles, excess plaster, and scratches or fractures and are highly polished.

■ **How are trimmed study models finished?**

Depending on the intended use of the models, casts are finished by smoothing the land area and tongue portion, filling voids, and smoothing with fine grit sandpaper. During the trimming procedure excess gypsum is removed from the tongue area, and nodules are removed from the teeth and soft tissue structures.

■ **Explain how casts are polished.**

When the casts are completely dried, they are placed in a medium thick soap solution for 15 to 20 minutes and then rinsed and allowed to dry. Once the cast is dry, it is rubbed with a clean dry cloth or paper towel to achieve a sheen.

The same procedure can be followed by using

a commercial gloss solution instead of soap, or the entire process can be eliminated by spraying lightly with a liquid plastic. Care must be taken not to make the plastic covering too thick.

■ **What are the four setting stages of self-curing acrylic?**

The setting stages of self-curing acrylic are wet, sticky, doughy, and final polymerization.

■ **Name the most common liners or spacers used when making an acrylic custom tray.**

The spacers most commonly used when making an acrylic custom tray are wax and asbestos.

■ **List the steps in the construction of an acrylic tray.**

With an indelible pencil, outline all areas to be included in the impression.

Adapt a spacer made of wax or asbestos to the model. The spacer provides adequate space for the impression material. On a quadrant tray this spacer includes the prepared tooth and two teeth anterior and posterior to this site. A full arch tray will include coverage of all teeth and may include the palatal area.

Block out undercuts with asbestos or wax.

Create "stops" by removing a small amount of the spacer from the occlusal surface of the most distal and mesial ends of the tray area. These stops will allow the tray to be seated in a firm position during the impression sequence.

Mix the acrylic material and adapt it over the spacer.

Press the acrylic firmly over the stop areas to assure adaptation to the model.

Trim excess material until the border of the tray meets the outline made in the first step.

Form a handle on the anterior of the tray.

Maintain pressure on the material until the acrylic achieves its initial set. Avoid forcing the material into the undercuts.

Remove the tray from the model. Remove the spacer, and smooth the peripheral borders on the lathe if necessary.

■ **Explain the purpose of a baseplate.**

Baseplates are devices constructed on models of an edentulous or partially edentulous patient. Baseplates are designed to hold various measuring devices in place during construction of a denture for a patient. Once the measurements have been obtained, the baseplate serves to support a bite rim into which denture teeth may be set in position for a "try in" before final processing of the denture.

■ **What materials are generally used for baseplates?**

Self-curing acrylic, vacuum polystyrene sheets, and shellac composition sheets are three commonly used baseplate materials.

■ **Describe the technique for constructing a shellac composition baseplate.**

Soak the cast in water prior to adaptation to prevent the heated baseplate from sticking to the model.

Draw a continuous waxed pencil line along the deepest part of the mucobuccal and mucolabial folds. On the posterior surface of the plate, draw a line from the small dimple in the palate (fovea palatine) to each hamular notch.

Place the baseplate material on the model, and begin softening the material with a Bunsen burner or heat gun.

On the maxilla adapt the baseplate to the palatal area first; on the mandible begin adaptation in the anterior region and progress posteriorly.

Moisten fingers in water to avoid burning.

For ease of adapting, warm the alveolar ridge areas, and adapt small sections at a time to prevent breakage.

Adapt the mucobuccal and mucolabial areas with a blunt instrument.

Trim the baseplate to the pencil line previously placed on the peripheral border. The baseplate may be warmed along the peripheral border, an inch or two at a time, and trimmed with scissors.

Return the trimmed baseplate to the model and readapt by heating with the Bunsen burner or heat gun. This procedure is repeated until the baseplate is completely trimmed and readapted.

The mandibular baseplate often requires reinforcement on the anterior lingual flange. To accomplish this reinforcement bend a piece of wire to fit the site, heat the wire, and embed it into the baseplate material.

Smooth all peripheral borders by using a heated blunt instrument—grinding stones on a lathe or a straight handpiece.

The finished shellac composition baseplate should have the following characteristics: (1) the peripheral border of the baseplate should be even with the marked peripheral border of the model; (2) the baseplate should be tightly adapted to the model; (3) the peripheral border should be rounded and free of sharp edges; and (4) the baseplate should be smooth and free of burn marks or smudges.

■ **Differentiate between a self-curing acrylic baseplate and a vacuum polystyrene baseplate.**

A vacuum polystyrene baseplate is constructed mechanically using a vacuum-molding machine. The self-curing acrylic baseplate is constructed of a custom-made acrylic tray but is more closely adapted to the final cast. In both procedures undercuts are blocked out, a spacer is applied, and a hole is placed in the maxillary lateral area. The criteria for each of these types of baseplates should be consistent with those described in the shellac baseplate technique.

■ **What is the purpose of an occlusal rim?**

The wax occlusal rim replaces the teeth when taking measurements for centric occlusion, lip line, muscular attachments, cuspid eminences, midline, and length and width of the denture teeth. It is also used to secure the artificial teeth in place for the wax "try-in."

■ **Describe the techniques for constructing a wax occlusal rim.**

Preconstructed wax bite rims may be purchased commercially, but it may be necessary to construct one for use of a baseplate. The basic procedure in wax occlusal rim construction includes the following steps:

Heat a sheet of baseplate wax, and roll it into a rope.

Press the roll into a firm rod, and gently stretch to increase its length. Reheating of the wax rod may be necessary.

Adapt the rod to the baseplate, bending the wax rod to achieve the form of the arch.

Press the rod while still warm onto a flat surface to flatten the occlusal surface.

Seal the rim to the baseplate with sticky wax using a hot spatula along the edges of attachment.

Fill in voids with scrap wax.

Smooth the surface with an alcohol torch, and polish the surface with cotton under running water.

A well-formed bite rim should have the following characteristics: (1) the bite rim should be uniform in width and symmetrically arranged on the baseplate; (2) the maxillary baseplate should have an approximate 10-degree tilt in the anterior and an anterior height of about 20 mm in the deepest portion; (3) the occlusal surface of the mandibular baseplate should be parallel from anterior to posterior and *not* tilted 10 degrees; (4) the buccal and lingual contour should be smooth; (5) all voids should be filled; and (6) the bite rim should be polished.

■ **Describe the procedure for polishing prosthetic appliances.**

Only areas of prosthetic appliances that do not touch tissue are polished. Areas not to be polished include the residual ridge, peripheral turns, post-dam, hamular notch areas, retromolar pad areas, and the frenum attachment areas.

For polishing prosthetic appliances brush wheels and a rag wheel are used with a slurry pumice. In addition tripoli and wet whiting can also be used.

Care should be taken in polishing a partial denture to avoid distortion of the metal clasps by catching them on a rag wheel. Care must also be taken not to burn or overheat the acrylic.

■ **Describe the core technique for repairing a denture.**

The parts of the denture are held together with sticky wax.

Toothpicks can be used to help stabilize the parts until the plaster core or index is made.

Dovetails are placed in the acrylic.

Repair acrylic is placed in the fracture lines after the wax has been removed, the core lubricated, and the denture pieces reassembled on the index.

The repaired denture is polished using the same method as that for a denture base.

■ **How is a denture tooth replaced?**

A determination of the tooth type must be made.

Porcelain teeth are removed by cutting acrylic away from the lingual surface.

The tooth can be removed with the fingers. If it is an acrylic tooth, it is carefully ground away.

The replacement tooth is held in place with sticky wax at the incisal angles.

The repair acrylic is processed by pressurizing for 30 minutes; however, cold-cure acrylic can also be used.

■ **Describe the markings placed on a final die impression.**

A ball-point or felt tip pen can be used to place guidelines for the location of dowel pins. They are placed on the surface of the impression in an area where the first pour will not obliterate them.

■ **Discuss the types, use, and placement of lubricating mediums used to separate mixes in a die.**

Commercial preparations as well as soap, petroleum jelly, and oil can be used successfully. The lubricating medium is placed on the exposed dowel pin and on an area of the first pour immediately over the removable crown. However, lubrication should not extend beyond the removable tooth.

■ **How does one determine the position of the dowel pin?**

Dowel pins are placed parallel to the long axis of the tooth in the exact center of the tooth. Care must be taken not to allow the die to sink to the bottom of the impression.

■ **What aids are available to help place dowel pins?**

Several commercial appliances are available for parallel placement of dowel pins during the set of the gypsum. Toothpicks can also be used. A toothpick is placed on the impression in a faciolingual direction and luted to stabilize it. The dowel pin is then rested against the toothpick to prevent it from leaning.

■ **Explain the purpose and position of the lock washers in relation to the dowel pin.**

Lock washers prevent the dual mixes of stone from separating. The washers are placed at least 5 mm mesial and distal to the dowel pin. Two lock washers are used. The rounded ends of cut paper clips may be used as substitutes for the lock washers.

■ **What materials are commonly used to make dies in elastomeric materials?**

Dies in elastomeric materials generally are made of improved stone, ceramics, epoxy resin material, or amalgam.

■ **List the steps in preparing a removable stone die.**

The impression is gently cleansed and dried.

Markings to indicate the exact center of the intended die are made with a ball-point or felt tip pen.

A small mix of type IV improved stone is made, preferably using a vacuum mixer.

The crowns of all of the teeth are poured to a point 3 to 5 mm apical to the gingival margins.

The dowel pin is placed and aligned precisely with the markings on the impression.

Lock washers are placed, and the material is allowed to set.

A humidor may be used to permit a slow set.

Separating medium is applied to the area of the die, and a small amount of beading wax is placed on the dowel pin tip to prevent it from being buried.

Contrasting colored stone is poured into the previously boxed impression just short of the dowel pin tip.

■ **Describe the separation and trimming of a die.**

After setting for 1 to 1½ hours the impression can be separated.

The dowel pin is exposed by removal of the beading wax.

A lab knife is used to trim the margins of the cast.

With an extra fine coping saw blade the stone is cut from the cervix to the base of the stone.

The die is removed by tapping it on the exposed dowel pin.

Excess stone is removed from the gingival margin of the die.

■ List the conditions for which a biteplane might be prescribed.

Biteplanes are used frequently in cases of temporomandibular joint dysfunction, periodontal trauma, and full mouth reconstruction when it is necessary for the bite to be opened.

■ Describe a biteplane.

Biteplanes are maxillary horseshoe-shaped removable acrylic appliances that are held in place with retention clasps on first molars. The bite plane may also have canine loops and labial arch wires. A flat or inclined plane surface may be added to the anterior region for directing teeth.

■ When are mouth protectors indicated?

Mouth protectors are widely used today by athletes involved in contact sports.

■ Describe a popular method for constructing custom-made mouth protectors.

All custom-made mouth protectors are made on a complete maxillary cast. The use of vinyl acetate or polyurethane sheets formed to the cast by a vacuum device is an efficient method of constructing a mouth guard.

MULTIPLE CHOICE QUESTIONS

1. Which of the following is frequently used for storing alginate impressions for less than 15 minutes?
   a. Open air
   b. A 100° F oven
   c. Submersion
   d. Cellophane
   e. Moist toweling
2. Undue kneading of impression compound while softening it in a water bath will:
   a. Volatilize important constituents
   b. Incorporate water into the surface
   c. Cause the compound to overheat
   d. Cause the compound to become too thin
3. The water:powder ratio for stone I is:
   a. 22 ml of water to 100 g of powder
   b. 22 g of powder to 100 ml of water
   c. 60 ml of powder to 100 g of water
   d. 30 ml of water to 100 g of powder
   e. 30 g of powder to 100 ml of water
4. The main function of the vibrator is to:
   a. Aid the flow of the plaster from one side to another
   b. Remove air bubbles already present in the material

   c. Aid in achieving a creamy consistency
   d. Provide stimulus
   e. Aid in bringing excess water to the surface
5. Which of the following should be done if water falls into a container of gypsum?
   a. Throw out all of the material in the container.
   b. Remove the entire top portion of powder.
   c. Save the affected material as a retarder.
   d. Remove all affected material immediately.
   e. Remove the lid so that the moisture can evaporate.
6. Overspatulation causes:
   a. The setting crystals to break up
   b. Additional strength in the mix
   c. Air bubbles to escape
   d. Increased surface porosity
   e. Elimination of lumps
7. If gypsum products are stored in a warm humid area:
   a. No detrimental effects will occur.
   b. The setting time will increase.

c. The setting time will decrease.

d. Setting expansion will increase.

e. The strength of the set product will increase.

8. The initial set of gypsum products is shown by:

a. The fingernail test

b. The temperature of the mix

c. The loss of gloss

d. The use of the Vicat needle

e. The extreme rigidity of the material

9. Before trimming, models should be soaked for:

a. 1½ minutes

b. 3 minutes

c. 5 minutes

d. 7 minutes

e. 10 minutes

10. The art portion of the model should be:

a. ⅛-inch thick

b. ¾-inch thick

c. ⅜-inch thick

d. ¼-inch thick

e. ⅝-inch thick

11. Buccal cuts on a model should begin at the:

a. Midline

b. Center of the canine

c. Distal of the canine

d. Center of the first premolar

e. Distal of the first premolar

12. Stone should be added to the die impression until the stone is:

a. Even with the teeth

b. 1 mm above the teeth

c. 4 mm above the teeth

d. 6 mm above the teeth

13. The custom tray for an edentulous model should extend:

a. 2 mm from the peripheral roll

b. 3 mm from the peripheral roll

c. 5 mm from the peripheral roll

d. To the deepest portion of the peripheral roll

e. 2 mm below the frenum

14. The custom tray should extend:

a. One tooth plus the proximal surface of the next tooth past the last preparation.

b. One tooth past the last preparation

c. One tooth plus the proximal surface of the next tooth past the last missing tooth

d. Two teeth past the last preparation

15. The placement of stops is necessary:

a. For the release of impression materials

b. For definite placement of the tray in the mouth

c. Only on the anterior portion of the tray

d. Only on the posterior portion of the tray

16. The height of the maxillary bite rim should be:

a 10 mm anteriorly

b. 15 mm anteriorly

c 20 mm anteriorly

d. 27 mm anteriorly

17. A dowel pin is used to:

a. Articulate models

b. Engage lock washers

c. Insert dies into a model

d. Fabricate bite rims

18. Dies may be made of:

a. Acrylic and stone

b. Stone and amalgam

c. Acrylic, stone, and alginate

d. Acrylic, stone, and amalgam

19. A sprue pin functions to:

a. Insert die into a model

b. Articulate models

c. Form a channel for molten metal

d. Support a class IV composite restoration

20. Baseplate wax is used to:

a. Construct baseplates

b. Construct wax patterns for inlays

c. Determine occlusal clearance

d. Form bite rims

SUGGESTED READINGS

Berliner, A.: Ligatures, splints, bite planes and pyramids: adjuncts in the treatment of periodontal disease, Philadelphia, 1964, J. B. Lippincott Co.

Craig, R. G., editor: Dental materials: a problem-oriented approach, St. Louis, 1978, The C. V. Mosby Co.

Craig, R. G., O'Brien, W. J., and Powers, J. M.: Dental materials: properties and manipulation, ed. 2, St. Louis, 1979, The C. V. Mosby Co.

O'Brien, W. J., and Ryge, G., editors: An outline of dental materials and their selection, Philadelphia, 1978, W. B. Saunders Co.

Phillips, R. W.: Elements of dental materials: for dental hygienists and assistants, ed. 3, Philadelphia, 1977, W. B. Saunders Co.

Torres, H. O., and Ehrlich, A.: Modern dental assisting, Philadelphia, 1976, W. B. Saunders Co.

Peterson, S. A., editor: The dentist and the assistant, ed. 4, St. Louis, 1977, The C. V. Mosby Co.

Answer sheet

Chapter 2	Chapter 3	Chapter 4	Chapter 5
1. c	1. e	1. d	1. b
2. a	2. d	2. c	2. d
3. b	3. c	3. c	3. c
4. b	4. d	4. d	4. b
5. c	5. b	5. c	5. c
6. a	6. c	6. d	6. a
7. b	7. a	7. d	7. d
8. c	8. c	8. c	8. a
9. c	9. a	9. d	9. d
10. b	10. b	10. c	10. b
11. a	11. c	11. d	11. a
12. c	12. c	12. b	12. e
13. c	13. b	13. c	13. c
14. a	14. b	14. a	14. e
15. c	15. b	15. d	15. e
16. b	16. c	16. b	16. c
	17. c	17. e	17. b
	18. a	18. c	18. e
	19. d	19. a	19. a
	20. c	20. a	20. a
	21. d	21. d	21. d
	22. b	22. a	22. d
	23. a	23. a	23. d
	24. c	24. c	24. a
	25. c	25. c	25. c
	26. c	26. c	26. b
	27. b	27. d	27. d
	28. e	28. b	28. d
	29. b	29. d	29. b
	30. c	30. c	30. a
	31. c	31. a	31. c
		32. c	32. b
		33. a	33. d
		34. d	34. d
		35. a	35. d
		36. c	36. b
		37. c	37. a
		38. c	
		39. b	
		40. d	
		41. b	
		42. a	

Chapter 6

1. c
2. c
3. e
4. e
5. b
6. a
7. e
8. d
9. e
10. e
11. e
12. e
13. e
14. e
15. a
16. c
17. a
18. b
19. e
20. c
21. c
22. a
23. a
24. c
25. c

Chapter 7

1. b
2. b
3. d
4. b
5. d
6. a
7. a
8. d
9. c
10. c
11. b
12. a
13. d
14. c

Chapter 8

1. d
2. a
3. b
4. d
5. c
6. b
7. b
8. d, c, a, g, e, b, h, f
9. a
10. a
11. c
12. a

Chapter 9

1. d
2. b
3. b
4. c
5. c
6. c
7. b
8. b
9. b
10. b
11. a
12. c
13. d
14. d
15. d
16. a
17. d
18. a
19. d
20. a
21. c
22. c
23. d
24. b
25. b
26. b
27. c
28. a
29. d
30. d
31. b
32. d
33. b

Chapter 10

1. a
2. d
3. c
4. d
5. a
6. d
7. c
8. a
9. b
10. a
11. b
12. c
13. a
14. b
15. b
16. d
17. b
18. a
19. c
20. b
21. c
22. b
23. d
24. c
25. d
26. c
27. c

Chapter 11

1. a
2. c
3. a
4. d
5. b
6. c
7. b
8. d
9. b
10. d
11. a
12. d
13. b
14. a
15. a
16. b
17. c
18. a
19. a
20. e
21. e
22. a
23. d
24. b
25. c
26. e
27. a
28. b
29. a
30. c
31. e
32. d

Chapter 12

1. b
2. a
3. c
4. c
5. b
6. a
7. d
8. b
9. c
10. b

Chapter 13

1. c
2. b
3. b
4. b
5. e
6. c
7. b
8. b
9. b
10. a
11. c
12. b

Chapter 14

1. d
2. b
3. d
4. a
5. c
6. d
7. b
8. a
9. b
10. c
11. a
12. b
13. d
14. d
15. c
16. a
17. d
18. a
19. c
20. b

Chapter 16

1. c
2. c
3. b
4. b
5. b
6. d
7. b
8. a
9. d
10. b
11. d
12. c
13. c
14. a
15. b
16. a
17. b
18. c
19. c
20. b
21. a
22. c
23. c
24. b
25. b
26. d
27. c
28. b

Chapter 17

1. c
2. b
3. d
4. c
5. b
6. a
7. d
8. d
9. b
10. c
11. b
12. a
13. e
14. a
15. d
16. c
17. d
18. a
19. b
20. b
21. c
22. d
23. b
24. a
25. b
26. b

Chapter 18

1. b
2. c
3. c
4. a
5. a
6. d
7. b
8. a
9. d
10. c
11. d
12. a
13. b
14. a
15. b
16. a
17. b
18. c
19. b
20. b

21. c
22. a
23. d
24. c
25. c
26. b
27. b
28. c
29. b
30. c
31. a
32. a
33. b
34. d
35. c
36. d
37. a
38. d
39. d
40. d
41. d
42. a
43. b
44. c
45. c
46. d
47. d
48. c
49. b
50. b
51. c
52. c
53. b

Chapter 19

1. c
2. d
3. c
4. b
5. b
6. d
7. c
8. c
9. b
10. c
11. b
12. a
13. d
14. a
15. d
16. c
17. a
18. e
19. a
20. b
21. d
22. a
23. c
24. a
25. c

Chapter 20

1. d
2. c
3. c
4. a
5. c
6. c
7. d
8. a
9. d
10. d
11. b
12. d
13. c
14. b
15. c
16. b
17. b
18. b
19. c
20. d
21. a
22. d
23. a

Chapter 21

1. a
2. c
3. c
4. d
5. c
6. d
7. b
8. a
9. a
10. b
11. c
12. c
13. c
14. b
15. c
16. c
17. b
18. b
19. c
20. d
21. d
22. b
23. d
24. a
25. d
26. b
27. a
28. c
29. d
30. d
31. c
32. d
33. c
34. b
35. c
36. c
37. b
38. d
39. a
40. b
41. c
42. d
43. c
44. b
45. a
46. d
47. b

Chapter 22

1. c
2. c
3. b
4. b
5. d
6. b
7. d
8. a
9. a
10. c
11. b
12. b
13. c
14. d
15. d
16. b
17. b
18. d
19. c
20. d
21. c
22. b
23. d

Chapter 23

1. d
2. b
3. d
4. c
5. b
6. d
7. a
8. a
9. a
10. d
11. d
12. b
13. a
14. a
15. b
16. d
17. a
18. d
19. d
20. b
21. c
22. b
23. a
24. c
25. e

26. e
27. a
28. b
29. c
30. a
31. d
32. d
33. c
34. a
35. b
36. d

Chapter 24

1. e
2. b
3. d
4. b
5. d
6. a
7. c
8. c
9. c
10. d
11. b
12. c
13. a
14. a
15. b
16. c
17. c
18. d
19. c
20. d